Visual Pathways

Documenta Ophthalmologica
Proceedings Series volume 27

Editor H.E. Henkes

Dr W. Junk Publishers   The Hague – Boston – London 1981

Visual Pathways
Electrophysiology and Pathology

Proceedings of the
18th I.S.C.E.V. Symposium
Amsterdam, May 18–22, 1980

Edited by
H. Spekreijse and P. A. Apkarian

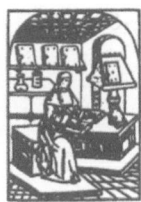

Dr W. Junk Publishers   The Hague – Boston – London 1981

Distributors:

for the United States and Canada

Kluwer Boston, Inc.
190 Old Derby Street
Hingham, MA 02043
USA

for all other countries

Kluwer Academic Publishers Group
Distribution Center
P.O. Box 322
3300 AH Dordrecht
The Netherlands

This volume is listed in the Library of Congress Cataloging in Publication Data

ISBN-13: 978-94-009-8658-9   e-ISBN-13: 978-94-009-8656-5
DOI: 10.1007/978-94-009-8656-5

Cover design: Max Velthuijs

© Dr W. Junk Publishers 1981
Softcover reprint of the hardcover 1st edition 1981

PREFACE

The XVIIIth ISCEV symposium was organized by the Netherlands Ophthalmic Research Institute and took place May 18–22, 1980, at the Wilhelmina Gasthuis in Amsterdam. The invited speakers and the theme "Electrophysiology and pathology of the visual pathways" were selected by a programme committee consisting of G.H.M. van Lith, D. van Norren, L.H. van der Tweel and H. Spekreijse. The success of a symposium depends not only on the topics selected but also on the clarity and quality of the presentations. In this respect it is a pleasure to acknowledge the four invited speakers for their clear and comprehensive presentations of recent research results.

My co-editor, P. Apkarian, and I wish to thank all participants for timely submission of the manuscripts and for prompt response to inquiries regarding editorial matters. Mr. Peters of Junk Publishers should be acknowleged for observing publication deadlines, thus ensuring that the proceedings will reach all participants prior to the next ISCEV meeting.

A word of thanks is also due to all those who helped to make the symposium a success, not only from a scientific but also from a social point of view. A special compliment should be expressed for the administrative manager of the Netherlands Ophthalmic Research Institute, Mr. Verbraak, for his excellent organization and for Miss Sweers for her secretarial assistance. Last but not least I wish to express my gratitude to Mrs. Bastiaenen, Mrs. Van der Tweel and Mrs. Spekreijse, who directed and actively participated in the social programme. The enthusiasm of the graduate students and of my colleagues at the Institute helped to ensure a fruitful meeting in a friendly atmosphere.

H. Spekreijse

CONTENTS

PART FIVE: BINOCULARITY

PART SIX: CENTRAL ASPECTS

LIST OF PARTICIPANTS

E. Adachi-Usami
Department of Ophthalmology
Chiba University School of Medicine
Inohana 1-8-1
280 Chiba
Japan

R. Alfieri
Faculté de Médecine
Place Henri Dunant
Boîte Postale 38
63001 Clermont-Ferrand
France

M. Anastasi
University Eye Clinic
Via Liborio Giuffré 13
I-90 127 Palermo
Italy

P.A. Apkarian
The Netherlands Ophthalmic Research
Institute
Department of Visual System Analysis
P.O. Box 6411
1005 EK Amsterdam
The Netherlands

P. N. Askelund
Kongens GT 27
7000 Trondheim
Norway

M.B. Baier
Max-Planck-Institut
Parkstrasse 1
D-6350 Bad Nauheim
Fed. Rep. of Germany

C. Barber
Medical Physics Department
Queens Medical Centre
Nottingham NG1 5DN
United Kingdom

M. Barris
Department of Ophthalmology
University of Florida
Gainesville, Florida 32610
U.S.A.

T. van den Berg
Laboratory of Medical Physics
University of Amsterdam
Herengracht 196
1016 BS Amsterdam
The Netherlands

K. van den Berge
Laboratory of Medical Physics
University of Amsterdam
Herengracht 196
1016 BS Amsterdam
The Netherlands

C.A. Bianchi
Via Santa Sofia 12
I-20122 Milano
Italy

W.M.R. Biersdorf
Department of Ophthalmology
University of South Florida
13000 N. 30th Street
Tampa, Florida 33612
U.S.A.

G.K. Bijl
Department of Neurophysiology
University of Groningen
Bloemsingel 16
9712 KZ Groningen
The Netherlands

L.D. Blumhardt
University Department of Neurology
Churchill Hospital, Headington
Oxford
United Kingdom

A. Bohár
Semmelweis Orvostudományi Egyetem
II. Szemklinika
Mária-ut 39
1085 Budapest
Hungary

M. Boiteux
Service Central de Biophysique et de
Médecine Nucléaire
Hôpital Lariboisière
2 Rue Ambroise-Paré
75010 Paris
France

N. Bonaventure
Laboratoire de Neurophysiologie
Centre de Neurochemie de CNRS
11 Rue Humann
67085 Strasbourg
France

G.H. Bresnick
Department of Ophthalmology
University of Wisconsin
Clinical Sciences Center FY/344
600 Highland Avenue
Madison, WI 53792
U.S.A.

J.R. Charlier
Service d'exploration fonctionelle de la
vision
C.H.R. de Lille
Place de Verdun
59000 Lille
France

D. Creel
Medical Center
Veterans Administration
Salt Lake City, Utah 84148
U.S.A.

S.J. Crews
Clinical Neurophysiology Unit
University of Aston and Birmingham
Birmingham
United Kingdom

G. Dagnelie
The Netherlands Ophthalmic Research
Institute
Department of Visual System Analysis
P.O. Box 6411
1005 EK Amsterdam
The Netherlands

J.T.W. van Dalen
Eye Clinic Wilhelmina Gasthuis
University of Amsterdam
Eerste Helmersstraat 104
1054 EG Amsterdam
The Netherlands

H. Dalens
Clinique Ophthalmologique
Hôpital Saint-Jacques
30, Place Henri Dunant
63000 Clermont-Ferrand
France

S.S. Declercq
Division of Ophthalmology
Stanford University Medical Centre
Stanford, CA 94305
U.S.A.

B. Degering
Augenklinik
Zentralkrankenhaus
St. Jürgenstrasse
D-2800 Bremen, F.R.G.

E. Dodt
Max-Planck-Institut
Parkstrasse 1
D-6350 Bad Nauheim
Fed. Rep. of Germany

C.E. Doggett
The University of Aston
Department of Ophthalmic Optics
Gosta Green
Birmingham B4 7ET
United Kingdom

G.T.M. van Dok-Mak
Spiegelenburghlaan 34
2111 BN Aerdenhout
The Netherlands

N. Drasdo
Neurophysiology Unit
Department of Ophthalmic Optics
University of Aston
Birmingham B4 7ET
United Kingdom

Á. Farkas
Semmelweis Orvostudományi Egyetem
II. Szemklinika
Mária-ul. 39
1085 Budapest
Hungary

G.A. Fishman
University of Illinois
Eye and Ear Infirmary
1855 W. Taylor Street
Chicago, Illinois 60612
U.S.A.

S. Fonda
Eye Clinic
University of Modena
Via Vivaldi 30
I-41100 Modena
Italy

A.B. Fulton
Department of Ophthalmology
Harvard Medical School
Children's Hospital Medical Center
300 Longwood Avenue
Boston, MA 02115
U.S.A.

N.R. Galloway
Department of Medical Physics and
Ophthalmology
Queens Medical Centre
Nottingham NG1 5DN
United Kingdom

R. Gemperlein
Zoological Institute of the
University of Munich
D-8000 Munich
Fed. Rep. of Germany

Y. Grall
Biophysique sensorielle
Hôpital Lariboisière
2, Rue Ambroise-Paré
75010 Paris
France

H.S. Graniewski-Wijnands
Academisch Ziekenhuis Leiden
Afdeling Oogheelkunde
Rijnsburgerweg 10
2333 AA Leiden
The Netherlands

A. Groneberg
Augenklinik der T.U.
Ismaingenstr. 20
D-8000 München
Fed. Rep. of Germany

G.F.A. Harding
Neurophysiology Unit
Department of Ophthalmic Optics
University of Aston in Birmingham
Birmingham B4 7ET
United Kingdom

J.R. Heckenlively
Jules Stein Eye Institute
800 Westwood Plaza
Los Angeles, California 90024
U.S.A.

K.A. Hellner
Department of Ophthalmology
University Hospital of Hamburg
Martinistrasse 52
D-2000 Hamburg 20
Fed. Rep. of Germany

H.E. Henkes
Oogziekenhuis
Schiedamse Vest 180
3011 BH Rotterdam
The Netherlands

G.L. van der Heijde
Department of Medical Physics
Vrije Universiteit
Van de Boechorststraat 7
Amsterdam
The Netherlands

G.E. Holder
Regional Department of Clinical
Neurophysiology
Brook General Hospital
Shooters Hill Road
Woolwich SE18 4LW
United Kingdom

J.W. Howe
The University of Newcastle upon Tyne
Department of Ophthalmology
The Royal Victoria Infirmary
Queen Victoria Road
Newcastle upon Tyne
United Kingdom

C. Huber
University Eye Clinic Zürich
Rämistrasse 100
CH-8091 Zürich
Switzerland

P. Jacobsson
University of Linköping
Department of Ophthalmology
University Hospital
S-581 85 Linköping
Sweden

P. Jonckheere
Academisch Ziekenhuis
Vrije Universiteit Brussel
Dienst Oogheelkunde
Laerbeeklaan 101
1090 Brussel
Belgium

J. Keller
Service Central de Biophysique et de
Medecine Nucleaire
Hôpital Lariboisiére
2, Rue Ambroise-Paré
75010 Paris
France

J.H. Kelsey
36 Weymouth Street
London W1N 3LR
United Kingdom

H.E. Kolder
Department of Ophthalmology
University of Iowa
Iowa City, Iowa 52242
U.S.A.

A.C. Kooijman
Kliniek voor Oogheelkunde
P.O. Box 30001
9700 RB Groningen
The Netherlands

M. Korth
Institut für Physiologie und Biokybernetik
der Universität Erlangen-Nürnberg
Universitätstrasse 17
D-8520 Erlangen
Fed. Rep. of Germany

H. Krauss
Jules Stein Eye Institute
800 Westwood Plaza
Los Angeles, California 90024
U.S.A.

C.J. Krüger
Augenklinik der
Mediz. Hochschule
Karl-Wiegert-Allee
D-3000 Hannover, F.R.G.

R.G.A. Langenhuysen
Nicolet Instrument B.V.
Korte Bergstraat 10
3811 ML Amersfoort
The Netherlands

E.R. Lapp
Max-Planck-Institut
Parkstrasse 1
D-6350 Bad Nauheim
Fed. Rep. of Germany

M. Lauricella
University Eye Clinic
Via Liborio Giuffré 13
I-90127 Palermo
Italy

T. Lawwill
301 East Muhammed Ali Boulevard
Louisville, Kentucky 40202
U.S.A.

G. Lennerstrand
Department of Ophthalmology
University Hospital
S-581 85 Linköping
Sweden

G.H.M. van Lith
Eye Department
Erasmus University Eye Hospital
Schiedamse Vest 180
3011 BH Rotterdam
The Netherlands

E.H. van der Marel
The Netherlands Ophthalmic Research
Institute
Department of Visual System Analysis
P.O. Box 6411
1005 EK Amsterdam
The Netherlands

J.l. Markoff
Department of Ophthalmology
1600 South Broad Street
Philadelphia, PA 19145
U.S.A.

M. Matsuhashi
Department of Ophthalmology
Keio University
35 Shinanomachi, Shinjuku-ku
Tokyo
160 Japan

W.P.M. Mayles
Guys Hospital
Department of Clinical Physics
St. Thomas Street
London SE1 9RT
United Kingdom

K.W. Mitchell
Department of Medical Physics
University of Newcastle upon Tyne
Royal Victoria Infirmary
Queen Victoria Road
Newcastle upon Tyne NE1 4LP
United Kingdom

M. Moschos
Athens University Eye Clinic
170 Messoghion Street
Cholargos-Athens
Greece

W. Müller
Medizinische Akademie Erfurt
Augenklinik
Nordhäuser Strasse 74
D-506 Erfurt
German Dem. Rep.

A. Neetens
Universiteit Antwerpen U.I.A.
Universiteitsplein 1
2610 Wilrijk
Belgium

G. Niemeyer
Department of Ophthalmology
Universitätsspital
CH-8091 Zürich
Switzerland

S.E. Nilsson
Department of Ophthalmology
University of Linköping
S-581 85 Linköping
Sweden

W.K. Noell
Neurosensory Laboratory
State University of New York at Buffalo
2211 Main Street
Buffalo, New York 14214
U.S.A.

D. van Norren
Institute for Perception TNO
Kampweg 5
3769 DE Soesterberg
The Netherlands

Y. Oguchi
Department of Ophthalmology
School of Medicine
Keio University
35 Shininomachi
Shinjuku-ku
Tokyo 160
Japan

A. Penne
Eye Clinic
University of Modena
Via Vivaldi 30
I-41100 Modena
Italy

J. Pokorny
University of Chicago
Eye Research Laboratory
937 E. 57 Street
Chicago, Illinois 60537
U.S.A.

F. Ponte
University Eye Clinic
Via Liborio Giuffré 13
I-90127 Palermo
Italy

V. Porciatti
Divisione Oculistica Spedali
Riuniti Livorno
I-57100 Livorno
Italy

A.M. Potts
Department of Ophthalmology
University of Louisville
301 E. Walnut Street
Louisville, KY 40202
U.S.A.

D. Regan
Department of Physiology and Biophysics
Gerard Hall, Halifax Infirmary
5303 Morris Street
Dalhousie University
Halifax, Nova Scotia B3J1B6
Canada

F.C.C. Riemslag
The Netherlands Ophthalmic Research
Institute
Department of Visual System Analysis
P.O. Box 6411
1005 EK Amsterdam
The Netherlands

R. Rix
Universitäts Augenklinik
Schwabachanlage 6
D-8520 Erlangen
Fed. Rep. of Germany

A. de Rouck
Victor Braeckmanlaan 68
B-9110 Ghent
Belgium

J. Röver
Universitäts Augenklinik
Killianstrasse 21
D-7800 Freiburg
Fed. Rep. of Germany

M.P. Rubinstein
The University of Aston in Birmingham
Neurophysiology Unit
College House, Gosta Green
Birmingham B4 7ET
United Kingdom

P. Salu
Academisch Ziekenhuis
Vrije Universiteit Brussel
Dienst Oogheelkunde
Laerbeeklaan 101
1090 Brussel
Belgium

A. Scarpatetti
Heinestrasse 17
CH-9008 St. Gallen
Switzerland

G. Schaubele
Universitäts Augenklinik
Killianstrasse 21
D-7800 Freiburg
Fed. Rep. of Germany

N.A.M. Schellart
Laboratory of Medical Physics
University of Amsterdam
Herengracht 196
1016 BS Amsterdam
The Netherlands

B. Schmidt
Augenklinik Klinikum Steglitz
Hindenburgdamm 30
1 Berlin 45
Fed. Rep. of Germany

J. Schmidt
Universitäts-Augenklinik
22 Robert Kochstrasse
D-5 Koln-Lindenthal
Fed. Rep. of Germany

XVI

E. Schmöger
Medizinische Akademie Erfurt
Augenklinik
Nordhäuserstrasse 74
D-506 Erfurt
German Dem. Rep.

R.P. Schuurmans
Max-Planck-Institut
Parkstrasse 1
D-6350 Bad Nauheim
Fed. Rep. of Germany

J.B. Siegfried
Pennsylvania College of Optometry
1200 West Godfrey Avenue
Philadelphia, Pennsylvania 19126
U.S.A.

P.A. Sieving
Eye & Ear Infirmary
University of Illinois
1855 W. Taylor St.
Chicago, Il. 60612
U.S.A.

H.W. Skala
Eye Foundation Hospital
University of Alabama in Birmingham
1720 Eighth Avenue South
Birmingham, Al. 35233
U.S.A.

V.C. Smith
Eye Research Laboratory
University of Chicago
937 E. 37 Street
Chicago, Illinois 60537
U.S.A.

S. Sokol
Department of Ophthalmology
New England Medical Center
171 Harrison Avenue
Boston, MA. 02111
U.S.A.

H. Spekreijse
The Netherlands Ophthalmic Research
Institute
Department of Visual System Analysis
P.O. Box 6411
1005 EK Amsterdam
The Netherlands

G. Stadler
Universitäts Augenklinik
Robert Kochstrasse 4
D-3550 Marburg/Lahn
Fed. Rep. of Germany

D.J. Stark
St. Andrews Neurosensory Unit
40 Annerley Road, Woolloongabba
Brisbane, Queensland
Australia

R.P. Stodtmeister
Universität Ulm
Abt. Für Augenheilkunde
Prittwitzstrasse 43
D-7900 Ulm
Fed. Rep. of Germany

L. Strzyzewski
Kreiskrankenhaus
Seilerweg 29
D-6430 Bad Hersfeld
Fed. Rep. of Germany

J. Tanabe
Max-Planck-Institut
Parkstrasse 1
D-6350 Bad Nauheim
Fed. Rep. of Germany

C. Teping
Abt. f. Augenheilkunde
Medizin. Fakultät
Rhein.-Westf. Techn. Hochschule
Goethestr. 27/29
D-5100 Aachen. F.R.G.

O. Textorius
University of Linköping
Department of Ophthalmology
S-581 85 Linköping
Sweden

A. Thaler
2. Universitäts Augenklinik
Alserstrasse 4
A-1090 Vienna
Austria

J.M. Thyssen
Department of Ophthalmology
Universiteit van Nijmegen
Geert Grooteplein 22
6525 GA Nijmegen
The Netherlands

XVII

K. Totsuka
2-7-27-101 Motoazabu
Minato-ku
Tokyo 106
Japan

R. Trau
Department of Ocular Electro-
physiology
A.Z., V.U.B.
Brussels, Belgium

G.L. Trick
College of Optometry
Ferris State College
Big Rapids, Michigan 49307
U.S.A.

L.H. van der Tweel
Laboratory of Medical Physics
University of Amsterdam
Herengracht 196
1016 BS Amsterdam
The Netherlands

S.M. Vijfvinkel-Bruinenga
Eye Department
Erasmus University Eye Hospital
Schiedamse Vest 180
3011 BH Rotterdam
The Netherlands

L.H. de Vries-Khoe
The Netherlands Ophthalmic Research
Institute
Department of Visual System Analysis
P.O. Box 6411
1005 EK Amsterdam
The Netherlands

E. Welinder
University of Linköping
Department of Ophthalmology
S-581 85 Linköping
Sweden

C.T. White
University of California Medical Center
Department of Pediatrics and
Ophthalmology
Mail code H-638-A
225 Dickinson Street
San Diego, California
U.S.A.

H.G.H. Wildberger
Universitäts Augenklinik Zürich
Stadelhoferstrasse 42
CH-8001 Zürich
Switzerland

N. Wioland
Laboratoire de Neurophysiologie
Centre de Neurochemie de CNRS
11 Rue Humann
67085 Strasbourg
France

K. Yanashima
Max-Planck-Institut
Parkstrasse 1
D-6350 Bad Nauheim
Fed. Rep. of Germany

M. Yuzawa
p/a Universiteit van Nijmegen
St. Radboud Ziekenhuis
Philips van Leydenlaan 15
6525 EX Nijmegen
The Netherlands

E. Zrenner
Max-Planck-Institut für
physiologische und klinische Forschung
Parkstrasse 1
D-6350 Bad Nauheim
Fed. Rep. of Germany

PART ONE

VISUAL PATHWAYS: BASIC ASPECTS

PROBLEMS ALONG THE COURSE OF THE SECOND VISUAL NEURON—GANGLION CELL TO LATERAL GENICULATE BODY

A.M. POTTS

(*Louisville, U.S.A.*)

ABSTRACT

The physiological problems connected with the distal visual pathway are determined by anatomical, hydrostatic, vascular, and toxicological conditions to mention but a few. A number of these problems have been solved with the help of electrophysiological methods, although virtually none of them are amenable to a non-invasive electrophysiological approach. A series of representative problems is treated with emphasis on conditioning factors and potential solutions.

INTRODUCTION

The ganglion cell-geniculate pathway is of prime importance for vision and its study is formidable.

1. It represents the course of a single neuron from cell body, through non-myelinated pressurized axon and myelinated less pressurized axon to synaptic terminal.
2. It represents the bottleneck of information transfer in the visual system from photoreceptor to consciousness.
3. Its physical location makes it virtually inaccessible to study by non-invasive techniques.
4. Invasion by disease is still unexplained on an anatomical and pathophysiological basis or juxtaposition of pathways is so close that these factors are meaningless in explanation of disease effects.

It is a discussion of these points which I wish to make during this presentation. I hope to substantiate the formidable nature of the optic nerve problem and to suggest that its investigation will require a number of invasive methods not yet attempted plus a combination of new and old non-invasive methods.

ANATOMY

Logically, one must begin at the ganglion cell which, because of the wide receptive field, we tend to think of as having widely extended dendrites as in the cat cell stained with horseradish peroxidase (Fig. 1). Recall that Polyak (1941), a meticulous morphologist, recognized five morphologically different ganglion cell types. Note, too, that the Golgi method used by Polyak was itself a selective stain and capriciously omitted cells stainable by other

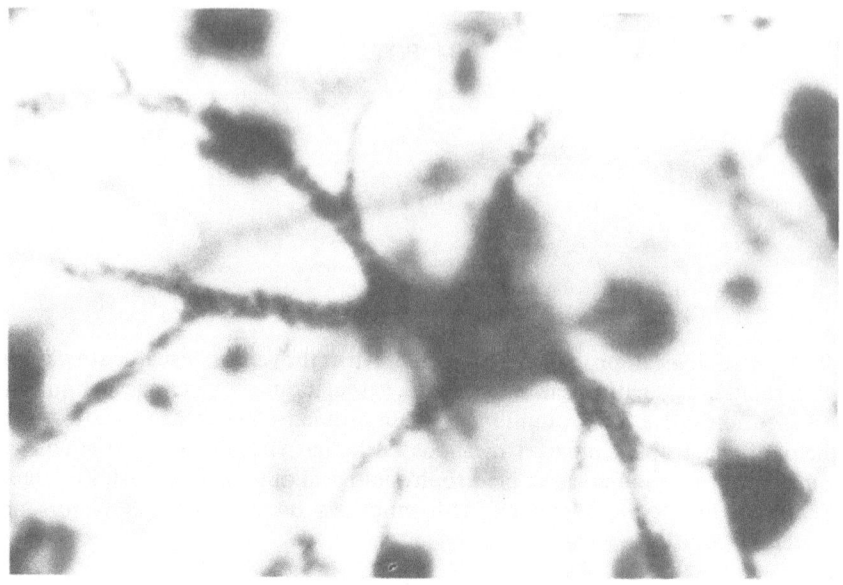

Fig 1. Cat ganglion cell stained retrograde with horseradish peroxidase.

techniques. However, there is no evidence that Golgi staining omits specific cell types selectively. One must remember that in the primate near the macula, ganglion cells are so crowded that a layer five cells thick is the rule. Short dendrites and small receptive fields are customary and one marvels how the fibers of the nerve fiber layer sort themselves out to begin their course to the optic nerve head (Fig. 2). The ophthalmoscope shows these fibers as glistening striae under favorable illumination, but only after reaching the lamina cribrosa and acquiring a myelin sheath does each fiber become easily identifiable by anatomical methods.

Epon sections and high power light microscopy after Trypan Blue allow each fiber to be identified in cross section and to be countable by a method which we have published in the past (Potts, Hodges, Shelman, Fritz, Levy & Mangnall 1972 a, b, c).

Results obtained by us on primates suggest that the nerve fiber count is;

Man	1,200,000
Rhesus Monkey	1,600,000

Unpublished results indicate further:

Cat	100,000
Pig	1,000,000

4

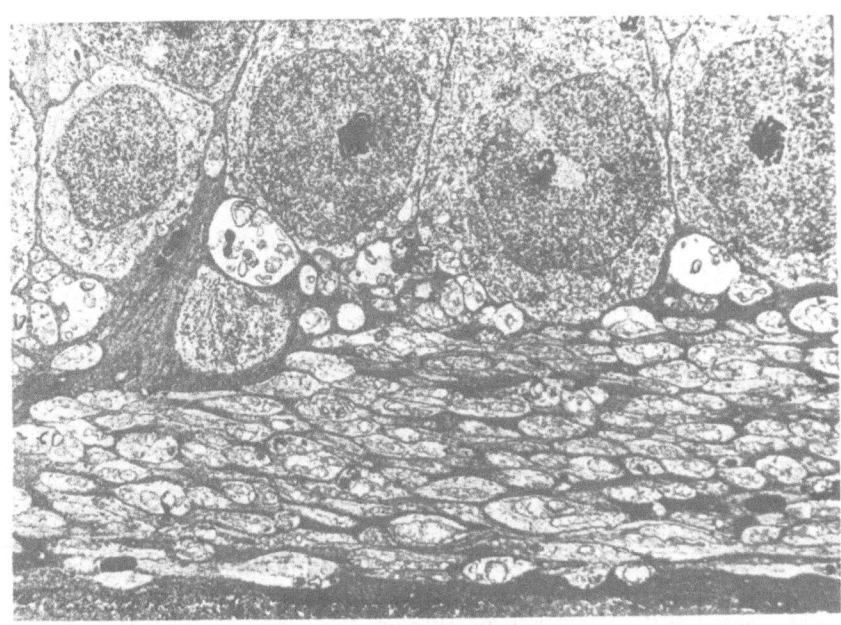

Fig. 2. Electron micrograph of ganglion cells near the fovea of the rhesus monkey together with unmyelinated fibers of the nerve fiber layer.

In the human eye, at least the estimate of the number of rods is 110 to 125×10^6 (Østerberg 1935). Thus the convergence factor in the human from receptor to nerve fiber averages 100 to 1.

At the proximal end of the tract, the lateral geniculate nucleus (LGN), the quantitative evidence is scanty and unreliable. On the grounds of estimated cell counts, the LGN has at least as many cells as the optic tract has fibers. In several lower animals connection of a single fiber to 5 to 10 LGN cells has been observed (Duke-Elder & Wybar, 1961).

Thus it is not unreasonable to designate the ganglion cell-geniculate tract as the bottleneck of the visual system. Small lesions of this tract are likely to cause large losses of information. Conversely, because of the small physical dimensions of the system, analyses by penetration with microelectrodes are unlikely to yield unequivocally useful information.

An additional anatomical fact which must be dealt with is the decussation of fibers at the chiasm. The crossing of fibers which supply the nasal halves of the retinas and the non-crossing of temporal fibers presumably facilitates the connection of binocularly driven cortical cells and aids stereopsis. The precise pathway taken by crossed and uncrossed fibers determines the details of visual field changes by pathological events in the neighborhood of the chiasm.

PHYSIOLOGY

Much of the information on the ganglion cell-geniculate tract has been derived from extracellular recordings with microelectrodes. Notable is the work of Kuffler (1952; 1953) and of Enroth-Cugell and co-workers (1966, et seq.). Kuffler demonstrated the center-surround organization of the receptive field of the cat ganglion cell. Stimulation of the central area caused a sharp increase in frequency of discharge of the cell. Stimulation of an approximately annular concentric surround caused inhibition of cell discharge. The opposite could be true, where light stimulus of the central area was inhibitory and stimulation of the surround was excitatory. These two categories of cells are most widely known as on-center and off-center cells.

The other major categorization of cat ganglion cells is into the categories *X-type* and *Y-type* by Enroth-Cugell and co-workers (1966, et seq.). X-cells have a sustained response to a step stimulus, Y-cells have a transient response. This is demonstrated with some ease by the use of gratings displaced over the cell center. One gets a sustained or transient response whether this is an 'on' or an 'off' response.

Direction sensitive ganglion cells have been demonstrated in the rabbit by Barlow & Levick (1964) and Levick (1965). Directional selectivity may be defined as cells responding best to motion of stimulus in one direction.

There are also orientation selective ganglion cells in the rabbit which have selectivity for a stimulus moved in either direction along a straight line.

In the rabbit Levick (1967) also found edge detectors. A bright or dark disc caused little effect passing through the receptive field of such a cell, but when it came to rest a discharge resulted.

For these latter physiological categories one must ask about the rabbit the same question one asked about the frog ganglion cells when these were described by Lettvin et al. (1959). How much of this retinal organization in the lower animal is a function assumed by the visual cortex in primates? The question yet to be answered is: How many distinct types of ganglion cells exist in man and the subhuman primates? In this question lies the more basic question: How many different types of messages are encoded in the frequency modulated spikes that pass along the optic nerve fibers? Under any circumstances there is a significant amount of pre-processing that is encoded in the ganglion cell spike even in the primate. We are not dealing with a simple relay station.

Fiber size, conduction rate, and function

The automated count of total fibers in an optic nerve cross section done in our laboratory also allowed for fiber area determination (Potts, Hodges, Shelman, Fritz, Levy & Mangnall 1972 b). The fiber diameters in the histograms of Figs. 1 and 2 of that paper (in units of $0.78\,\mu$, not 0.24 as stated in the paper) are axoplasmic diameters and do not include myelin. There is no bimodal or polymodal distribution of fiber diameters. In both rhesus monkey and in human optic nerves the size histogram resembles a skewed distribution curve. When the circumfoveal area is destroyed by photocoagulation, only fibers of the smallest diameters disappear (Potts, Hodges, Shelman, Fritz Levy & Mangnall, 1972 c). Nevertheless the majority of fibers of even these small diameters survive. Similar distribution curves are present for the cat and the domestic pig (Potts unpublished). In no case are there two or more size distribution peaks.

However, when one returns to electrophysiological measurements there is some evidence that X-cells (sustained, tonic, Type II) have axons with a relatively slow conduction time and Y-cells (transient, phasic, Type I) have axons with a faster conduction time. According to Fukada (1971) the range of conduction times is 10 m/sec to nearly 70 m/sec. Although there is much overlap in the 30 m/sec range, Fukada's Fig. 8B clearly shows that there are distinctly different conduction rate distribution curves for X-fibers and Y-fibers. For clinical implications see below.

Non-invasive physiology

The whole point of ISCEV is emphasis on methods which can be applied to the human patient in a clinical situation. The information obtained from the invasive anatomical and physiological methods described above is invaluable in helping our thinking about non-invasive approaches but the problems of the latter are formidable.

To begin, the electroretinogram bears no detectable contribution from the ganglion cell layer. Measurements at the front of the globe contribute nothing to our knowledge of ganglion cell-geniculate function.

Secondly, extradural measurements in the orbit have yielded nothing of importance so far. To get intraorbital electrical responses, one must penetrate the dural sheath and this is hardly practical as a routine clinical procedure.

This leaves study of the visually evoked response (VER). Since the optic nerve must be intact for normal VER, optic nerve defects are reflected in the VER. However, the many strictures that concern the VER in general apply to its use in study of the optic nerve.

1. Many structures contribute to the integrity of the VER.
   a. The outer retinal layers must be functional. Many photoreceptor ± bipolar cell diseases betray themselves by their typical ophthalmoscopic picture and can be eliminated. However some diseases such as rod dystrophies and cone dystrophies do not.
   b. The optic radiations and the calcarine cortex must be healthy. Additional image processing goes on at the lateral geniculate and at the cortex. Hubel and Wiesel (1962) have shown the presence of 'complex' and 'hypercomplex' cells. They postulate that the output of these cells represent two levels of synergy of the output of groups of simple center-surround cells. Thus measurements at the occipital pole reflect further processing, and disease of the more proximal neural structures can mask or can simulate optic nerve disease. Since 'complex' cells are stimulated specifically by bars of light or dark, much attention is now being paid to spatial modulation of stimuli. Bar patterns with sine or square wave profiles and reversing checkerboard stimuli reflect this outlook.
2. The inter-individual variation of the VER is so great that its use in bilateral disease is unreliable. The soundest use of the VER is in unilateral disease where the known healthy side can act as control.

3. Macular vision is very strongly represented in the VER. This fact which has been remarked on numerous times by us and by others (Potts & Nagaya 1965) makes the VER an excellent measure of foveal and macular function and a poor measure of peripheral function. Thus, there is no practical way to use the VER in determination of the visual field with the accuracy of some of the determinations described below. However, two approaches to visual field determination should be mentioned. One of these is the use of hemi- and quadrant-field stimulation particularly in the hands of Biersdorf and his group (Biersdorf 1974). The other is the use of the scotopic VER as in the hands of Adachi-Usami et al. (1978). Although responses could be obtained with annular stimuli of 20° radius by the latter authors, the times required to complete a measurement were impractical, and even so, use of less than a 360° annulus caused rapid loss of response.

OPTIC NERVE DISEASE

Glaucoma

Perhaps the major optic nerve disease in terms of incidence is glaucoma. After the measurement of intraocular pressure, the single most important determination is that of the visual field. Dynamic and static perimetry can give pathognomonic findings. The next most important determination is examination of the nerve head ophthalmoscopically for pallor and cupping. Recent attempts to quantify this examination are beginning to meet with success. The work of the late Gerald Portney (1976) on measurement of cupping is worthy of notice. A characteristic attempt to quantify pallor is that of Nagin & Schwartz (1980) using a color slide of the fundus and photoelectric photometry.

Attempts have been made to use the VER in the detection of glaucoma (Sokol, Domar, Moskowitz & Schwartz 1980; Sonty & Schwartz 1980). The first group of authors showed that in patients with proved glaucoma the first major positive component of the pattern reversal VER had significantly longer latency than that of ocular hypertensives or of normals. The application to individual cases was questionable. However in asymmetric pressure difference between the two eyes or in asymmetric glaucoma (field loss in one eye only), the significant latency difference found may be more useful.

However, the major interest in glaucoma is still concentrated on psychophysical methods. Tests using the Arden sinusoidal contrast gratings are proving equivocal for glaucoma detection (Hsu-Winges, Stamper & Sopher 1980; Ozaki, Levy & Bonney 1980). However there are refinements of the Enoch static perimetry technique which are claimed to differentiate between pre-laminar and post-laminar lesions of the optic nerve (Fitzgerald, Enoch & Temme 1980 a, b).

Of more than passing interest is the report by Tyler (1980) of a dip in modulation sensitivity at 30–40 Hz for a 5° flickering field. This dip was found centrally and 20° peripherally in glaucoma patients and in ocular hypertensives, not in normals. Lower and higher frequencies showed no such loss in sensitivity. This phenomenon is presumably a generalized retinal phenomenon and might be explored electrophysiologically.

Demyelinating and other inflammatory disease

A portion of demyelinating disease of the optic nerve (how large a portion is still unknown) is characterized by central scotoma. Particularly when the effect is unilateral there is a marked diminution of VER amplitude to a small target or a textured reversal target resolved normally by the macula. This type of phenomenon was demonstrated by Van Lith & Mak (1974). More generally observed is the delay in the VER impulse in optic neuritis of demyelinating disease and from other causes. Here there need not be a central scotoma (Halliday, McDonald & Mushin 1972).

Tumors

There are a large number of ways in which intraorbital intracanalicular, intracranial, and particularly circumsellar tumors can affect optic nerve and optic tract. Primary tumors of the ganglion cell-geniculate pathway may also occur. Electrophysiological methods are virtually last in diagnostic usefulness. Dependence is greatest on visual field findings and on radiological findings. Conventional tomography and computerized axial tomography are most informative. Where homonymous hemianopsia is present, delay in latency of major VER components can be observed (Kooi & Marshall 1979).

TOXIC PHENOMENA

Methanol

In a study of methanol and its oxidation products, Praglin et al. (1955) showed that the optic nerve discharge measured by an intradural needle was abolished by an adequate dose of formaldehyde in the cat and the rabbit. However, the b-wave of the electroretinogram was abolished simultaneously. Thus, although the optic nerve is the primary target in methanol poisoning and although formaldehyde is the immediate oxidation product of methanol, there is evidence that the pre-ganglion cell pathway may be affected in this acute experiment. We cannot differentiate between direct effect on the optic nerve and effect on receptor-bipolar-Müller cell structures.

Ethanol

The acute effects of ethanol administration of the VER have been measured in humans. The light flash generated VER shows longer latency (Müller & Haase 1967) and decrease in amplitude (Lewis, Dustman & Beck 1970; Rhodes, Obitz & Creel 1975). Using pattern reversal stimuli, Van Lith & Vijfvinkel-Bruinenga (1978) found both decreased amplitudes and increased latency of major VER components after administration of the equivalent of 70 ml of absolute ethanol. Once again, one cannot be certain that the effect is a direct one on optic nerve and not one on other parts of the retina and visual pathway.

Quinine

In quinine poisoning one sees retinal edema with cherry-red spot, dilation of the pupil, early loss of vision and frequent permanent constriction of peripheral visual fields. Typically there is late depression of the b-wave of the ERG (e.g. François, Verriest & De Rouck 1967). However, early measurement of the non-invasive VER may be expected to give a more reliable answer about optic nerve disease. We have developed a model for quinine poisoning in the cat (Potts, Wheeler & Hope, unpublished) and will have more to communicate on this subject in the future.

Pentavalent arsenicals

Since the time that electrophysiological studies have become practical, pentavalent arsenicals are used in man for trypanosomiasis and in chickens and pigs to promote growth. Unpublished work from our laboratory (Wheeler and Potts) has demonstrated depression of occipital cortical response in cats given acetarsone. As with quinine the typical pattern of visual field loss in humans is peripheral constriction. Much study remains to be done in order to characterize the nature of changes in the ganglion cell-geniculate pathway. The existence of a typical visual field change suggests specificity of action and such a study should be well worth while.

CONCLUSION

To summarize, the ganglion cell-geniculate pathway is highly important for vision since it represents the bottle-neck for visual information as it travels from photoreceptor to occipital cortex. This compression of information channels in an extremely tight bundle makes the pathway susceptible to a wide variety of disease entities. The inaccessibility of the pathway makes isolation of its function by non-invasive methods virtually impossible. When overall methods such as visually evoked response are utilized to obtain information on optic nerve function, the most rigorous precautions must be taken to rule out effects from other portions of the visual system.

ACKNOWLEDGEMENT

Supported in part by USPHS Research Grant Numbers EY 01704 and EY 01591 from the National Eye Institute, National Institutes of Health, Bethesda, Maryland: by the L. L. Sinton Trust Research Grant and by the Unrestricted Research Grant from Research To Prevent Blindness, Inc., New York, New York.

REFERENCES

Adachi-Usami, E., Misago, M. & Kanayama, N. Electro-perimetry by means of the scotopic VECP. In: Electrodiagnosis, toxic agents and vision. 15th ISCEV Symposium (Ed. J. François & A. De Rouck) Junk, The Hague. (Doc. Ophthal. Proc. Series, Vol. 15) 179–187 (1978).

Barlow, H.B. & Levick, W.R. Retinal ganglion cells responding selectively to direction and speed of image motion in the rabbit. J. Physiol. 173: 377–407 (1964).

Biersdorf, W.R. Cortical evoked responses from stimulation of various regions of the visual field. In: 11th ISCERG Symposium (Ed. E. Dodt & J.T. Pearlman) (Doc. Ophthal. Proc. Series, Vol. 4) Junk, The Hague. 249–255 (1974).

Duke-Elder, Sir S. & Wybar, K.C. The anatomy of the visual system. In: System of Ophthalmology, Vol. 2 (Ed. Sir S. Duke-Elder). Kimpton, London. 605–606 (1961).

Enroth-Cugell, C. & Robson, J.G. The contrast sensitivity of retinal ganglion cells of the cat. J. Physiol. 187: 517–552 (1966).

Fitzgerald, C.R., Enoch, J.M. & Temme, L.A. Different functional changes recorded in open-angle glaucoma and anterior ischemic optic neuropathy. Invest. Ophthalmol. Vis. Sci. (Suppl.). 125 (1980a).

Fitzgerald, C.R., Enoch, J.M. & Temme, L.A. Kinetic perimetry (in the plateau region of the field) as a sensitive indicator of visual fatigue or saturation-like defects in retrobulbar anomalies. Invest. Ophthalmol. Vis. Sci. (Suppl.). 92 (1980b).

François, J., Verriest, G. & De Rouck, A. Étude des fonctions visuelles dans deux cas d'intoxication par la quinine. Ophthalmologica 153: 324–335 (1967).

Fukada, Y. Receptive field organization of cat optic nerve fibers with special reference to conduction velocity. Vision Res. 11: 209–226 (1971).

Halliday, A.M., McDonald, W.I., & Mushin, J. Delayed visual evoked response in optic neuritis. Lancet 2: 982–985 (1972).

Hsu-Winges, C., Stamper, R.L. & Sopher, M. Arden contrast sensitivity testing in normals, glaucoma suspects and chronic glaucoma patients. Invest. Ophthalmol. Vis. Sci. (Suppl.). 84 (1980).

Hubel, D.H. & Wiesel, T.N. Receptive fields, binocular interaction and functional architecture in the cat's visual cortex. J. Physiol. 160: 106–154 (1962).

Kooi, K.A. & Marshall, R.E. Visual evoked potentials in central disorders of the visual system. Harper and Row, Hagerstown, Maryland (1979).

Kuffler, S.W. Neurons in the retina: organization inhibition and excitation problems. Cold Spring Harbor Symp. Quart. Biol. 17: 281–292 (1952).

Kuffler, S.W. Discharge patterns and functional organization of mammalian retina. J. Neurophysiol. 16: 37–68 (1953).

Lettvin, J.Y., Maturana, H.R., McCulloch, W.S. & Pitts, W.H. What the frog's eye tells the frog's brain. Proc. Inst. Radio Eng. N.Y. 47: 1940–1951 (1959).

Levick, W.R. The mechanism of directionally selective units in the rabbit's retina. J. Physiol. 178: 477–504 (1965).

Levick, W.R. Receptive fields and trigger features of ganglion cells in the visual streak of rabbit retina. J. Physiol. 188: 285–308 (1967).

Lewis, E.G., Dustman, R.E. & Beck, E.C. The effects of alcohol on visual and somatosensory evoked responses. Electroenceph. clin. Neurophysiol. 28: 202–205 (1970).

Müller, W. & Haase, E. Das Verhalten der corticalen Antwort unter Alkoholeinwirkung. Graefes Arch. Ophthal. 173: 108–113 (1967).

Nagin, P.A. & Schwartz, B. Image processing in the measurement of optic disc pallor. Invest. Ophthalmol. Vis. Sci. (Suppl.). 275 (1980).

Østerberg, G.A. Topography of the layer of rods and cones in the human retina. Acta. Ophthal., Suppl. 6 (1935).

Ozaki, K., Levy, N.S. & Bonney, R.C. Responses to the Arden modulation transfer function plates in normal eyes with optically altered visual acuity. Invest. Ophthalmol. Vis. Sci. (Suppl.) 125 (1980).

Polyak, S. The Retina. University of Chicago Press, Chicago (1941).

Portney, G.L. Photogrammetric analysis of the three dimensional geometry of normal and glaucomatous cups. Trans. Am. Acad. Ophthalmol. Otolaryngol., 81: 239–246 (1976).

Potts, A.M. & Nagaya, T. Studies on the visual evoked response. I. The use of the 0.06 degree red target for evaluation of foveal function. Invest. Ophthalmol. Vis. Sci. 4: 303–309 (1965).

Potts, A.M., Hodges, D., Shelman, C.B., Fritz, K.J., Levy, N.S. & Mangnall, Y. Morphology of the primate optic nerve: I. Method and total fiber count. Invest. Ophthalmol. Vis. Sci. 11: 980–988 (1972a).

Potts, A.M., Hodges, D., Shelman, C.B., Fritz, K.J., Levy, N.S. & Mangnall, Y. Morphology of the primate optic nerve: II. Total fiber size distribution and fiber density distribution. Invest. Ophthalmol. Vis. Sci. 11: 989–1003 (1972b).

Potts, A.M., Hodges, D., Shelman, C.B., Fritz, K.J., Levy, N.S. & Mangnall, Y. Morphology of the primate optic nerve: III Fiber characteristics of the foveal outflow. Invest. Ophthalmol. Vis. Sci. 11: 1004–1016 (1972c).

Praglin, J., Spurney, R. & Potts, A.M. An experimental study of electroretinography: I. The electroretinogram in experimental animals under the influence of methanol and its oxidation products. Am. J. Ophth. 39: 52–62 (1955).

Rhodes, L.E., Obitz, F.W. & Creel, D. Effect of alcohol and task on hemispheric asymmetry of visually evoked potentials in man. Electroenceph. clin. Neurophysiol. 38: 561–568 (1975).

Sokol, S., Domar, A.D., Moskowitz, A. & Schwartz, B. Pattern VEP latency and contrast sensitivity in glaucoma. Invest. Ophthalmol. Vis. Sci. (Suppl.). 84 (1980).

Sonty, S. & Schwartz, B. Visually evoked potentials in evaluation of glaucoma and ocular hypertension. Invest. Ophthalmol. Vis. Sci. (Suppl.). 142 (1980).

Tyler, C.W. Notch loss of temporal frequency sensitivity in glaucoma and ocular hypertension. Invest. Ophthalmol. Vis. Sci. (Suppl.). 124 (1980).

Van Lith, G.H.M. & Mak, G.T.M. A quantitative evaluation of the VECP in optic neuritis. In: 11th ISCERG Symposium (Ed. E. Dodt & J.T. Pearlman) (Doc. Ophthal. Proc. Series, Vol. 4) Junk, The Hague. 375–386 (1974).

Van Lith, G.H.M. & Vijfvinkel-Bruinenga, S. Optic neuropathy due to alcohol abuse and evoked cortical potentials. In: Electrodiagnosis, toxic agents and vision. 15th ISCEV Symposium (Ed. J. François & A. De Rouck) (Doc. Ophthal. Proc. Series, Vol. 15) Junk, The Hague, 221-225 (1978).

Authors' address:
Department of Ophthalmology
University of Louisville
301 E. Walnut Street
Louisville, Kentucky 40202 U.S.A.

12

ETHAMBUTOL MAINLY AFFECTS THE FUNCTION OF RED/GREEN OPPONENT NEURONS

E. ZRENNER & C.J. KRÜGER

(*Bad Nauheim & Frankfurt/M., F.R.G.*)

ABSTRACT

In patients with ocular defects caused by the tuberculostaticum ETHAMBUTOL the spectral data obtained under selective chromatic adaptation with psychophysical and electrophysiological methods clearly indicate that signals of all three types of spectrally different cones are present in the visual cortex; however, the signs of color-opponent interactions between the individual cone mechanisms are lacking. Therefore it becomes evident that ETHAMBUTOL mainly affects the function of red/green antagonistic neurons. This method of investigation in patients as described here permits differentiation between toxic alterations affecting the cone receptor and their direct pathways to the visual cortex from those disturbing the action of color-antagonistic mechanisms, upon which chromatic as well as spatial coding strongly relies.

INTRODUCTION

Visual defects caused by toxic agents often affect color vision as one of the first clinical symptoms. In acquired color vision deficiencies, the receptors and the various post-receptor neurons might be affected in very different manners. It therefore appears useful to apply psychophysical and electrophysiological tests for differentiating between defects in receptor and post-receptor processing of chromatic signals. The spectral sensitivity of the receptors themselves is mainly defined by pigment absorption; yet spectral sensitivity functions of post-receptor neurons are changed considerably by inhibitory mechanisms which exhibit themselves best in the so-called color-opponent neurons. The typical color-opponent spectra as recorded in single cells (Wiesel & Hubel 1966; De Valois, Abramov & Jacobs 1966; Gouras 1968; Gouras & Zrenner 1979), of monkey retina and geniculate can also be demonstrated in human cortical processing, psychophysically (King-Smith & Carden 1976) as well as electrophysiologically (Zrenner 1976, 1977; Jankov 1978) in the visually evoked cortical potential (VECP). In order to find out which functions in the human visual system are most affected by toxic agents, we determined the spectral sensitivity functions on various back-grounds in patients with normal and with defective color vision by psycho-physical and electrophysiological methods. The experiments revealed that ETHAMBUTOL, a commonly used tuberculostatic drug, mainly affects opponent processing in red/green color-opponent neurons, while signals of the three spectrally different types of cones are still present at the visual cortex.

METHOD AND MATERIALS

EOG: After 30 min of dark adaptation ($0.1 \, cd/m^2$) the patient was light adapted for 15 min ($310 \, cd/m^2$). Eye movements between two fixation marks, alternatively once per 2 seconds presented in a visual angle of $40°$, were recorded with Beckman silver-silver-chloride electrodes attached to the left and right of each eye. The responses were amplified (DC) one hundredfold and registered with a Y-T pen recorder. Averaged from recordings of several eye movements, normal values of the EOG light peak ranged between 180% and 250% of the baseline value which had been obtained after 25 min of dark adaptation (for additional information see Zrenner, Langhof, Welt & Kojima 1976).

ERG: A Xenon arc lamp (XBO 150 W, Osram) provided two beams, one for test lights of 100 ms duration, the other for steady adapting lights. The illuminance was controlled by neutral density filters, the spectral bands by Schott filters (BG 28, OG 5). Ganzfeld illumination was obtained with a diffusing acrylic disk in front of the Henkes ERG electrode. The potentials were amplified, filtered (band-pass $0.1 - 300$ Hz) and averaged ($n = 8-16$) by a Nicolet computer (Model 1072). The scotopic b-wave was elicited after 20 min of dark adaptation with blue test flashes. The photopic a- and b-wave were recorded in the presence of a blue steady adapting light (2.2 log td) and orange test flashes (for details see Hoffmann, Zrenner & Langhof 1978). The second oscillatory potential (OP_2) was measured under photopic con-ditions and filtered (band-pass 100–300 Hz) similarly to the method used by Kojima & Zrenner (1978). The voltage vs. log intensity functions (V-log I) were considered normal if they did not fall outside the ± 1 standard deviation range obtained in a sample of 16 normal observers.

VECP: Diffuse flashes were provided by a Grass photostimulator (PS 2) viewed at a distance of 30 cm. Checker board patterns were presented on a TV-screen (Medelec Generator). The check size could be varied from $4'$ to $80'$, the test field size from $5°$ to $11°$ of visual angle. The VECP were recorded with a gold disk cup electrode, 3 cm above the inion (right earlobe as reference); the potentials were amplified, filtered (band-pass 0.1 to 30 Hz) and averaged with a Nicolet computer (Model 1072). Normal observers showed a latency of the first positive peak (PI) for flash stimulation between 100–125 ms; a maximum of the VECP amplitude occurred for a check size of $20'$ during foveal stimulation, whereas with parafoveal stimulation the maximum shifted to a check size of $50'$.

PSYCHOPHYSICAL DATA

A two channel Maxwellian-view optical system was used to present a homogeneous circular test target ($4°$ in diameter) on a background of $11°$ in diameter. In the test beam a monochromator (Jobin Yvon H.10) and a variable neutral density wedge were used, both controlled by a PDP 11/40 computer as described by Zrenner & Baier (1978). The spectral characteristics of the background beam were controlled by narrow band interference filters (Schott AL, half bandwidth 20 nm) of red (623 nm), blue/green (487 nm), purple (422 + 630 nm) or yellow (577 nm) appearance. Increment spectral sensitivity curves were obtained after 5 min of adaptation to a particular background. For each of 26 wavelengths (400–650 nm) the computer set the neutral density wedge at its maximum density and decreased it by 0.5 log unit steps until the subjects indicated by pressing a pushbutton that they saw the test flash (TF) of 400 ms duration. Depending on the subject's response the computer program subsequently incremented the TF intensity up or down by only 0.1 log unit until a total of 8 TFs were presented. The threshold was calculated from these data according to the procedure described by Little (1974).

Case reports

Case 1: A female patient (A.W., age 49) took a total of 200 g Ethambutol over a period of eight months as treatment for tuberculosis of the urinary tract. As shown in Fig. 1, her visual acuity decreased to 0.3 (OD) and 0.2 (OS). Except for a slightly pale appearance of the optic discs, the fundus was normal. Visual fields determined by Goldmann perimetry were concentrically narrowed in both eyes. The Haitz campimeter revealed a small central scotoma for all colors. Confusion in the Farnsworth-Munsell 100 Hue test (F.M. 100 Hue) occurred mainly along the deutan and protan axes with a large total error score in both eyes (488 OD and 544 OS). The electro-ophthalmological investigation (Fig. 2) revealed a normal EOG with the light peak reaching a ratio of 254% of the baseline value. The scotopic and photopic ERG were completely normal. In the VECP (Fig.2, right) the first positive peak had a latency near 140 ms and was thereby delayed by about 20 ms when evoked by diffuse flashlight stimuli. Stimulation with checkerboard patterns of various size in the central $5°$ of the retina showed pathological responses of reduced amplitude, except for squares of $36'$ in visual angle; stimulation of peripheral retinal parts, with the foveal region blanked out, evoked normal responses.

Case 2: A male patient (D.J., age 36) having taken 400 g Ethambutol over eight months showed very similar symptoms; investigated the same way as Pat. A.W., his visual field showed concentric narrowing to the central $30°$; total central scotoma for colored stimuli in the central $10°$ (Haitz) and highly increased confusions in the F.M. 100 Hue test were noted (total error score 1024 OS and 920 OD). The fundus appeared normal. In this patient, electrophysiological findings also revealed a normal photopic and scotopic ERG,

15

PAT.. A.W. (age 49) VA: OD 0.3 OS 0.2

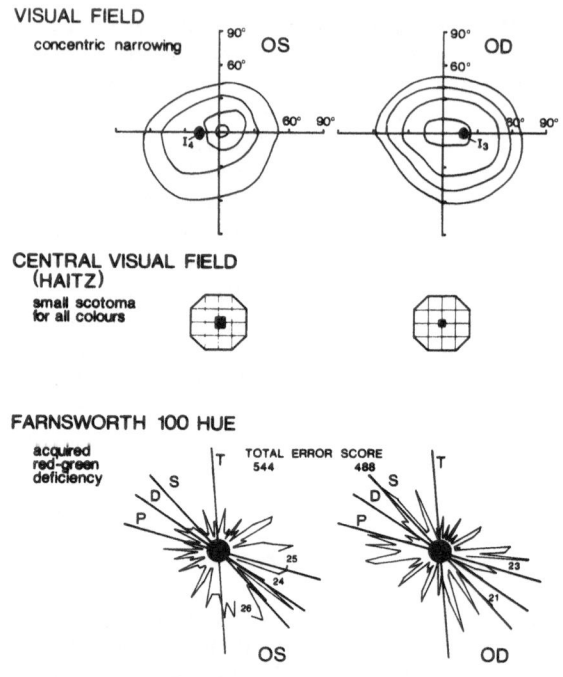

Fig. 1. Top: Visual fields determined with Goldmann-perimetry (white test targets, III₄, I₄, I₃, I₂). Center: Recognition of colored (white, yellow, blue, red, green) stimuli in the central field (10°), according to Haitz. Bottom: Farnsworth-Munsell 100 Hue test including the maximum-error axes for protanopes (P), deuteranopes (D), tritanopes (T) and for scotopic vision (S).

with normal oscillatory potentials: VECP responses were considerably delayed with the first positive peak occurring 160 ms after the onset of diffuse light stimulation.

RESULTS

In Fig. 3 spectral sensitivity functions of our standard sample (4 normal trichromatic observers) are shown, including mean and standard deviation. Either the psychophysical threshold (left) or a VECP amplitude criterion (right) was used to determine spectral sensitivity to monochromatic lights between 400 nm and 650 nm. The spectral sensitivity of the three cone mechanisms was selectively isolated by the appropriate chromatic background (upper half of Fig. 3). This method was introduced by Stiles (1959) and Wald (1964) and turned out to be useful for clinical applications (Marré 1972). In the presence of strong yellow adaptation light (577 nm, triangles) the observer's spectral sensitivity is determined by the blue sensitive

16

PAT.: A.W. (age 49)   VA: OD 0.3   OS 0.2

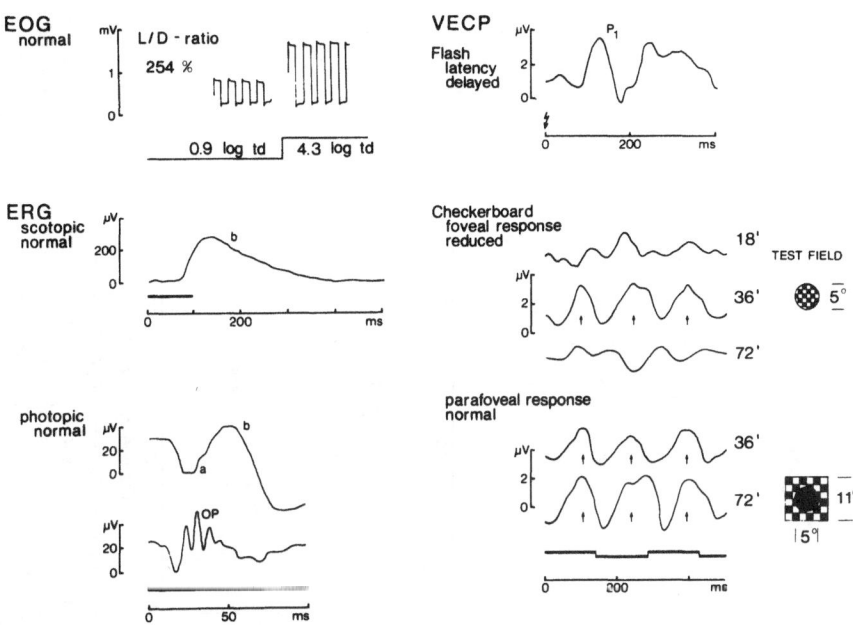

Fig. 2. Electro-ophthalmological findings in Pat. A.W. *Left:* EOG-recordings (top) during the 25th minute of dark adaptation (baseline value, 680 μV) and during the 8th minute of light adaptation (light peak, 1730 μV). The step in illumination from 0.9 log td to 4.3 log td is given below the EOG recordings. Scotopic ERG (center), elicited by a blue test light (3.1 log td). Photopic ERG (bottom), a-wave, b-wave and oscillatory potential (OP) recorded during adaptation to blue light of 2.2 log td, elicited by orange test flashes with a pupillary radiant intensity of 5.6 log I_p (nW/sr). *Right:* Averaged VECP recordings (n = 128). *Top:* Responses elicited by diffuse white test flashes of $10^{6.2}$ lm/sr, presented twice per second. *Center:* Foveal responses, elicited by checkerboard stimuli subtending a central 5° test field; size of the squares as indicated beside each record in minutes of visual angle; contrast 80%, 7 pattern reversals per second. *Bottom:* Parafoveal responses, elicited by a test field of 11° with the central area of 5° blanked out.

cone mechanism (B), during purple adaptation (422 + 630 nm, dots) by the green sensitive system (G) and during blue-green adaptation (487 nm, squares) by the red sensitive cone (R). The three functions mainly resemble the Stiles (1959) π_1, π_4 and π_5 functions (solid lines), peaking near 440, 540 and 570 nm.

In contrast, in the presence of strong white background (Fig. 3, lower half, 5.500° K, 3.7 log td), the spectral sensitivity of a normal trichromatic observer follows a three-peaked function (triangles), with a peak near 440, 530 and 610 nm. Only the action of color-opponent neurons can shift the peaks to longer and shorter wavelengths and produce a pronounced sensitivity-decrease in between the peaks. These dips at 575 nm and 490 nm therefore resemble a sensitive indicator for the function of color-opponent mechanisms (Zrenner 1976, 1977; Jankov 1978).

17

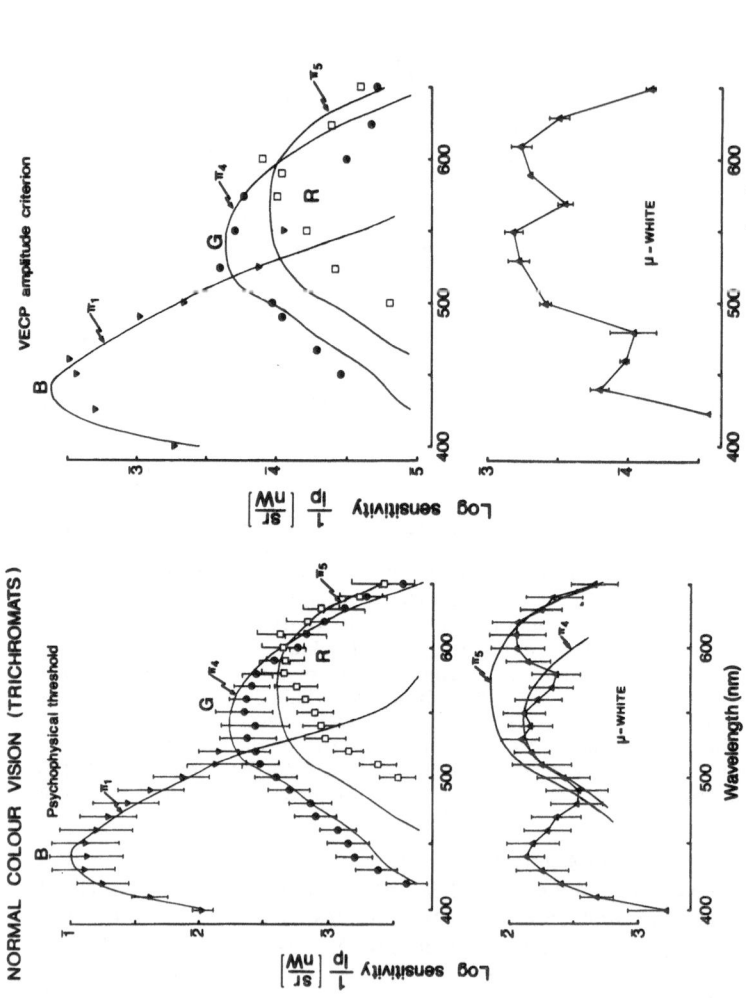

Fig. 3 Upper half: Chromatically separated spectral sensitivity functions of the three cone mechanisms (B, G, R) in normal trichromats. Data points fitted to corresponding Stiles (1959) π functions (solid lines). *Left:* Psychophysical increment threshold measurements (mean and S.D. of 4 observers), obtained during chromatic adaptation to monochromatic yellow (triangles; 574 nm, 3.3 log td), purple (dots; 422 + 630 nm, 4.1 log td) and blue-green light (squares; 487 nm, 3.9 log td). *Right:* Corresponding action spectra obtained by VECP amplitude criterion (mean of three observers), criteria varied individually between 2 μV and 4.5 μV. Retinal illumination of the three adapting lights was 4.9 log td. *Lower half:* Three-peaked spectral sensitivity functions, obtained during adaptation to white light of 3.7 log td. *Left:* Psychophysical threshold measurements (mean and S.D. of 12 trichromats). *Right:* Action spectrum, determined by VECP amplitude criteria (2 μV and 4 μV) in 2 trichromats.

Thus, the function of the three spectrally different receptors (Fig. 3, upper half) as well as the influence of color-opponent neurons (Fig. 3, lower half) producing a three-peaked spectral sensitivity function can be clearly demonstrated in the psychophysical thresholds (Fig. 3, left) as well as in cortical electrical signals (Fig. 3, right) of the human visual system. Since blue sensitive cones are rare in the human retina and have small electrical responses of long latency it is difficult to reveal the blue sensitive mechanism by an electrical criterion (Zrenner & Kojima 1976).

The corresponding tests, performed on the two patients treated with ETHAMBUTOL, are shown in Fig. 4 and 5. Despite their heavily disturbed

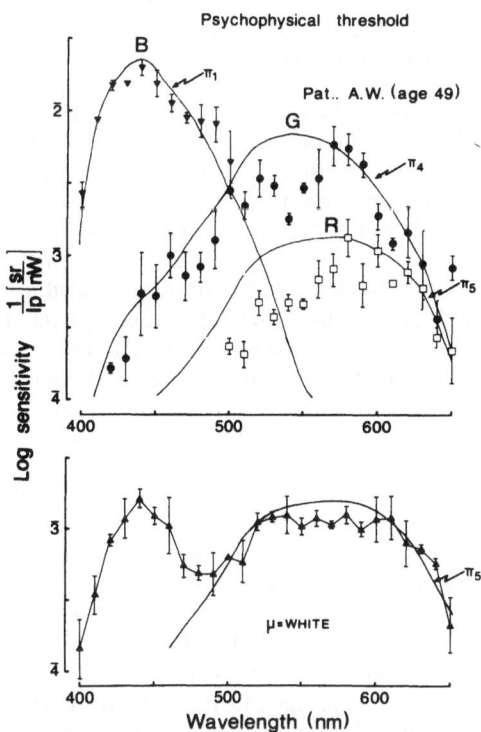

ACQUIRED COLOUR VISION DEFECT

Fig. 4. Spectral sensitivity functions in patient A.W., suffering from acquired color vision defect, caused by Ethambutol. *Top:* Psychophysical increment threshold measurements of the three cone mechanisms (B, G, R). *Bottom:* The spectral sensitivity function determined in presence of strong white adapting light (3.7 log td), lacking the sensitivity decrease at 575 nm, seen in normals (Fig. 3). Each data point represents mean of two measurements, matched to Stiles (1959) π functions. Recording and stimulus conditions as described in Fig. 3.

19

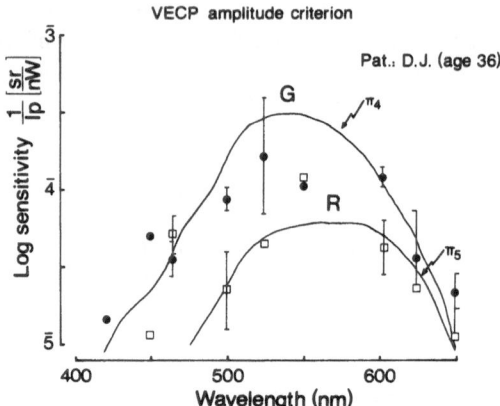

VECP amplitude criterion

Pat.: D.J. (age 36)

Fig. 5. Action spectra of the two long-wavelength cone mechanisms (G, R), determined by a VECP amplitude criterion in Pat. D.J.

color vision, all three receptor mechanisms can be clearly distinguished in the psychophysical threshold measurements (upper half of Fig. 4) as well as by a VECP amplitude criterion, at least for the red and green sensitive mechanism (Fig. 5); however, on a white background (Fig. 4, bottom) these patients showed an altered spectral sensitivity function. Even though the blue sensitive mechanism was clearly revealed, the long wavelength region appeared broadband and single-peaked. The pronounced dip at 575 nm, seen in normal trichromats (Fig. 3, bottom left), was completely lacking; it mainly resembled the Stiles π_5 function, or at least a *synergistic* action between the red and green mechanism. Consequently, in these patients the *antagonistic* interactions between the green and the red sensitive mechanism seem to be lacking, while the receptors, including their individual pathways up to the visual cortex and perceptual areas, are not affected. Only when the dominant red and blue sensitive mechanism is considerably weakened or suppressed by strong purple light (Fig. 5, dots) can the green sensitive mechanism provide some opponent action on the red mechanism as indicated by the dip at 550 nm. Apparently, even with purple adapting light, the green sensitive mechanism is not dominant enough to determine the threshold throughout the entire spectrum, as seen in normals. The absolute sensitivity is reduced by 0.3–0.8 log units, an observation made already by Adachi-Usami, Kellermann & Makabe (1974) in the VECP of ETHAMBUTOL patients.

While the psychophysical data are more of an indicator of the presence or absence of subtractive interaction at visual threshold, the action of opponency in the suprathreshold range can only be shown in the V-log I functions of the VECP. To serve as a routine clinical measurement, this was performed only for the critical wavelength at 575 nm (Fig. 6), where the dip in the spectral sensitivity function is most pronounced in normals. On the x-axis the data were scaled in such a manner that the radiant intensities required for producing a threshold sensation at 620 nm (where *only* the red mechanism is active) are equal for normals (open squares) and for the

20

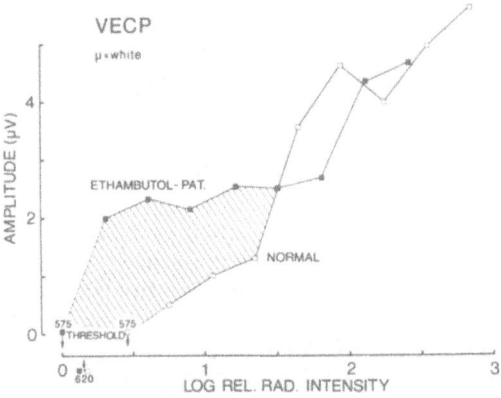

Fig. 6. Amplitude of the first positive peak of the VECP, plotted against the pupillary radiant intensity of monochromatic test lights (575 nm) during adaption to white light (4.2 log td) in the Ethambutol-patient A.W. (filled squares) and in a normal trichromat (open squares). The data are scaled on the x-axis, so that the psychophysical thresholds (arrows) at 620 nm are equal for both observers.

ETHAMBUTOL patient (A.W.). In the presence of white backgrounds (4.2 log td) and with flashes of long duration (400 ms), the patient's (A.W.) threshold was about 0.2 log units *lower* at 575 nm than at 620 nm (arrows at the x-axis).

This is qualitatively the case also in a Stiles π_5 function. The thresholds of normal observers, however, are about 0.3 log units *higher* at 575 nm than at 620 nm, due to the antagonistic interactions in a normal observer (Fig. 3, bottom). When the radiant intensity is increased, both V-log I functions initially rise over a range of about 0.5—0.7 log units (hatched area). Ultimately, however, the patient's V-log I function also turns to the right by more than 1 log unit, indicating an increasing action of color-opponent processing between the two long wavelength sensitive cone mechanisms. At high test light intensities, too, the patient's data match those of normals in which color-opponency was acting already from the psychophysical threshold on. Consequently, color-opponent neurons are acting despite the damage caused by ETHAMBUTOL, but only at quite suprathreshold levels. It is not surprising, then, that patient A.W., having stopped ETHAMBUTOL for half a year, performs perfectly on the normal Panel D-15, while on the desaturated version, large confusions still occur along the red/green deficiency axis. In the period from Sept. 15, 1979 to May 9, 1980, she also improved on the matching range on the Nagel Anomaloscope, still showing deutan-like matches (D). The error score on the F.M. 100 Hue test decreased from 488 to 292 and 544 to 328 for the right and left eye, respectively. In the psychophysical threshold measurements, few changes occurred; probably a more pronounced peak at the red end of the spectrum. Also the visual acuity gradually increased to 0.6 OD and 0.4 OS, similar to the time course of recovery described by Weder (1972).

The data on the second patient (D.J.) strongly support the findings in

21

patient A.W. in all aspects. In this patient, too, both long wavelength mechanisms were present up to the visual cortex as the action spectra obtained by VECP threshold measurements indicated (Fig. 5).

DISCUSSION

In acquired color vision deficiencies caused by ETHAMBUTOL, the toxicity of this drug apparently does not manifest itself so much at the receptor level, since the ERG is normal and all three fundamental cone mechanisms remained unaltered up to the visual cortex. However, the signs of color-opponent interactions are lost in the spectral data on white backgrounds. It becomes very clear that ETHAMBUTOL mainly affects the function of those cells which provide the antagonistic interaction between red and green sensitive neurons on which *color-opponent* processing vitally depends (Zrenner 1979).

According to Pahlitzsch & Tiburtius (1969), in histological investigations of the human eye, only an edema of the optic nerve disk was reported. Gross, Eule & Hager (1973) suggest that in severe cases, toxic damage might also occur at the retinal level; candidates for being affected by ETHAMBUTOL in the early stages of the visual system would be the horizontal cells and/or the amacrine cells connecting the pathway of red and green sensitive cones and thereby providing color-opponent processing, which is revealed in retinal ganglion cells. Still, the loss of color-opponent processing may have taken place at higher levels of the visual system as well. Very high dosages (1300–1600 mg/kg/day applied in rhesus monkey (Schmidt 1966) caused demyelinization of the optic nerve. This would point to a loss of color-opponency due to pooling the information normally carried in individual, well isolated fibers of the optic nerve. Such a high, only experimentally applied dosage, however, is far above the critical therapeutic level 25 mg/kg/day (Leibold 1966; Orou, Sideroff & Schnabel 1972) which nevertheless still causes damage of visual function in about 0.5 to 1.5% of the patients (Pau & Wahl 1972; Thaler, Heilig, Heiss & Lessel 1974). The pathological latency seen in the VECP indicates that at least in early stages of *cortical* processing of visual stimuli the defect manifests itself very clearly.

Interestingly, the action of the green sensitive cone mechanism seems to be more strongly affected than that of the red sensitive one, judging from the spectral sensitivity functions and the performance on the Nagel anomaloscope. This is less surprising since the red sensitive cones functionally dominate in the fovea (Zrenner & Gouras 1979). ETHAMBUTOL probably affects the function of foveal elements to a higher degree than the perifoveal ones; this becomes evident in the Haitz test, since scotomata for green stimuli occur earlier than those for red ones (Stärk 1972). The fact that mainly the green sensitive system's function is affected would also fit Köllner's (1912) law, according to which those deutan-like defects should be caused by damage in the optic pathway. However, this rule is not unequivocally accepted, as exceptions commonly occur (Jaeger, Lux, Grützner & Jessen 1961). According to Grützner (1966; 1972) and Verriest (1974) the position of the neutral band gives additional information about the site of the defect. Patient A.W.'s neutral bands were broad and positioned around 500 nm, while all colors longer than 520 nm were reported as appearing more or less orange ('like fire' according to A.W.) while those shorter than 480 nm appeared bluish.

The damage is, with exceptions (Reimers 1972) neither necessarily complete nor irreversible; strong chromatic stimuli show color-opponent processing also in these patients; color vision and visual acuity improved after stopping the intake of ETHAMBUTOL. The neutral bands, as revealed by a color naming procedure (rather than by a matching experiment) therefore undergo considerable variations which are difficult to quantify. The F.M. 100 Hue test is of great value in estimating changes during the period of observation, in accordance with the findings of Trusciewicz (1975).

ETHAMBUTOL apparently causes a retrobulbar neuritis and thereby only secondarily a red/green color vision defect as it becomes evident in previous clinical reports (first by Carr & Henkind 1962; for a list of subsequent literature, see Verriest 1974 and Pokorny, Smith, Verriest & Pinckers 1979). The damage affecting particularly the function of color-opponent neurons might be a common feature of many types of retrobulbar neuritis, when combined with demyelinization and color vision defects.

The clinically applied electrophysiological and psychophysical tests described here permit the detection of signals of all three types of spectrally different cones up to the visual cortex; moreover, it allows clear differentiation between the *loss* of a receptor mechanism and a *defect* in the neuronal interaction between these cones in the human visual system.

ACKNOWLEDGEMENTS

We are very greatful to Mrs. M. Baier for her dedicated technical assistance in all phases of this study and to Prof. Dr. E. Dodt and R.P. Schuurmans for stimulating discussions of this project.

REFERENCES

Adachi-Usami, E., Kellermann, F.J. & Makabe, R. Visuell evozierte Antworten bei Patienten mit Ethambutol-Schäden. Ber. Dtsch. Ophthalmol. Ges. 72: 181–185 (1974).

Carr, R.E. & Henkind, P. Ocular manifestation of Ethambutol. Toxic amblyopia after administration of an experimental antituberculotic drug. Arch. Ophthal. 67: 566–571 (1962).

De Valois, R.L., Abramov, I. & Jacobs, G.H. Analysis of response patterns of LGN cells. J. Opt. Soc. Am. 56: 966–977 (1966).

Gouras, P. Identification of cone mechanisms in monkey ganglion cells. J. Physiol. 199: 533–547 (1968).

Gouras, P & Zrenner, E. Enhancement of luminance flicker by color-opponent mechanisms. Science 205: 587–589 (1979).

Gross, V., Eule, H. & Hager, G. Auswertung einer Toxizitätsstudie bei intermittierender Ethambutol-Medikation. Klin. Mbl. Augenheilk. 163: 17–22 (1973).

Grützner, P. Über erworbene Farbensinnstörungen bei Sehnervenerkrankungen. Graefes Arch. Ophthalmol. 169: 366–384 (1966).

Grützner, P. Acquired color vision defects. In: Handbook of Sensory Physiology, (Ed. H. Autrum, R. Jung, W.R. Löwenstein, D.M. Makay & H.L. Teuber) Springer, New York. VII/4: 643–659 (1972).

Hoffmann, M.L., Zrenner, E. & Langhof, H.J. Die Wirkung der Pupille als Apertur- und Bildfeldblende auf die verschiedenen Komponenten des menschlichen Elektroretinogramms. Albrecht v. Graefes Arch. klin. exp. Ophthal. 206: 237–245 (1978).

Jaeger, W., Lux, P., Grützner, P. & Jessen, K.H. Subjektive und objektive spektrale Helligkeitsverteilung bei angeborenen und erworbenen Farbensinnstörungen. In R. Jung (ed.): Neurophysiologie und Psychophysik des visuellen Systems. Symposium Freiburg/Br. Springer, Berlin. p. 199–208 (1961).

Jankov, E. Spektralsensitivität der off-Antwort in menschlichen VECP bei verschiedenfarbiger Adaptation. Albrecht v. Graefes Arch. klin. exp. Ophthal. 206: 121–133 (1978).

King-Smith, P.E. & Carden, D. Luminance and opponent-color contributions to visual detection and adaptation and to temporal and spatial integration. J. Opt. Soc. Am. 66: 709–718 (1976).

Köllner, H. Die Störungen des Farbensinnes. Karger, Berlin. (1912).

Kojima, M. & Zrenner, E. Off-components in response to brief light flashes in the oscillatory potential of the human electroretinogram. Albrecht v. Graefes Arch. klin. exp. Ophthal. 206: 107–120 (1978).

Leibold, J.E. The ocular toxicity of Ethambutol and its relation to dose. Ann. N.Y. Acad. Sci. 135: 904–908 (1966).

Little, R.E. A mean square error comparison of certain median response estimates for the up-and-down method with small samples. J. Am. Statist. Assoc. 69: 202–206 (1974).

Marré, M. Clinical examination of the three color vision mechanisms in acquired color vision defects. In: Acquired color vision deficiencies In. Symposium, Ghent. 1971. Karger, Basel. (Mod. Probl. Ophthal. 11) 224–227 (1972).

Orou, F., Sideroff, G. & Schnabel, F. Frequenzuntersuchungen von Opticuserkrankungen im Rahmen der Myambutol-Behandlung. Klin. Mbl. Augenheilk. 161: 601–603 (1972).

Pahlitzsch, H. & Tiburtius, H. Augenuntersuchungen bei Behandlung mit dem neuen Tuberculostaticum Ethambutol-dihydrochlorid. Klin. Mbl. Augenheilk. 154: 228–232 (1969).

Pau, H. & Wahl, M. Myambutol-Schädigung des Auges. Ber. Dtsch. Ophthalmol. Ges. 72: 176–181 (1972).

Pokorny, J., Smith, V.C., Verriest, G. & Pinckers, A.J.L.G. Congenital and acquired color vision defects. Grune and Stratton, New York (1979).

Reimers, D. Irreversible Augenschäden durch Ethambutol. Prax. Pneumol. 26: 445–449 (1972).

Schmidt, I.G. Central nervous system effects of Ethambutol in monkeys. Ann. N.Y. Acad. Sci. 135: 759 (1966).

Stärk, N. Toxische Sehnervenschädigung durch Myambutol. Med. Klin. 67: 913–916 (1972).

Stiles, W.S. Colour vision: the approach theory increment threshold sensitivity. Proc. Nat. Acad. Sci. USA 45: 100–114 (1959).

Thaler, A., Heilig,P., Heiss, W.D. & Lessel, M.R. Toxische Schädigung des nervus opticus durch Ethambutol. Klin. Mbl. Augenheilk. 165: 660–664 (1974).

Trusciewicz, D. Farnsworth 100-Hue Test in diagnosis of Ethambutol-induced damage to optic nerve. Ophthalmologica 171: 425–431 (1975).

Verriest, G. Recent advances in the study of the acquired deficiencies of color vision. Fondazione 'Giorgio Ronchi' XXIV. Firenze (1974).

Wald, G. The receptors of human color vision. Science 145: 1007–1017 (1964).

Weder, W. Myambutolschäden des Sehnerven. Ber. Dtsch. Ophthalmol. Ges. 72: 172–175 (1972).

Wiesel, T.N. & Hubel, D.H. Spatial and chromatic interactions in the lateral geniculate body of the rhesus monkey. J. Neurophysiol. 29: 1115–1156 (1966).

Zrenner, E. Evidence of colour opponency as detected by the visually evoked cortical potential (VECP). Pflügers Arch. Suppl. 365: R 48 (1976).

Zrenner, E. Influence of stimulus duration and area on the spectral luminosity function as determined by sensory VECP measurements. In: (Doc. Ophthal. Proc. Series Vol. 13) 14th ISCERG Symposium Louisville 1976 (ed. T. Lawwill) Junk, The Hague 21–30 (1977).

Zrenner, E. Die Verarbeitung von farbigen Reizen der Primaten retina. Klin. Mbl. Augenheilk. 174: 654–656 (1979).

Zrenner, E. & Baier, M. Einsatz eines Prozeßrechners für on-line Untersuchungen der lichtinduzierten elektrischen Antwort des menschlichen Auges. EDV in Medizin und Biologie 9: 41–46 (1978).

Zrenner, E. & Gouras, P. Cone opponency in tonic ganglion cells and its variation with eccentricity in rhesus monkey retina. Invest. Ophthalmol. Vis. Sci. (Suppl.) 18: 77 (1979).

Zrenner, E. & Kojima, M. Visually evoked cortical potential (VECP) in dichromats. Mod. Probl. Ophthal. 17: 241–246 (1976).

Zrenner, E., Langhof, H.J., Welt, R. & Kojima, M. Elektro-ophthalmologische Beobachtungen zum Verlauf einseitiger tapetoretinaler Dystrophie. Klin. Mbl. Augenheilk. 169: 331–337 (1976).

Authors' addresses:
Dr. E. Zrenner
Max-Planck-Institut für
Physiologische und Klinische Forschung
Parkstr. 1
D – 6350 Bad Nauheim, F.R.G.

Dr. C.J. Krüger
Augenklinik der Mediz, Hochschule
Karl-Wiechert-Allee 9
D-3000 Hannover, F.R.G.

CHROMATIC SIGNALS IN THE VISUAL PATHWAY OF THE DOMESTIC CAT

R.P. SCHUURMANS & E. ZRENNER

(*Bad Nauheim, F.R.G.*)

ABSTRACT

Recordings from the cornea (ERG) and optic nerve (ONR) in the arterially perfused cat eye as well as in vivo from the visual cortex (VECP) revealed a rod (500 nm) mechanism and two clearly distinct cone mechanisms with sensitivity maxima near 460 and 560 nm, when strong selective chromatic adaptation was applied. However, the action spectra obtained during the first seconds of dark adaptation had a sensitivity maximum near 510 nm and came spectrally close to a rod action spectrum. It became apparent that a 510 nm mechanism was present during strong purple adaptation light, when rods were clearly saturated. This mechanism was able to follow flicker as high as 38 c/s; it could be found in the cone dominated VECP recordings; in the ERG it produced cone-like responses of short latency with pronounced a-waves and off-responses; it showed steep V-log I functions, different from rods, and followed the cone branch of the dark adaptation curve. Its spectrum could not be matched by any weighted addition of a 460 nm and 560 nm pigment nomogram. Apparently in cat under photopic conditions, besides a 460 and a 560 nm cone mechanism, a 510 nm mechanism is active which differs in many respects from rods. When strong white or yellow adapting lights are used, opponent-like interactions between these three mechanisms can be demonstrated.

INTRODUCTION

In the analysis of the visual system's function, cats have been widely used as experimental animals. However, the cat's ability to discriminate wavelengths was questioned for a long time. Behavioral studies of the cat's spectral sensitivity function consistently revealed a scotopic luminosity function with a peak near 500 nm (Gunter 1952; La Motte & Brown 1970; Loop 1971). The data on the cat's photopic vision are very inconsistent; apparently stimuli must subtend a large visual angle to reveal abilities of color discrimination in behavioral studies on cat (see Loop, Bruce & Petuchowski 1979). On the other hand, determinations of the cat's spectral sensitivity functions by electroretinographical recordings indicated that at least two cone processes are active under photopic conditions (Rabin, Mehaffey & Berson 1976), one of which, in many respects, resembles rods (Zrenner & Gouras 1979). Granit (1950) and more recently Ringo et al. (1977) and Saunders (1977) showed that cat retinal ganglion cells have input not only from rods, but also from three separate cone systems with peak sensitivity near 450–460, 510–530 and 560–590 nm. Interactions between the short and long wavelength sensitive cone mechanism were shown by Pearlman and Daw (1970) in recordings of color-opponent cells in the cat's corpus geniculatum laterale.

In the present study, during selective chromatic adaptation, we recorded action spectra at three sites of the cat's visual system: From the cornea and the optic nerve in the arterially perfused eye as well as in vivo, from the visual cortex. In particular we established interactions between the three different mechanisms which are active under photopic conditions and differentiated them from rods.

MATERIALS AND METHODS

In the arterially perfused cat eye, as described by Gouras & Hoff (1970), Niemeyer (1975), Zrenner & Gouras (1979), the electroretinogram (ERG) and the optic nerve response (ONR) were recorded simultaneously by silver-silverchloride electrodes from the cornea and with a suction electrode from the trunk of the optic nerve, respectively (Schuurmans & Niemeyer 1978); 51 enucleated eyes were perfused through the ophthalmociliary artery with an oxygenated tissue culture medium, kept at body temperature (37.5°C) inside a heated chamber. Furthermore, in 12 experiments on the intact animal, visually evoked cortical potentials (VECPs) were recorded under Nembutal anaesthesia from the left hemisphere, the ipsilateral eye being covered by a black eye patch. After trepanation of the skull, a silver-silverchloride electrode was positioned beneath the dura at the area striata A (see Doty 1958). The light evoked electrical responses were amplified (Mod. Tönnies), filtered (bandpass 1–300 Hz), monitored on an oscilloscope (Tektronix 5000) and averaged by a Nicolet 1070 computer (n = 64 or 128). In order to rule out influences from anaesthesia, recordings were made during the steady-state, when latencies showed variations no greater than 1.0–1.5 ms. Amplitudes of 'on' and 'off' responses were measured from the first negative through to the subsequent positive peak.

Two beams originating from a Xenon arc lamp (Osram, 150 W) were used for light stimulation; one served as a-test-beam with calibrated, narrow-band interference (half-width 20 nm) and neutral filters; the other served as an adaptation beam with cut-off filters (Jena OG 515 and BG 23) and a purple, two-band interference filter for selective chromatic adaptation (422 + 630 nm, half-band widths of 23 and 46 nm, respectively). The purple, yellow (OG 515) and blue (BG 23) adaptation lights were 3.6, 4.5 and 4.0 log units above the b-wave threshold for rods, respectively. The energy E (Quanta $\cdot$ $s^{-1} \cdot \mu m^{-2}$) of the narrow band stimuli was measured at the retinal level by a calibrated photodiode (United Detector Technology, UDT). Corrections were made for preretinal absorption according to the functions given for cat by Dodt & Walther (1958a).

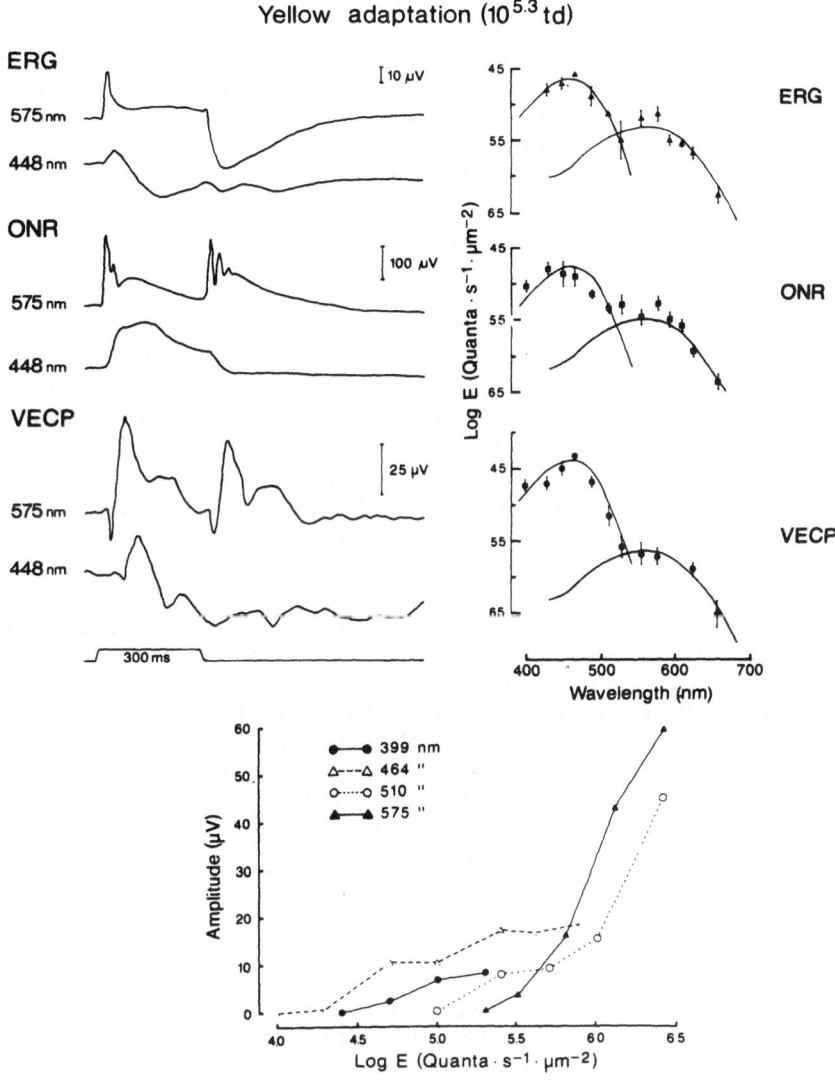

Fig. 1. Original recordings (left), V-log I functions (below) and action spectra (right) obtained during strong yellow adaptation lights ($10^{5.3}$ td) for the ERG (triangles), ONR (squares) and VECP (dots). The data points were fitted by two Dartnall nomograms (solid lines) with peak sensitivity near 460 and 560 nm. The electrical responses to 448 and 575 nm test lights exemplify the typical differences between the two cone mechanisms at all three sites of the visual system. The amplitudes of the VECP plotted against irradiance E for four wavelengths show two different slopes, reflecting the short and long wavelength sensitive cone mechanisms, respectively. Calibrations are given beside each record. Mean values and standard deviations are indicated by filled symbols and vertical bars, respectively.

RESULTS

Fig. 1 shows the responses (left) and action spectra (right) obtained for the ERG, ONR and VECP recordings during strong yellow adaptation as well as the voltage versus log intensity (V-log I) functions for the VECP (Fig. 1, below). The spectral sensitivity functions were based on constant amplitude criteria of $3\,\mu V$, $5\,\mu V$ and $10\,\mu V$ for the ERG (triangles), ONR (squares) and VECP (dots), respectively. The data points were fitted by two Dartnall (1953) pigment nomograms, one having its maximum at 460 nm, the other at 560 nm (solid lines). At intensities between 0.1 and 0.5 log units above threshold, only the short wavelength sensitive cone mechanism responded to a 448 nm test light, while at 575 nm only the long wavelength sensitive cone mechanism was active. The electrical responses to these two light stimuli revealed remarkable differences at all three sites of the visual system which can be characterized as follows: The short wavelength sensitive cone mechanism has a longer latency than the long wavelength sensitive cone mechanism; its optic nerve response consists of a predominantly tonic discharge; it lacks a positive off-effect, typical for the long wavelength sensitive cone mechanism; its flat V-log I functions saturate at much smaller amplitudes. Taken as a whole, these characteristics are typical for the blue sensitive cone mechanism in mammals (Gouras 1970; Zrenner & Gouras 1979). Moreover, a paradoxical transient decrease in sensitivity for the short wavelength sensitive cone mechanism can be observed immediately after extinction of the yellow light adaptation. This is shown in Fig. 2. Every 19 seconds a yellow adaptation light was switched off for 3 seconds. Test stimuli of different wavelengths were applied immediately before (A) extinction of the adaptation light, and 400 (B), 1,400 (C) and 2,400 (D) ms thereafter. The changes in the sensitivity of the different cone mechanisms are evidenced by the action spectra, recorded 400 ms after the offset of the adaptation light (Fig. 2, left, open symbols). The solid lines represent two Dartnall nomograms with maxima at 460 and 560 nm, fitted to the data points obtained during yellow adaptation (filled circles). While the sensitivity of the long wavelength sensitive cone mechanism increased continuously after the extinction of the adaptation light, that of the short wavelength mechanism paradoxically decreased by about 0.6 ± 0.2 log units at 448 nm (arrows). Under identical stimulus conditions a similar change in sensitivity could also be found for the optic nerve response, but not for the simultaneously recorded b-wave. In the latter case, rods dominated the responses; apparently only after a pre-adaptation to white light, bleaching rods to a large extent, a similar paradoxical sensitivity decrease to short-wavelength lights can be found (Valeton & Van Norren 1979). The transient sensitivity change indicates that the blue sensitive cone mechanism's sensitivity is controlled not only by the quanta absorbed by the blue receptors but also by a mechanism with a different spectral sensitivity (Mollon & Polden 1977). The action spectrum recorded 2,400 ms after the long wavelength sensitive cone's recovery (open symbols in Fig. 2, right) did not resemble any of the two action spectra recorded during the yellow adaptation nor any combination of these; with a sensitivity maximum near 510 nm it came close to a rod action spectrum.

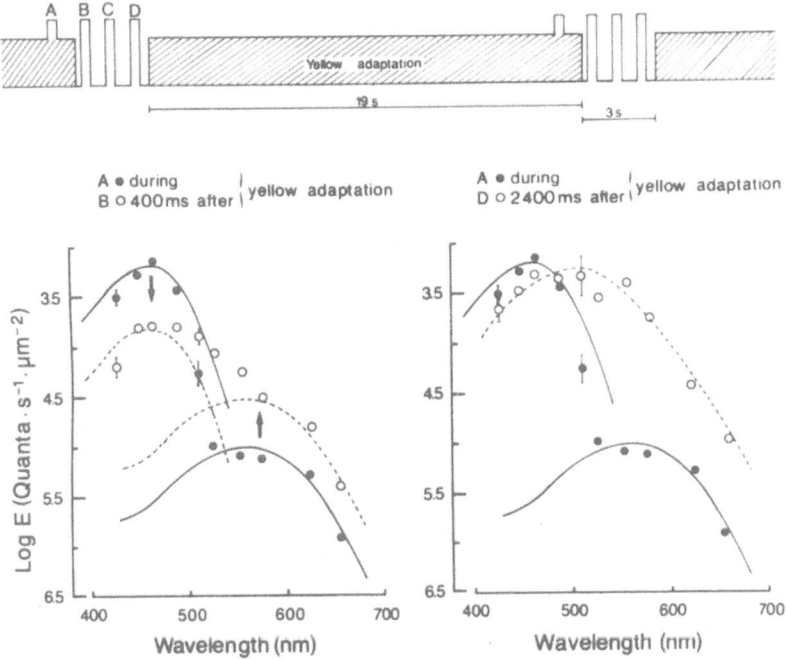

Fig. 2. VECP action spectra obtained by constant threshold response criteria during (A, filled symbols), 400 ms (B, left, open symbols) and 2,400 ms (D, right, open symbols) after the offset of a yellow adapting light. A schematic drawing of the stimulus sequence is shown on top of the figure. A, B, C and D indicate light stimuli presented before, as well as 400, 1,400 and 2,400 ms after extinction of the adaptation light. After 400 ms the sensitivity of the 560 nm cone mechanism increases but that of the 460 nm mechanism decreases (arrows). The action spectrum recorded after 2,400 ms cannot be matched by a 460 or 560 nm pigment nomogram (solid lines) nor by any combination of these. Having a maximum near 510 nm (broken line) it came close to a rod action spectrum.

However, responses mediated by rods can be recorded in the cone dominated VECP only under strictly scotopic conditions and after several minutes of dark adaptation (Huber & Adachi-Usami 1972; Kojima & Zrenner 1977; 1980). They are not likely to contribute to the response occurring already three seconds after extinction of this strong yellow light. This indicates that at least two long wavelength sensitive cone mechanisms participate in generating the cat's VECP during recovery after strong light adaptation. The question arises, whether this middle wavelength cone could be the *third* cone mechanism, recorded in cat ganglion cells (Granit 1950; Ringo, Wolbarsht, Wagner, Crocker & Amthor 1977).

In order to separate the 460 nm and the 560 nm cone mechanism from this middle wavelength mechanism a strong purple background adaptation of 3.5 log td was applied. On top of Fig. 3 (left) the transmittance of this purple filter is shown. It consists of a short and long wavelength band at 422 and 630 nm, respectively. The VECP action spectrum obtained by a 25 μV

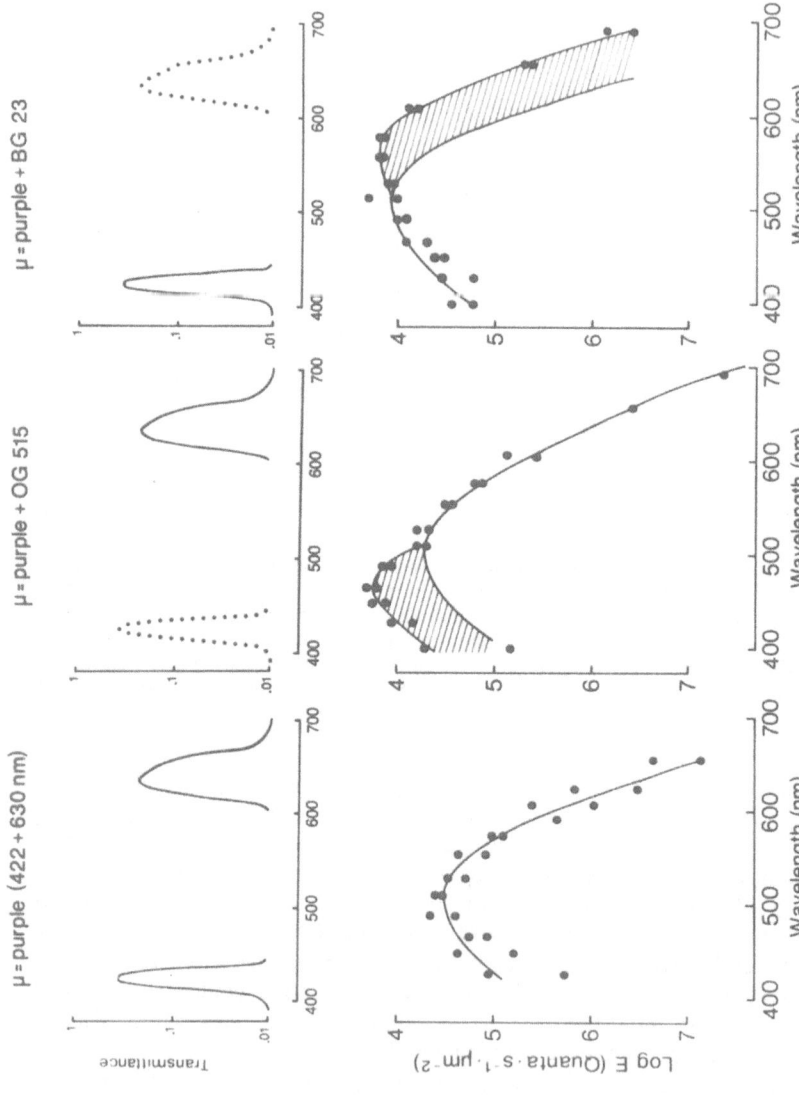

Fig. 3. Action spectra obtained by a VECP amplitude criterion in presence of strong purple adapting lights (left). The transmittance of the purple filter is shown at the top. The corresponding VECP action spectrum fitted a 510 nm pigment nomogram. Adding a OG 515 or BG 23 filter (center and right) which blocks the dotted part of the purple filter results in red and blue adaptation lights, respectively. Correspondingly the sensitivity of the 460 nm and 560 nm cone mechanism increased (hatched areas), the 510 nm mechanism being still present.

criterion during this purple adaptation fairly fitted a Dartnall nomogram with a maximum sensitivity at 510 nm. The recordings elicited by stimuli of all wavelengths showed univariant responses. Adding an additional orange (OG 515) adaptation filter (Fig. 3, center), resulted in a monochromatic 'red' adaptation since the short wavelength band of the purple filter (dotted) was blocked by the orange filter; consequently, the short wavelength sensitive cone mechanism's sensitivity increased (hatched area), the 510 nm function still being present. The responses in the short wavelength branch of the function were slow, lacked a positive off-effect and had a long implicit time, typical for the blue cone mechanism.

On the other hand, when the long wavelength band of the adapting filter was blocked by a blue/green filter (BG 23) the sensitivity of the 560 nm cone increased (hatched area in Fig. 3, right), so that it almost superceded the 510 nm mechanism. Obviously a third mechanism with a maximum sensitivity near 510 nm was active under photopic conditions at which also the 460 and 560 nm cone mechanism can be recorded in the VECP.

In order to investigate the extent to which rods are involved in forming this mechanism, we recorded V-log I functions for a 510 nm test light in the ONR as well as in the ERG at various levels of purple adaptation (Fig. 4). When after 30 min of dark adaptation the purple adaptation was increased by small steps (as indicated beside each function in log td), the slopes of the curve gradually flattened; however, in a typical rod-fashion, they did not adapt, i.e., did not show a shift of the V-log I functions; their half-saturation point stayed at about 2.7 log Quanta $\cdot$ s^{-1} $\cdot$ μm^{-2}. The saturation point was not determined in all V-log I functions in order not to change the state of adaptation by strong test lights. From 3.5 log td purple adaptation on, a second mechanism with a steeper V-log I function emerged, which can be seen also in a prominent change of the response itself (inset figures) when the test light was changed from 4.9 to 6.2 log E, going along the V-log I function. A pronounced a-wave preceeded the b-wave which had a short implicit time. The ERG as well as the optic nerve response exhibited a fast off-effect not seen at lower intensity levels.

Interestingly, the action spectrum of this response which emerged after complete saturation of rods also peaked at 510 nm, as indicated in Fig. 5, completing the data shown in the lower right portion of Fig. 4. Even after the break in the V-log I function's slope from rods to cones as can be seen in the b-wave of the ERG, 510 nm lights were most effective in the ERG as well as in the ONR (upper half). At these high adaptation and intensity levels, the ERG exhibited a fast off-response (lower left), not present at low intensities (3.5 to 5.0 log E), where rods are active. In the optic nerve response (Fig. 5, right) which is 1–2 log units more sensitive than the b-wave of the ERG, the 510 nm test light was again the most sensitive wavelength for the on- as well as for the off-responses. Therefore, with purple adaptation, a photopic 510 nm mechanism determined the responses even in the rod dominated retina of the cat. Moreover, this 510 nm mechanism could easily follow flicker rates up to 38 c/s (Fig. 6), which is not at all typical for rods. A good temporal resolution of the cat's cone mechanisms up to at least 40 c/s was found in behavioral experiments (Loop, personal communication) as well as

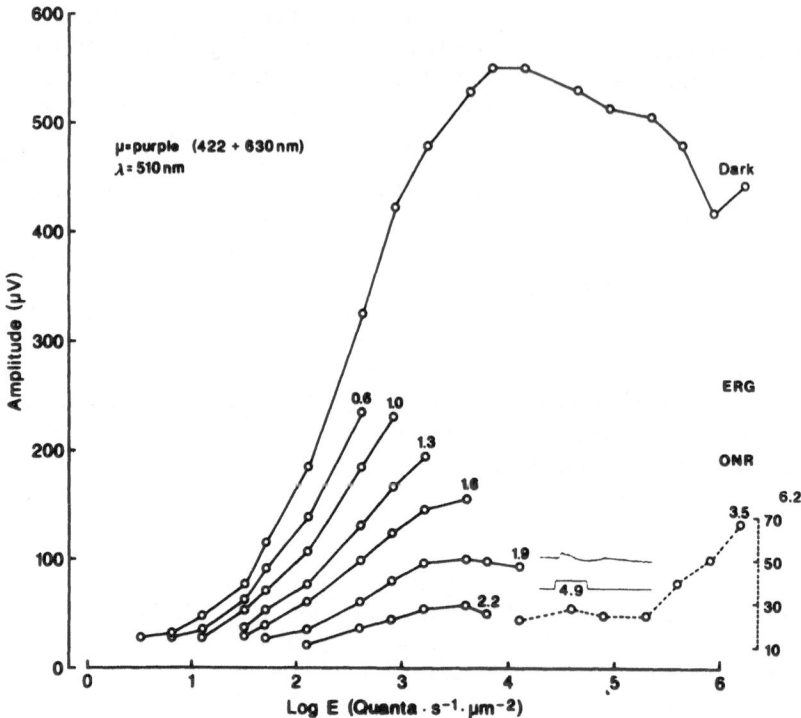

Fig. 4. Amplitude vs. log intensity curves recorded with a 510 nm test light for the b-wave of the ERG at various levels of purple adaptation as indicated in log td beside each function. Responses during purple adaptation of 3.5 log td (broken line, corresponding to the ordinate on the right hand side) are shown for the ERG and ONR at 4.9 and 6.2 log irradiance E, respectively.

in recordings of horizontal (Grüsser 1979) and ganglion cells (Enroth 1952; Dodt & Enroth 1954; Grüsser & Creutzfeldt 1957; Enroth-Cugell & Shapley 1973) in the cat's retina. During purple adaptation, 510 nm stimuli needed the least energy to provoke even the largest response amplitudes at 38 c/s. The action spectrum on the right shows a close fit of the flicker data with a linear addition of a 510 nm and a 560 nm Dartnall nomogram. Interestingly, in the dark adaptation curve obtained by ERG threshold measurements after strong purple adaptation, a cone/rod break was observed after 8 minutes. However, the spectrum obtained during the initial cone-phase again showed a 510 nm mechanism. Such breaks in the dark adaptation curve without concurrent changes in the spectral characteristics were observed by Dodt & Elenius (1960) in rabbit and, under certain conditions, also in cat.

DISCUSSION

In the cat's visual system under photopic conditions a 510 nm receptor mechanism is active besides the 460 nm and 560 nm cone mechanism which have

34

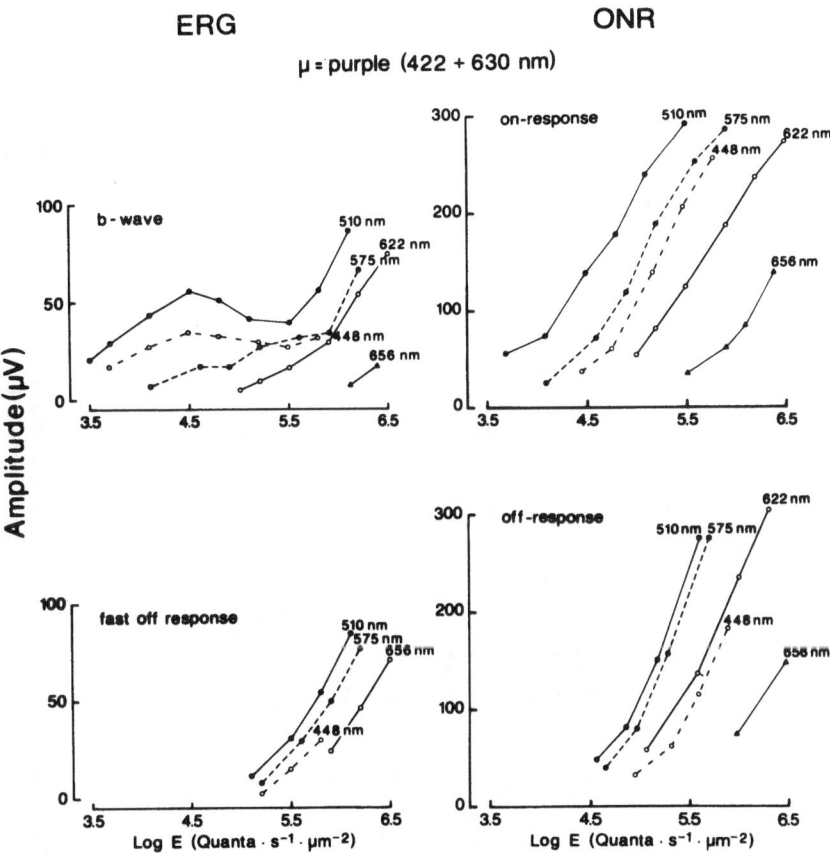

Fig. 5. Amplitudes of the ERG and ONR vs. log irradiance recorded during strong purple adaptation at five different wavelengths. At threshold, rods determine the response for the b-wave. At high intensities, the ERG and ONR exhibit fast off-effects, typical for cones. In the ONR and ERG 510 nm test lights determine the responses, at all levels of stimulus strength, before and after the break in the V-log I function.

been well studied in single cells (Granit 1950) and ERG (Zrenner & Gouras 1979; Rabin et al., 1976) as well as in the optic nerve and VECP (Schuurmans & Zrenner 1979). A photopic mechanism with such spectral characteristics is also found in other mammals such as rabbit (Dodt & Walther 1958b). Even though the 510 nm mechanism action spectrum is almost undiscernably close to that of rods, its functional properties in almost all respects resemble those of cones; it works at adaptation levels, where rods are clearly saturated; it produces cone-like responses (with typical a-waves, b-waves of short implicit time and positive off-responses); it shows steep V-log I functions, while rods show much flatter ones at high adaptation levels; its spectrum cannot be matched by any weighted addition of 460 and 560 nm pigment nomograms; it follows flicker rates up to about 40 c/s, not observed in the ERG of rods; it follows the cone branch of the dark adaptation curve up to eight minutes,

36

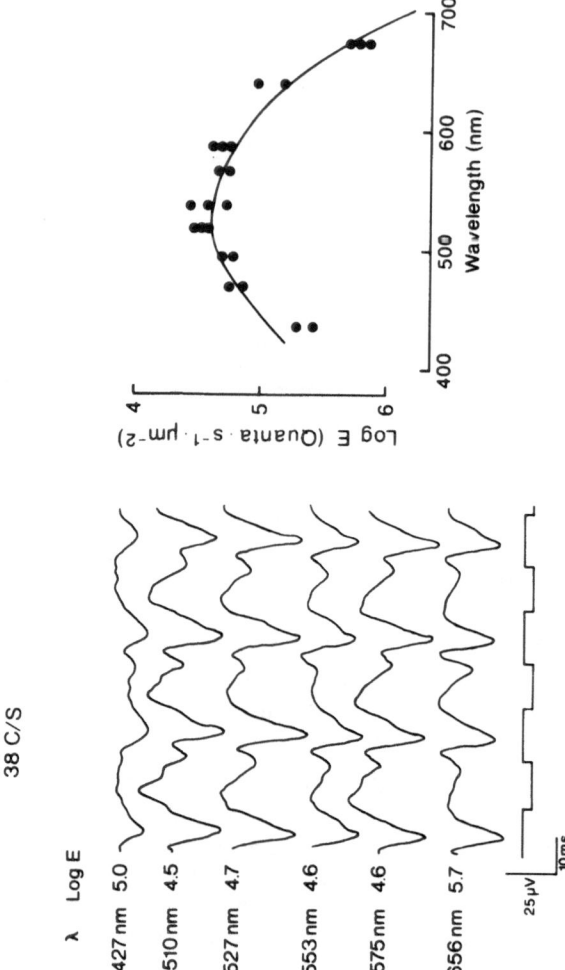

Fig. 6. ERG responses during strong purple adaptation to light stimuli of different wavelengths presented at a flicker rate of 38 c/s. The data points of the corresponding action spectrum shown on the right are fitted with a linear addition of a 510 and 560 nm pigment nomogram. Calibration is indicated on the lower left.

when rods begin to determine the threshold; it can easily be recorded in the cone dominated VECP responses, when a purple adapting light is applied.

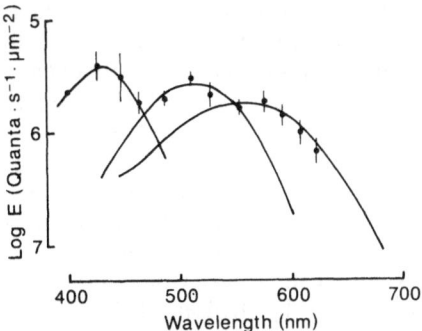

Fig. 7. The action spectrum obtained by a 15 μV amplitude criterion for the ONR during adaptation to strong (4.6 log td) white light exhibits a three peaked function with maxima near 435, 510 and 560 nm. The solid lines represent a 560 nm Dartnall nomogram (right), a weighted linear subtraction (see text) of a 510 and a 460 nm nomogram (center) and a weighted linear subtraction of a 460 nm and 510 nm nomogram (left). The sensitivity of the 460 nm cone mechanism is shifted to shorter wavelengths and its action spectrum is narrowed indicating color-opponent interactions.

An indication that rods could behave like cones comes from the work of Conner & MacLeod (1977), who showed in man that rods (as evidenced by their spectral sensitivity, their dark adaptation as well as directional-sensitivity properties) abruptly change their temporal frequencies at high luminances permitting the detection of rapid flicker. The same kind of data is presented by Green and Siegel (1975) in a study on the critical flicker frequency in the all-rod skate retina.

However, we do not want to commit ourselves by calling the receptors subserving this mechanism rods or cones, since these terms are mainly ana-tomical. Clear evidence that the spectral data of this 510 nm mechanism are not produced by any additive or subtractive combination of the 560 and 460 nm cone mechanisms is given in Fig. 7. The function obtained by a 15 μV amplitude criterion in the ONR during strong white adaptation (4.6 log td) clearly shows three peaks at 560 nm, 510 nm and 435 nm, separated by dips at 550 nm and 470 nm. Apparently *three individual,* spectrally different receptor mechanisms are active during strong white light adaptation. This is in agreement with Donner's (1950) observation that there are three groups of optic fibres distinguishable by the temporal characteristics of their spike-frequency maxima elicited by red, green and blue lights.

The question, whether these mechanisms interact with each other in a color-opponent manner, is difficult to answer without recordings from single cells. However, spectral data obtained on bright white backgrounds can give strong evidence for such interactions, both psychophysically (Sperling & Harwerth 1971; King-Smith & Carden 1976) as well as in electrical sum potentials (Padmos & Graf 1974; Van Norren & Baron 1977 and Zrenner 1977). The action spectrum in the long wavelength region of Fig. 7 is best fitted by a 560 nm Dartnall nomogram, while for the middle wavelength part a 510 nm spectrum fits especially well after a linear subtraction of

37

$1\alpha_{510} - 0.25\alpha_{460}$, where α indicates the corresponding Dartnall nomogram, according to the method described by Sperling & Harwerth (1971). In the short wavelength region the sensitivity maximum occurs at 435 nm. This shift of the peak by 25 nm to shorter wavelengths and the narrowing of the spectral branch can only be produced by an opponent interaction. The best fit for the short wavelength part can be obtained by a linear subtraction of $1\alpha_{460} - 1\alpha_{510}$, which indicates that on white background particularly the 510 nm mechanism interacts with the 460 nm mechanism. The lack of an obvious antagonistic interaction between the 560 and 510 nm mechanism observed in the optic nerve recording points to a retinal circuitry which must be different from the classical opponent one shown in monkey by Wiesel & Hubel (1966). De Valois et al. (1966), Gouras (1968) and Gouras & Zrenner (1979). However, as shown by Krüger (1979), even color non-selective cells can be assumed to mediate the detection of heterochromatic stimuli. On the other hand, opponent interactions between the 460 nm and the long wavelength sensitive mechanisms are shown in the ERG by Zrenner & Gouras (1979), in ganglion cell recordings by Cleland & Levick (1974) and in the c-laminae of the corpus geniculatum laterale by Pearlman & Daw (1970) as well as by Wilson & Stone (1975). Furthermore, it is indicated in our data by the paradoxical decrease in threshold found for the 460 nm cone's sensitivity after extinction of a yellow adapting light as well as by the narrowing and shift of the 460 nm maximum to shorter wavelengths during strong white background adaptation.

Considering the paucity of blue sensitive cones and the fact that opponency in the cat's visual system occurs mainly when the 460 nm cone mechanism is involved, color-opponency in cat retinal ganglion cell is expected to be less common. We cannot prove that the cat perceives color, since the perception of color demands higher order cortical functions; however, we could clearly demonstrate that the 510 nm mechanism is a good candidate for providing cat with trichromatic vision, since it is present from the receptor layer on, up to the neurons which generate the responses in the cat's visual cortex.

ACKNOWLEDGEMENTS

The authors wish to thank Prof. Dr. E. Dodt and Dr. J. Tanabe for their stimulating discussions and Miss M. Klein for excellent technical assistance.

REFERENCES

Cleland, B.G. & Levick, W.R. Properties of rarely encountered types of ganglion cells in the cat's retina and an overall classification. J. Physiol. 240: 457–492 (1974).

Conner, J.D. & MacLeod, D.I.A. Rod photoreceptors detect rapid flicker. Science 195: 698–699 (1977).

Dartnall, H.J.A. The interpretation of spectral sensitivity curves. Brit. Med. Bull. 9: 24–30 (1953).

De Valois, R.L., Abramov, I. & Jacobs, G.H. Analysis of response patterns of LGN cells. J. Opt. Soc. Am. 56: 966–977 (1966).

Dodt, E. & Elenius, V. Change of threshold during dark adaptation measured with orange and blue light in cats and rabbits. Experientia 16: 313 (1960).

Dodt, E. & Enroth, Ch. Retinal flicker response in cat. Acta Physiol. Scand. 30: 375–390 (1954).

Dodt, E. & Walther, J.B. Netzhautsensitivität, Linsenabsorption und physikalische Lichtstreuung. Der skotopische Dominator der Katze im sichtbaren und ultravioletten Spektralbereich. Pflügers Arch. 266: 167–174 (1958a).

Dodt, E. & Walther, J.B. Photopic sensitivity mediated by visual purple. Experientia 14: 142 (1958b).

Donner, K.O. The spike frequencies of mammalian retinal elements as a function of wave-length of light. Acta Physiol. Scand. Suppl. 21: 1–59 (1950).

Doty, R.W. Potentials evoked in cat cerebral cortex by diffuse and by punctiform photic stimuli. J. Neurophysiol. 21: 437–464 (1958).

Enroth, Ch. The mechanism of flicker and fusion studied on single retinal elements in the dark-adapted eye of the cat. Acta Physiol. Scand. Suppl. 27: 1–67 (1952).

Enróth-Cugell, Ch. & Shapley, R.M. Adaptation and dynamics of cat retinal ganglion cells. J. Physiol. 233, 271–309 (1973).

Gouras, P. Identification of cone mechanisms in monkey ganglion cells. J. Physiol. 199: 533–547 (1968).

Gouras, P. Electroretinography: Some basic principles. Invest. Ophthal. 9: 557–569 (1970).

Gouras, P. & Hoff, M. Retinal function in an isolated, perfused mammalian eye. Invest. Ophthal. 9: 388–399 (1970).

Gouras, P. & Zrenner, E. Enhancement of luminance flicker by color-opponent mechanisms. Science 205: 587–589 (1979).

Granit, R. The organization of the vertebrate retinal elements. In: Ergebnisse der Physiologie, biologischen Chemie und experimentellen Pharmakologie (Ed. O. Krayer, E. Lehnartz, A.v. Muralt & F.H. Rein. Springer, Berlin. 31–70 (1950).

Green, D.G. & Siegel, I.M. Double branched flicker fusion curves from the all-rod skate retina. Science 188: 1120–1122 (1975).

Grüsser, O.-J. Cat ganglion-cell receptive fields and the role of horizontal cells in their generation. In: The Neurosciences (Ed. F.O. Schmitt & F.G. Worden) MIT Press, Cambridge. 247–273 (1979).

Grüsser, O.-J. & Creutzfeldt, O. Eine neurophysiologische Grundlage des Brücke-Bartley-Effektes: Maxima der Impulsfrequenz retinaler und corticaler Neurone bei Flimmerlicht mittlerer Frequenzen. Pflügers Arch. 263: 668–681 (1957).

Gunter, R. The spectral sensitivity of dark-adapted cats. J. Physiol. 118: 395–404 (1952).

Huber, C. & Adachi-Usami, E. Scotopic luminosity curve as obtained by the visual evoked response in man. Experientia 28: 1045–1046 (1972).

King-Smith, P.E. & Carden, D. Luminance and opponent-color contributions to visual detection and adaptation and to temporal and spatial integration. J. Opt. Soc. Am. 66: 709–717 (1976).

Kojima, M. & Zrenner, E. Local and spatial distribution of photopic and scotopic responses in the visual field as reflected in the visually evoked cortical potential (VECP). In: 14th ISCERG Symposium (Ed. Th. Lawwill). Junk, The Hague (Doc. Ophthal. Proc. Ser. Vol. 13) 31–40 (1977).

Kojima, M. & Zrenner, E. Determination of local thresholds in the visual field by recording the scotopic visually evoked cortical potential in man. Ophthalmic Res. 12: 1-8 (1980).

Krüger, J. Responses to wavelength contrast in the afferent visual systems of the cat and the rhesus monkey. Vision Res. 19: 1351–1358 (1979).

La Motte, R.H. & Brown, J.L. Dark adaptation and spectral sensitivity in the cat. Vision Res. 10: 703–716 (1970).

Loop, M.S. An investigation of the scotopic luminosity function in the cat employing a modified conditioned suppression technique. Unpublished master's thesis. Florida State University, Tallahassee (1971).

Loop, M.S., Bruce, L.L. & Petuchowski, S. Cat color vision: The effect of stimulus size, shape and viewing distance. Vision Res. 19: 507–513 (1979).

Mollon, J.D. & Polden, P.G. An anomaly in the response of the eye to light of short wavelengths. Phil. Trans. R. Soc. Lond. B 278: 207–240 (1977).

Niemeyer, G. The function of the retina in the perfused eye. Docum. Ophthal. 39: 53–116 (1975).

Padmos, P. & Graf, V. Colour vision in rhesus monkey, studied with subdurally implanted cortical electrodes. In: 11th ISCERG Symposium (Ed. E. Dodt & J.T. Pearlman). Junk, The Hague (Doc. Opthal. Proc. Ser. Vol. 4) 307–314 (1974).

Pearlman, A.L. & Daw, N.W. Opponent color cells in the cat lateral geniculate nucleus. Science 167: 84–86 (1970).

Rabin, A.R., Mehaffey III, L. & Berson, E.L. Blue cone function in the retina of the cat. Vision Res. 16: 799–801 (1976).

Ringo, J., Wolbarsht, M.L., Wagner, H.G., Crocker, R. & Amthor, F. Trichromatic vision in the cat. Science 198: 753–755 (1977).

Saunders, R. McD. The spectral responsiveness and the temporal frequency response (TFR) of cat optic tract and lateral geniculate neurons: Sinusoidal stimulation studies. Vision Res. 17: 285–292 (1977).

Schuurmans, R.P. & Niemeyer, G. Effects of strychnine on light-evoked electrical responses in the perfused eye of the cat. Ophthalmic Res. 10, 336 (1978).

Schuurmans, R.P. & Zrenner, E. The short and long wavelength sensitive cone mechanisms in the cat's visual system: ERG, optic nerve and VECP recordings. Pflügers Arch. Suppl. 382: R 47 (1979).

Sperling, H.G. & Harwerth, R.S. Red-green cone interactions in the increment-threshold spectral sensitivity of primates. Science 172: 180–184 (1971).

Valeton, J.M. & van Norren, D. Retinal site of transient tritanopia. Nature 280: 488–490 (1979).

Van Norren, D. & Baron, W.S. Increment spectral sensitivities of the primate late receptor potential and b-wave. Vision Res. 17: 807–810 (1977).

Wiesel, T.N. & Hubel, D.H. Spatial and chromatic interactions in the lateral geniculate body of the rhesus monkey. J. Neurophysiol. 29: 1115–1156 (1966).

Wilson, P.D. & Stone, J. Evidence of W-cell input to the cat's visual cortex via the C laminae of the lateral geniculate nucleus. Brain Res. 92: 472–478 (1975).

Zrenner, E. Influence of stimulus duration and area on the spectral luminosity function as determined by sensory and VECP measurements. In: 14th ISCERG Symposium (Ed. Th. Lawwill). Junk, The Hague (Doc. Ophthal. Proc. Ser. Vol. 13) 21–30 (1977).

Zrenner, E. & Gouras, P. Blue-sensitive cones of the cat produce a rodlike electroretinogram. Invest. Ophthalmol. Visual Sci. 18: 1076–1081 (1979).

Authors' address:
Max-Planck-Institute for
Physiological and Clinical Research
Parkstr. 1
D – 6350 Bad Nauheim

EARLY WAVELETS IN THE VECP

J.B. SIEGFRIED & J. LUKAS

(Philadelphia & Aberdeen Proving Ground, U.S.A.)

ABSTRACT

Utilizing a Maxwellian view optical system to present light flashes to the right eye, electroretinograms (ERG) and visual evoked cortical potentials (VECP) were recorded from normal subjects. The first 120 mS post flash onset was examined. A series of 5 VECP wavelets were recorded with implicit times of 50, 72, 82, 90 and 101 mS, at the highest radiance used. Recordings of ERG in the same experimental session revealed a series of 3 wavelets with implicit times of 23, 30, and 38 mS. It is concluded that the VECP wavelets are not volume conducted from the retina, and probably represent initial arrival of visual information at the cortex or subcortical activity.

INTRODUCTION

The human visual evoked cortical potential (VECP) recorded from the occipital region of the scalp exhibits photopic characteristics under photopic conditions of stimulation (Siegfried 1971; Siegfried 1978), strongly emphasizes the contribution from the fovea (Riggs & Wooten 1972), and is exquisitely sensitive to spatial (pattern) characteristics of the stimulus. (Siegfried 1975). Most quantitative studies of the VECP have examined components with implicit times of 80–300 mS which average 5–20 μV in amplitude and are of under 100 Hz frequency. These components are almost certainly of intracortical origin. A few experiments (Cobb & Dawson 1960; Cracco & Cracco 1978; Tsuchida, Kawasaki, Fujimura & Jacobson 1973) have drawn attention to the existence of early, initial components of the VECP, which consist of 3–5 wavelets, each approximately 1 μV in amplitude. Cracco & Cracco (1978) report VECP wavelets with peaks occurring at very short implicit times (21, 30, 39 and 52 mS), whereas those reported by others (Cobb & Dawson 1960; Tsuchida, Kawasaki, Fujimura & Jacobson 1973) occur after approximately 40 mS. We describe early visual wavelets which have been recorded on our laboratories, and compare them to similiar wavelets ('oscillations') in the electroretinogram (ERG).

Doc. Ophthal. Proc. Series, Vol. 27, ed. by H. Spedreijse & P.A. Apkarian   41

© *1981 Dr W. Junk Publishers, The Hague/Boston/London*

MATERIAL AND METHODS

The VECP was recorded by means of an electrode (Grass Inst. Co., gold) affixed to the scalp in the midline approximately 2 cm anterior to the occipital protuberance (inion), referenced to the left ear lobe, with subject ground on the right ear lobe. ERG activity was recorded by means of a platinum electrode in contact with the inferior portion of the cornea (Cummings & Kaluzne 1978), referenced to the upper middle of the forehead. Inter-electrode skin impedance was maintained below 5,000 ohms. Amplification was by means of battery operated differential units (Grass Inst. Co., Model P-15), operated in cascaded pairs to achieve sufficient gain. Although a number of band pass settings was investigated, in these experiments optimum available settings were 100 Hz to 1,000 Hz for ERG wavelets and a window peaking at 100 Hz (6 dB/octave roll off) for VECP wavelets. Amplified potentials were led to a DEC LAB 8/e computer for signal averaging utilizing a 120 mS analysis time. Sampling frequency was 2,083 Hz for each channel. Therefore the frequency response of the recording system was effectively limited by the amplifier pass band settings. Some of the amplified electrical activity was also recorded, in parallel, on FM magnetic tape for subsequent additional analysis. Subjects were housed within a light proof and electromagnetically shielded room. They viewed the flashing stimulus in Maxwellian view with the right eye, the left eye being patched. In order to minimize spurious electromyographic (EMG) signals, subjects were placed in the supine position on a padded surgical table. The light beam subtended 25° visual angle, and included an incomplete cross-hairs to aid fixation. The head was additionally stabilized by means of a dental impression wax bite board, containing an impression of only the two front upper teeth. Flashes of 20 mS duration were presented at a frequency of 3 Hz and 200 (ERG) or 500 (VECP) responses were averaged. The highest stimulus radiance employed produced a retinal illuminance of 1.94×10^5 Trolands. Neutral density filters were inserted into the light path to achieve a 3 log unit range of retinal illuminance. Subjects were undergraduate students who had normal vision.

RESULTS

Fig. 1 illustrates the behavior of ERG and VECP wavelets in response to a series of light radiances. Three main positive (downward) wavelets are seen in the ERG, with implicit times of 23, 30, and 38 mS in the topmost record. The simultaneously recorded VECP exhibits 5 negative (upward) wavelets, with implicit times of 50, 72, 82, 90, and 101 mS. in the topmost record. Experiments utilizing an analysis time of 450 mS and a slower flash rate verified that additional VECP wavelets were not present past the initial 120 mS. Choosing as arbitrary reference points the first ERG and VECP wavelets, their implicit times increase with decreasing illuminance from 23 mS to 37 mS (ERG) and from 50 mS to 88 mS (VECP). These curves

42

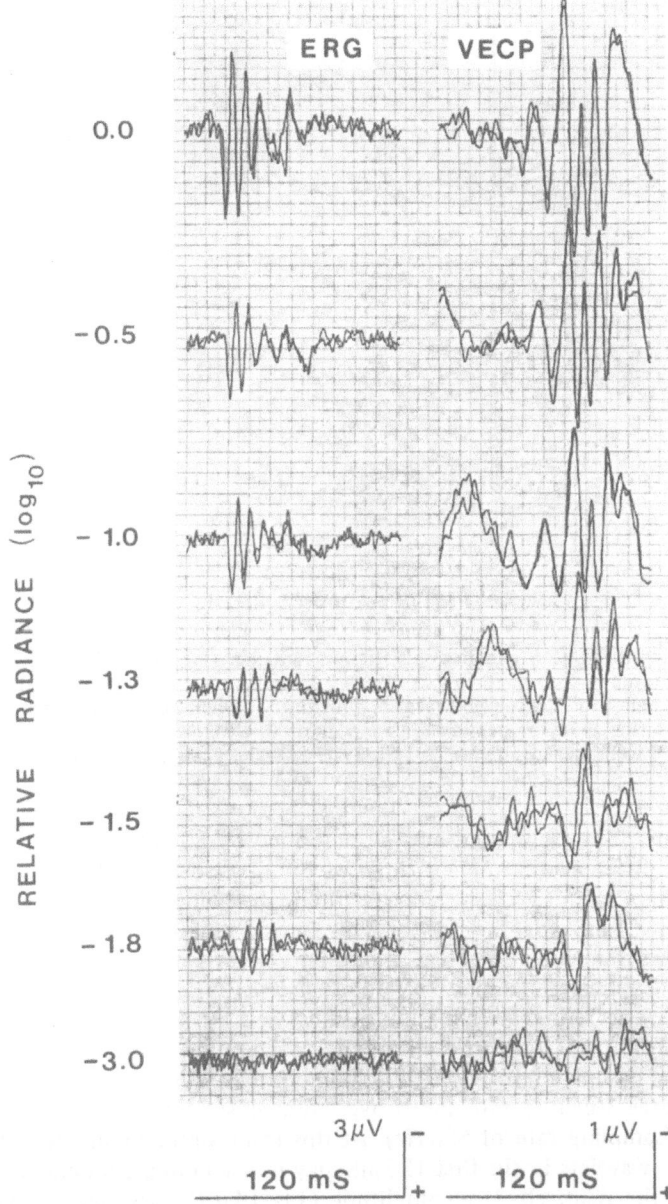

Fig. 1. Wavelets in ERG (left column) and VECP (right column). Relative radiance (log$_{10}$) is indicated on the left hand side. Each pair of ERG tracings (2 consecutive averages superimposed) is based on 200 flash presentations, and is recorded with a pass band setting of 100 Hz to 1,000 Hz. Each pair of VECP tracings is based on 500 flash presentations, and is recorded with a pass band centered on 100 Hz (6 dB/octave roll off). In both columns negativity at the active electrode (cornea or occipital scalp) is upward.

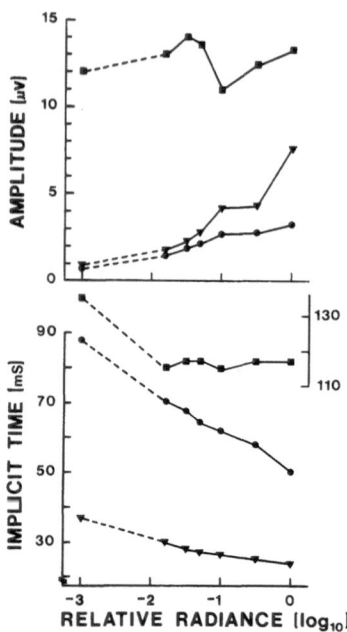

Fig. 2. Top: Amplitude as a function of relative radiance ($\log_{10}$) of the first major positive-negative deflection of the VECP slow component ($P_1 - N_1$) (squares), and VECP (circles) and ERG (triangles) wavelets. Bottom: Implicit time as a function of relative radiance ($\log_{10}$) of first major negative peak of VECP slow component (squares), N_1, VECP first wavelet peak, (circles), and ERG first wavelet peak, (triangles).

are not parallel, but each could be well described by a linear function (Fig. 2). Thus, the difference in implicit times of the first wavelet in the ERG and the VECP ranges from a low of 27 mS at the highest illuminance employed, to a high of 51 mS for the lowest illuminance employed. Peak-to-peak amplitude measurements also reveal similar curves for ERG and VECP wavelets. Amplitudes increase from $1.0\,\mu V$ to $7.6\,\mu V$ (ERG), and from $0.7\,\mu V$ to $3.3\,\mu V$ (VECP) as retinal illumination is increased by 3.0 log units. These curves relating implicit time and amplitude to stimulus radiance for VECP wavelets were compared to those obtaining in VECP slow wave activity. Fig. 3 illustrates VECP records taken over an analysis time of 450 mS from flash onset, (sampling rate of 556 Hz). At this resolution and analysis time, suggestions of wavelets in the first 120 mS may be seen but are unremarkable compared to the relatively large amplitude ($11-14\,\mu V$) slow wave activity. In addition, heavy contamination of the records by alpha activity, and associated photic driving exists in the records. When the amplitude of $P_1 - N_1$, and implicit time of N_1 are plotted as a function of stimulus radiance, they are characterized by the lack of clear trend.

The repetition frequency of ERG wavelets has been shown to be relatively constant, independent of changes in stimulus conditions (Babel, Stangos, Korol & Spiritus 1977). Over the range of retinal illuminances employed in

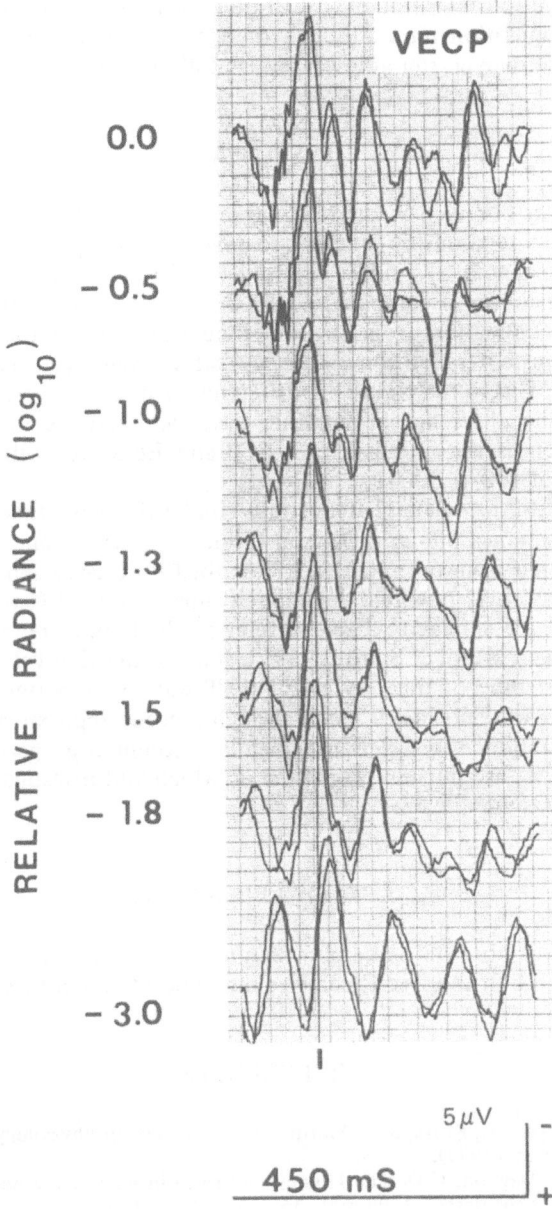

RELATIVE RADIANCE ($\log_{10}$)

0.0

– 0.5

– 1.0

– 1.3

– 1.5

– 1.8

– 3.0

VECP

5 µV

450 mS

Fig. 3. VECP recordings obtained with a 450 mS analysis time and a pass band setting of 1 Hz to 1,000 Hz. Two consecutive averages of 200 flashes are presented super-imposed for each value of radiance. The first 120 mS of the responses is indicated by the vertical line at the bottom.

45

these experiments, for the ERG the mean inter-wavelet time is 7.2 mS, or 139 Hz repetition rate. For the VECP the mean inter-wavelet time is 9.8 mS, or 102 Hz repetition rate, although there was some tendency for the inter-wavelet time to be greater at lower levels of illuminance.

DISCUSSION

Early wavelets observed in these VECP records exhibit the following properties: 1) linear relationship of peak-to-peak amplitude and implicit time to retinal illuminance; 2) similar amplitude to ERG wavelets; 3) substantially greater implicit times compared to ERG wavelets ruling out the possibility of volume conduction from the inner nuclear layer of the retina; and 4) relatively constant repetition frequency, whose value (102 Hz), is less than that for the ERG (139 Hz). This difference in repetition frequencies is not caused be the difference in amplifier pass band settings, as essentially the same differences are found when VECP and ERG are both recorded with a pass band of 100–1,000 Hz.

These VECP wavelets share certain similarities with those of Tsuchida, et al. (1973), and Cobb and Dawson (1960). However, some of the implicit times measured from occipital leads described by Cracco and Cracco (1978) (21, 30, 39, 52 mS) resemble the implicit times of our ERG wavelets (23, 30, 38 mS), and are similar to ERG wavelet implicit times reported by others (Babel, Stangos, Korol & Spiritus 1977). It is possible that volume conduction accounts for some of the very early VECP wavelets reported by others. We have not seen wavelets in our records which precede approximately 40 mS.

The generation of wavelets is evidently a common property of the visual system, and we are pursuing experiments which will investigate the relations between ERG and VECP wavelets.

ACKNOWLEDGEMENT

Partial support for this research was provided by The Pennsylvania Lions Sight Conservation and Eye Research Foundation to John B. Siegfried.

REFERENCES

Babel, J., Stangos, N., Korol, S., & Spiritus, M. Ocular electrophysiology. Georg Thieme, Pub., Stuttgart. (1977).

Cobb, W.A. & Dawson, G.D. The latency and form in man of the occipital potentials evoked by bright flashes. J. Physiol., 152, 108–121, (1960).

Cracco, R.Q. & Cracco, J.B. Visual evoked potentials in man: early oscillatory potentials. Electroencephal. clin. Neurophysiol. 45: 731–739. (1978).

Cummings, R.W. & Kaluzne, S.J. An improved electrode for electroretinography: design and standardization. Amer. J. Optom. Physiol. Optics. 55: 719–724 (1978).

Riggs, L.A. & Wooten, B.R. Electrical measures and psychophysical data on human vision. In Handbook of Sensory Physiology, Vol. VII/4, Visual Psychophysics (ed. D. Jameson & L.M. Hurvich) Springer. Verlag Pub. New York 690–752 (1972).

Siegfried, J.B. Spectral sensitivity of human visual evoked cortical potentials: a new method and a comparison with psychophysical data Vis. Res., 11: 405–417 (1971).

Siegfried, J.B. The effects of checkerboard pattern check size on the VECP. Bull. Psychon. Soc. 6: 306–308 (1975).

Siegfried, J.B. VECP: its spectral sensitivity. In: Visual Psychophysics and physiology (Ed. J.C. Armington, J. Krauskopf & B.R. Wooten). Academic Press, New York. 257–267 (1978).

Tsuchida, Y., Kawasaki, K., Fujimura, K., & Jacobson, J.H. Isolation of faster components in the electroretinogram and visually evoked response in man. Amer. J. Ophthalmol. 75: 846–852 (1973).

Authors' addresses:
J.B. Siegfried
Pennsylvania College of Optometry
Neuro-visual Sciences Tract
1200 West Godfrey Avenue
Philadelphia, PA 19126, U.S.A.

J. Lukas
Behavioral Research Directorate
U.S. Army Human Engineering Laboratory
Aberdeen Proving Ground, Maryland, U.S.A.

EARLY COMPONENTS OF THE VISUAL EVOKED POTENTIAL IN MAN

Are they of sub-cortical origin?

G.F.A. HARDING & M.P. RUBINSTEIN

(*Birmingham, England*)

ABSTRACT

Stimulus and analysis parameters have been adjusted to provide optimum conditions for producing and recording the early components of the flash VEPs. A visual evoked potential of mean latency P20-N26-P34 has been recorded in 93% of normal subjects maximally from an electrode position slightly posterior to the Rolandic/Sylvian fissure and around the upper mastoid process.

This potential is topographically separated from the lid ERG and the occipital VECP. Monocular stimulation shows abolition of the ERG ipsilateral to occlusion but bilateral reduction of the amplitude of the P20-N26-P34 potential, indicating that the wave is independent of the ERG and optic nerve and must be arising from a post-chiasmal site.

Patients with homonymous hemianopia of both cortical and subcortical origin, and bitemporal hemianopia have been studied and the results obtained are consistent with potentials arising from a post-chiasmal but infra-cortical site. In view of these results and those of the topographical studies indicating a non-retinal and non-optic nerve origin we have entitled these components 'visual evoked subcortical potentials' (VESPs).

INTRODUCTION

The early components of the visual evoked potential, that is components before 50 milliseconds latency, are poorly documented due to their minute amplitude, inter-subject variability and poor repeatability under the standardised experimental conditions used for eliciting the visual evoked cortical potential. (Desmedt 1977).

Surprisingly, early components of the visual evoked potential are often mentioned by early evoked potential workers and can often be seen in their early crude averaged records. Cobb and Morton (1952), Ciganek (1961) and Cobb and Dawson (1960) all show these low amplitude components. These early workers all used high intensity flash stimuli and the reduction in use of this technique may explain the loss of interest in early components.

The earliest specific description of a short latency visual evoked potential

Doc. Ophthal. Proc. Series, Vol. 27, ed. by H. Spekreijse & P.A. Apkarian   49

© *1981 Dr W. Junk Publishers, The Hague/Boston/London*

was that of Van Hasselt (1972), who recorded a potential occurring at 10 milliseconds latency of maximal amplitude around the ear and mastoid and only obtainable in four out of ten subjects. He concluded that this potential arose from structures peripheral to the optic chiasma since it was only clearly recorded ipsilateral to the stimulated eye, and suggested that since the latency was longer than the 'a' wave of the ERG, it was probable that the potential arose from the optic nerve.

Cracco and Cracco (1978) recently described oscillatory potentials at around 100 cycles per second recorded from a wide scalp distribution of electrodes all referred to the ear-lobes. These components had latencies between 9—24 milliseconds and were of maximal amplitude in the mid-line and parasaggital recording locations. They suggested that on the basis of present information the potentials probably ranged from those originating in the ERG and optic nerve, to additional potentials arising in the lateral geniculate body, optic radiation or the cortex.

The possibility that some of the early components of the visual evoked potential were of sub-cortical origin first attracted us in 1978. Our work on the auditory evoked brain stem potentials convinced us of the possibility of recording visually evoked sub-cortical potentials by far-field techniques.

In 1978 a pilot study was carried out on a small group of normal volunteer controls. By increasing the number of responses averaged to bright stroboscopic flashes by multi-channel recording from a variety of cephalic sites we eventually identified a small, less than 3 microvolt complex, recorded by far-field techniques. This complex consisted of a positive wave at 22 milliseconds, a negative at 27 milliseconds and a positive wave at 35 milliseconds (Harding 1979) and appeared to be located around the mid-temporal region. It was essential to topographically define this component and to demonstrate its independence from both the scalp recorded electroretinogram or ERG and its associated oscillatory potentials and also from the visually evoked cortical potential.

MATERIALS AND METHODS

Observations were made on thirty normal young volunteers, 16 male and 14 female, mean age 23.2 years. All had visual acuities of 6/6 or better. The subjects were seated in a dimly-lit room and flash stimulation delivered by a Grass PS22 Photo-stimulator ranged from 1363 to 9661 nits. A PDP8E computer was used to simultaneously average eight channels of responses to 500 stimuli which were usually presented at a rate of 6 per second, although slower presentations have been used. The band-pass of the equipment was 66—700 Hz. Since the photo-stimulator produced an audible 'click', control trials were performed with white noise delivered through earphones and with the lamp occluded.

Investigation of commonly used cephalic reference sites revealed that any site anterior to the vertex was markedly contaminated by flash-evoked ERG and both the earlobe and mastoid were highly active at latencies around 20—40 milliseconds. Indeed, it may be that the active nature of this reference

50

site may be responsible for some so-called early components of the visual evoked cortical potential.

In our investigations of possible reference sites we found that the vertex electrode Cz was relatively inactive at early latencies. It is, of course, well known that the vertex site is highly active at later latencies and indeed many late nonspecific components of both the auditory and visual evoked potentials are maximal at this site. The vertex site has the added advantage that it is approximately equidistant from a temporal chain of active recording sites. Since the anterior-posterior location of the source of the signal would be determined from this chain and since the amplitude of the signal is partially proportional to the inter-electrode distance, this constituted a major advantage in using the vertex reference. (Fig. 1) All the electrode positions were

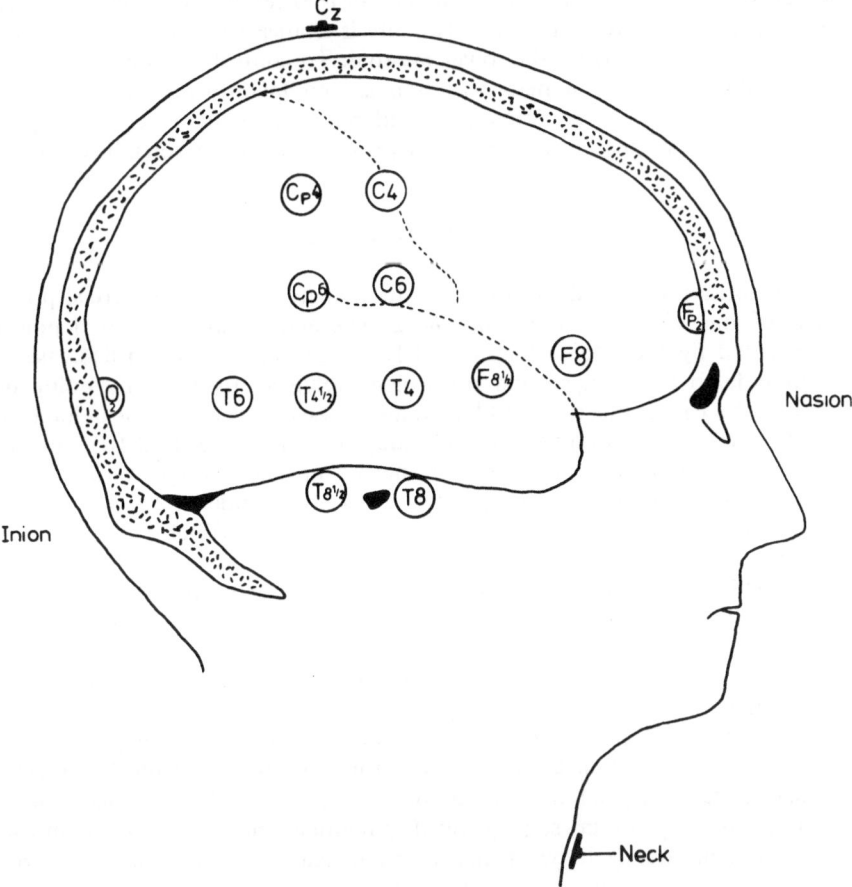

Fig. 1. Scalp distribution of electrodes used in topographical study of the visually evoked sub-cortical potential, consisting of an anterior-posterior chain and two transverse chains of electrodes. Most electrodes are placed according to the International 10/20 System but electrodes CP4, CP6, T4$\frac{1}{2}$, T8$\frac{1}{2}$, C6, T8 and F8$\frac{1}{2}$ are additional electrodes placed midway between the standard placements. The vertex (Cz) and the neck electrodes are used as the common reference.

determined according to the International 10/20 System, using additional half distance electrodes.

In the anterior-posterior study half distance electrodes were placed at F8½ and T4½. For the study of the transverse distribution additional electrodes were placed at C6, CP4, and CP6, that is, midway between the central and parietal positions and T4½ and T8½. (Fig. 1).

Unfortunately, in the study of the transverse distribution of the amplitude of the potential, it is impossible to find a site for the reference electrode that is both inactive and equidistant from all recording electrodes. Obviously, both the frontal and occipital poles, which are equidistant from the electrodes, are highly active and therefore it was decided to use inactive reference sites which were not equidistant from all members of the electrode chain. To obtain direct comparability with the anterior-posterior study the vertex was again used as one reference site. This site is nearest the centrorolandic electrodes and furthest from the lower mastoid. To control for this factor as far as possible, the anterior neck was used as a comparator reference site. This site was found to be completely uncontaminated by the electroretinogram and is, of course, nearer to the lower electrodes than to the rolandic ones.

RESULTS

The anterior-posterior distribution of the visually evoked sub-cortical potentials of the VESPs is shown in Fig. 2. The activity at the frontal pole is dominated by the ERG which is widely distributed, but which decreases in amplitude to a trough around the Rolandic-Sylvian fissure. At a point just behind the ear, at electrode T4½ a triphasic wave is seen. The mean latencies of this wave are positive 20.1 (± 2.03), negative 26.3 (± 2.10), positive 33.9 (± 1.87) milliseconds, and its mean amplitudes positive to negative 1.6 (± 0.78) and negative to positive 2.3 (± 0.99) microvolts. It does not occur at similar latencies to any components of the visual evoked cortical potential recorded at the occiput (Oz). When the lamp was occluded similar potentials could not be recorded. When trials were performed with white noise delivered through earphones a clear response to the photic stimulus was elicited.

Although the VESP is of a different latency to that of known myogenic components, control trials were performed with subjects relaxed and also maintaining high muscular tension as monitored by the on-going EEG. Neither of these actions altered the amplitude or latency of the VESP. This visual evoked potential was successfully recorded in 28 of the 30 subjects. Unlike auditory brain stem evoked potentials there was no significant difference in latency between males and females. In nine subjects the trial-retrial repeatability was tested over a period of between 1 and 12 months. (Fig. 3.). The mean variability in latency over time is relatively small being 1.11 milliseconds for the P20 wave, 1.88 milliseconds for the N26 wave and 1.11 milliseconds for the P34 wave.

The variation in amplitude is far greater although only two scores are shown since the amplitude measures are made peak to peak, that is, P20—N26

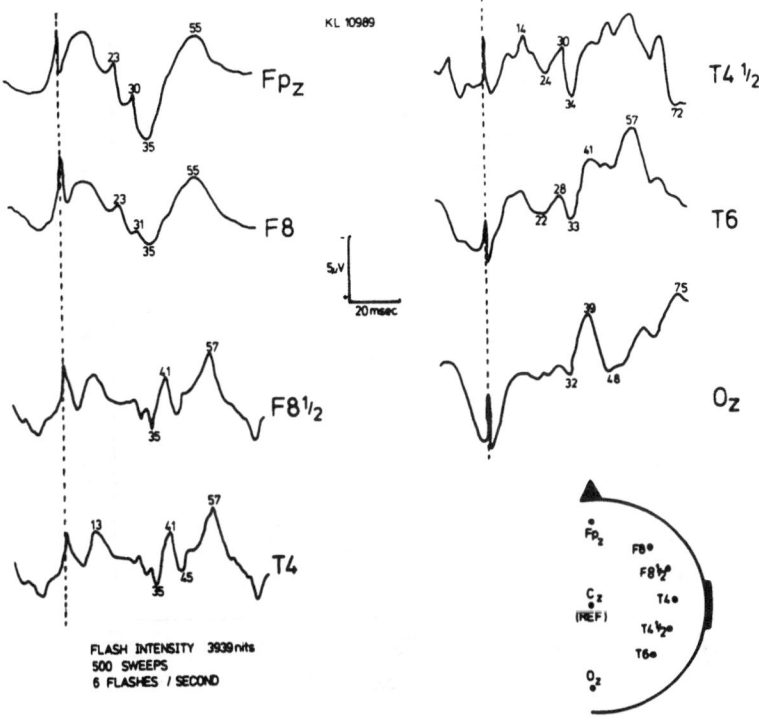

Fig. 2. Distribution of potentials recorded in an anterior-posterior chain of electrodes from frontal to occipital pole all referred to the vertex (Cz). The activity of the frontal pole (Fpz) shows the inverted ERG and its oscillatory potentials, and each subsequent site shows the decreasing amplitude of these components. At T4½ however, the VESP consisting of a P24, N30, P34 complex appears and this reduces in amplitude at more posterior sites and almost disappears at the occipital pole (Oz) which shows the N39, P48, N75 components of the VECP.

and N26–P34. Peak to peak measures of amplitude are more liable to variation and variation in background noise will also affect the averaged amplitude and reduce its repeatability.

In the transverse topographical study, the amplitude of the VESP was maximal at sites below the temporal electrode chain and at a point with, but behind the pinna, that is, around the mastoid process at electrodes T4½ and T8½. This finding was irrespective of whether the vertex or neck electrode sites are used. (Fig. 4). This would indicate that inter-electrode distance was not a confounding factor.

Since the VESP is recorded bilaterally, it is possible that the response might be related to the ERG and the oscillatory potentials. However, the topographical distribution of the VESP contrasts markedly with that of the scalp recorded ERG when referred to the same vertex site. (Fig. 5).

The amplitude of the ERG as recorded at half gain by a Gold Foil electrode (Channel 1) is markedly reduced when recorded at sub-lid, nasal,

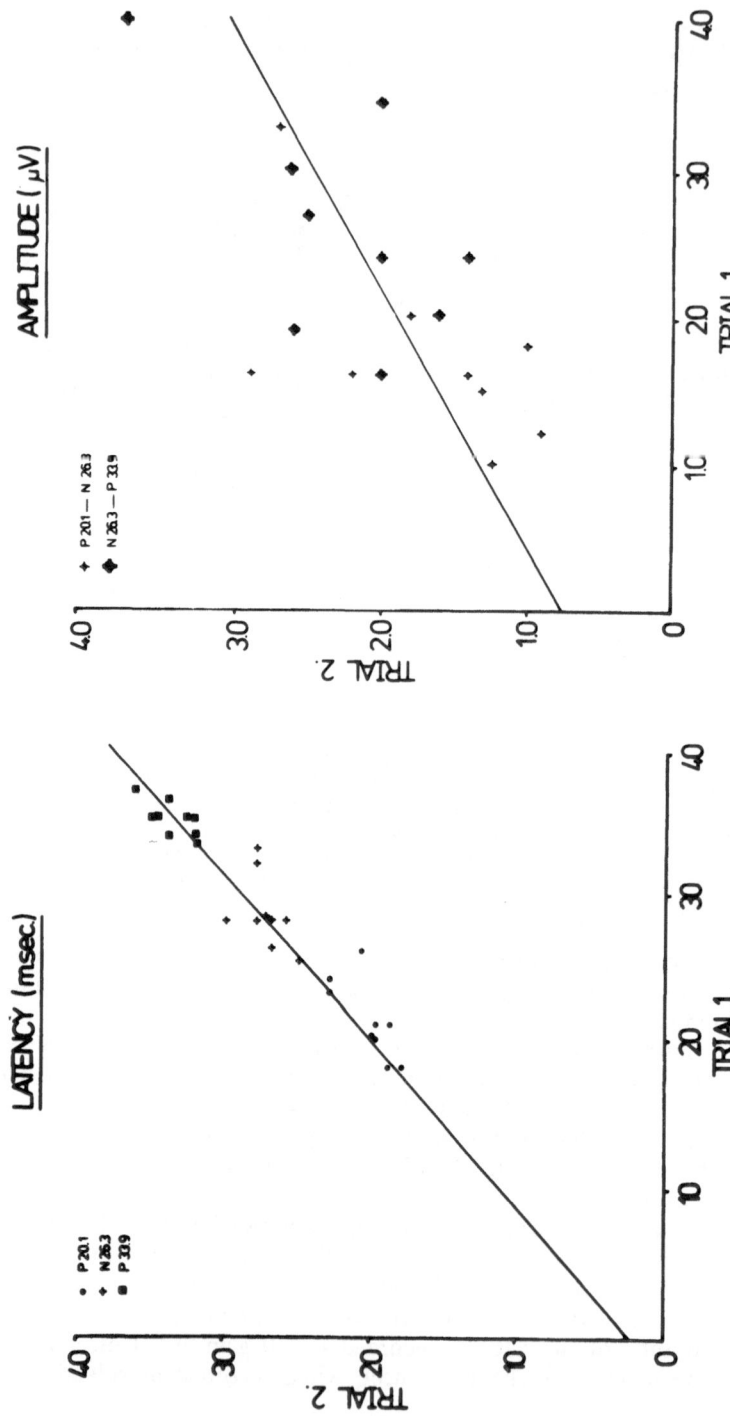

Fig. 3. Scattergram of trial-retrial repeatability of VESP latency and amplitude over periods of between 1 and 12 months. The regression line of y (trial 2) on x (trial 1) is calculated and considered as a 'best-fit' line.

54

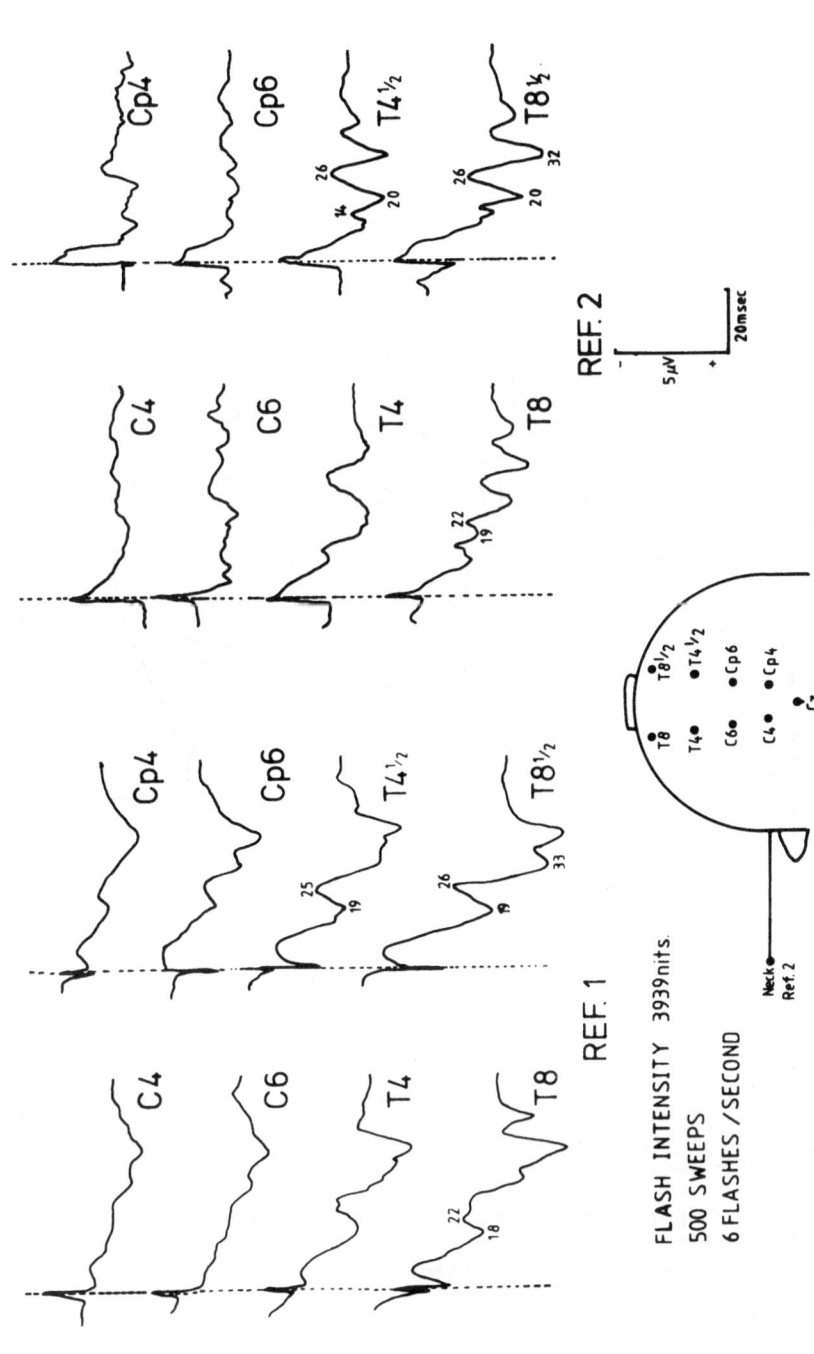

Fig. 4. Topographic distribution of potentials recorded in transverse chains of electrodes referred to vertex (Ref. 1) and to an anterior neck site (Ref. 2) as a comparator. Using either reference, the amplitude of the VESP is shown to be maximal at (or around) electrode T8½, that is, an area level with the cochlea but behind the external auditory meatus.

55

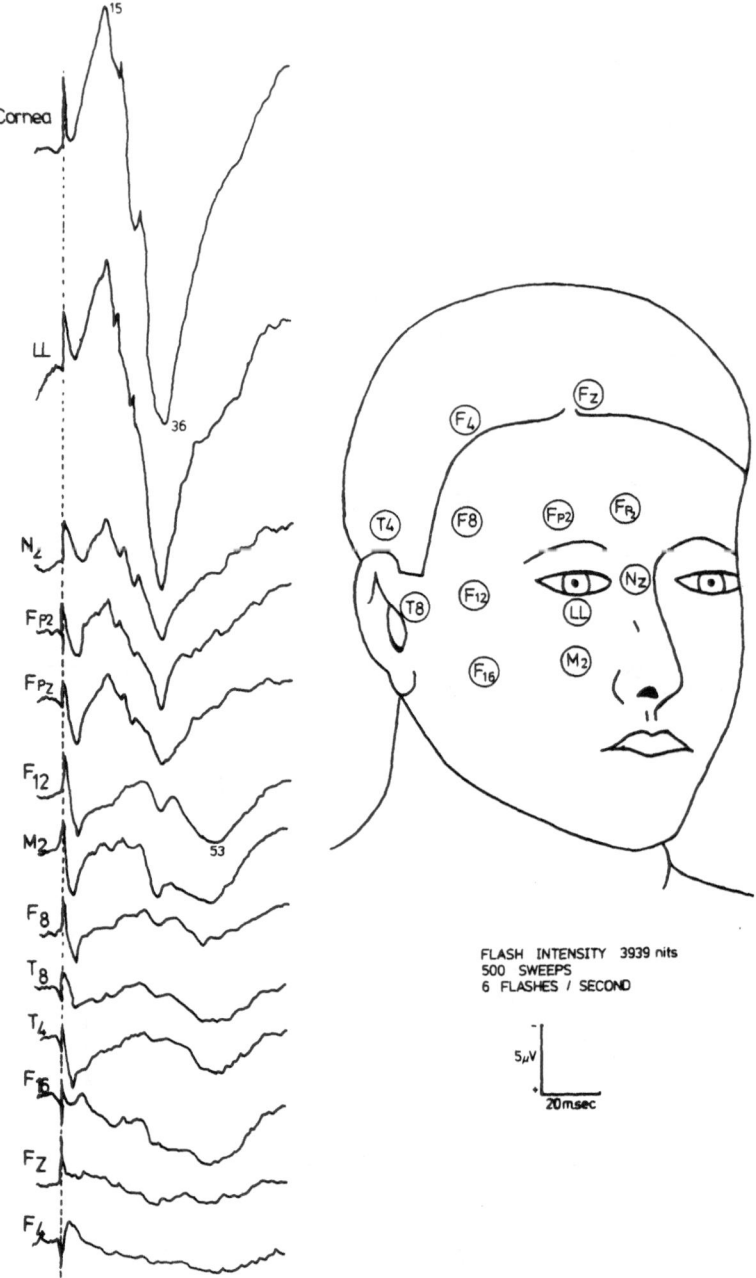

Fig. 5. Facial and scalp topography of electroretinogram in one subject. All electrodes are referred to the vertex (Cz) and recordings made in accordance with EEG convention (Positive at Grid 1. downwards). The corneal signal is recorded at half gain from a Gold Foil Electrode, with a peak of the 'a' wave at 15 milliseconds and a peak of the 'b' wave at 36 milliseconds. The amplitude of the signal rapidly decreases as cornea-electrode distance increases. At electrodes T8 and T4, the ERG is almost absent, only a vestigial 'b' wave appearing as a slight deflection.

frontal pole and frontal sites. The reduction is even more marked at fronto-temporal sites and at the electrodes where the VESP is maximal, that is, electrodes T4 and T8 the ERG is almost non-existant. During simultaneous recording with all electrodes referred to the vertex (Cz) it can be seen that the latency of the 'b' wave of the ERG contrasts with latency of the VESP, (Fig. 6). The former having a peak positive latency of 39 milliseconds and

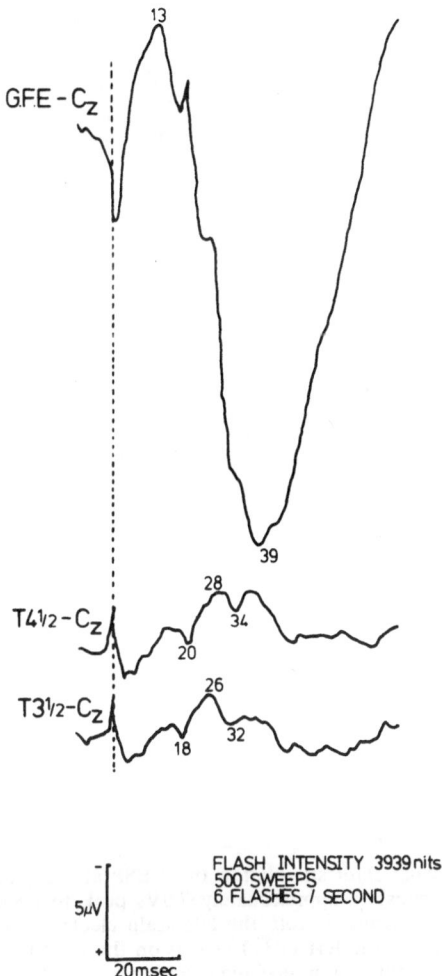

FLASH INTENSITY 3939 nits
500 SWEEPS
6 FLASHES / SECOND

Fig. 6. Simultaneous recording of the electroretinogram and VESP. The peak of the ERG 'a' wave is seen at 13 milliseconds and that of the 'b' wave at 39 milliseconds. The VESP was seen bilaterally at T4$\frac{1}{2}$ and T3$\frac{1}{2}$ at latencies unrelated to those of the ERG in its oscillatory potentials.

the latter latencies of positive 18–20, negative 26–28 and positive 32–34. Neither do the latencies and morphology of the oscillatory potentials of the ERG appear to coincide with the VESP.

Equally, if the VESP were part of the oscillatory potentials of the ERG or arose from the optic nerve, when stimulation is changed from binocular to monocular the response should reduce ipsilateral to the occluded eye.

It can be seen that in Fig. 7, although the ERG potential on the scalp is

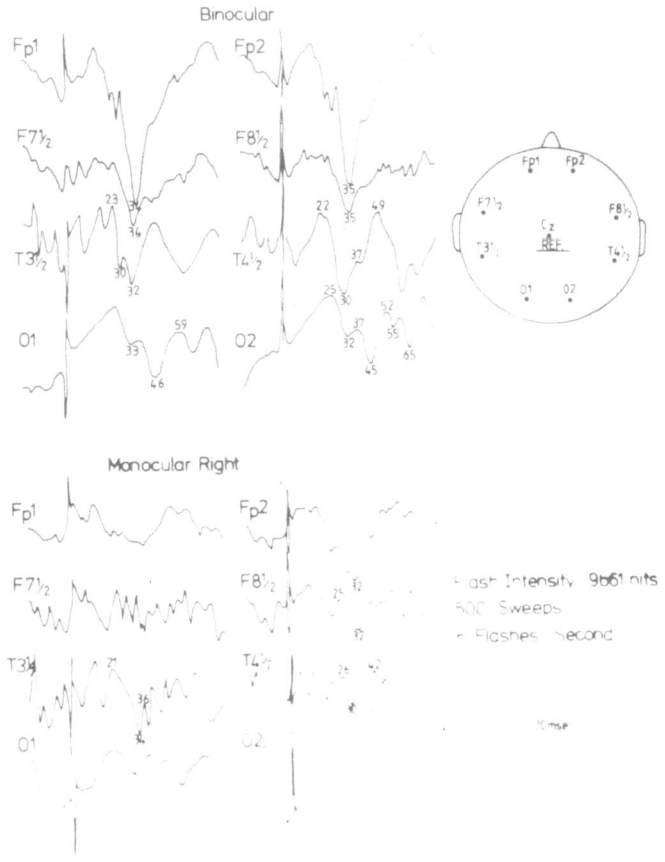

Fig. 7. During binocular flash stimulation the VESP at N23, P32 is seen bilaterally at T3½ and T4½ and equal to approximately 7 uVs peak to peak. When the left eye is occluded the ERG is reduced from the left scalp electrodes (Fp1 and F7½) but the VESP is still present at the left (T3½) as it is on the right (T4½). Similar findings are obtained when the right eye is occluded, with a reduced VESP recorded bilaterally contrasting with an ipsilateral reduction of the ERG.

reduced ipsilateral to the eye which is occluded, the VESP, which in this individual is early at negative 23, positive 32, is reduced bilaterally. These results can only be explained by the response arising from a post-chiasmal site.

We have begun to study patients with lesions of the visual pathway using these techniques. A recent patient presented with a right homonymous hemianopia following a vascular disturbance of the basilar and posterior cerebral arteries. The patient was fully conscious and was dysarthric. There was a clear right homonymous hemianopia, horizontal nystagmus on lateral gaze to either side, and a mild right sided facial weakness. There was bilateral ataxia of all four limbs which was more evident on the right than the left, the tendon reflexes were brisk and the plantors were flexor. CAT scan showed global atrophy involving the left cerebral hemisphere and also the cerebellum. The visual fields are shown in Fig. 8 together with the visual evoked cortical potential. Using flash stimulation and our standard montage it can be seen that the VEP is partly reduced contralateral to the field defect and phase-reversals and amplitudes differ between the two sides.

If the VESP does arise from a thalamic or post-thalamic site it should be reduced on the side of the head contralateral to the field defect. This is clearly demonstrated in Fig. 9 in which the component is absent or markedly reduced on the left, that is, contralateral to the right homonymous hemianopia. In patients with a recent cortical deficit, the VESP should remain preserved. We have investigated a child with cortical abnormality who presented with sudden loss of co-ordination of right limbs and head movements and reduced amplitude of the EEG over the left hemisphere. Unfortunately, due to the young age of the patient accurate field studies could not be obtained. The VESPs were well maintained bilaterally and showed clear components (Fig. 10). The visual evoked cortical potential however showed a clear reduction over the left hemisphere of both the P1 and P2 components. Such a finding would suggest cortical involvement without involvement of subcortical visual pathways.

The final patient was a 66 year old lady with bitemporal hemianopia. The CAT scan showed a large supra-sellar cystic space occupying lesion with expanded pituitary fossa and erosion of the floor and posterior clinoids. The VESP is clearly reduced over the right cerebral hemisphere on left eye stimulation with flash. On right eye stimulation the converse is seen with reduction over the left hemisphere (Fig. 11).

We have compared the VESP to visual evoked cortical responses obtained by pattern-reversal of half the visual field using a 56 minute checkerboard. When the left half field of the left eye was stimulated no response was obtained. Stimulation of the nasal field however produced a clear response of higher amplitude over the left hemisphere. When the temporal half field of the right eye was stimulated no cortical response was seen whereas the nasal field produced a clear response.

DISCUSSION

The visual evoked sub-cortical potential elicited under our standardised conditions appears to be a relatively stable phenomenon recorded in 93% of normal subjects.

The potential is of low amplitude but the confidence limits for test-retest

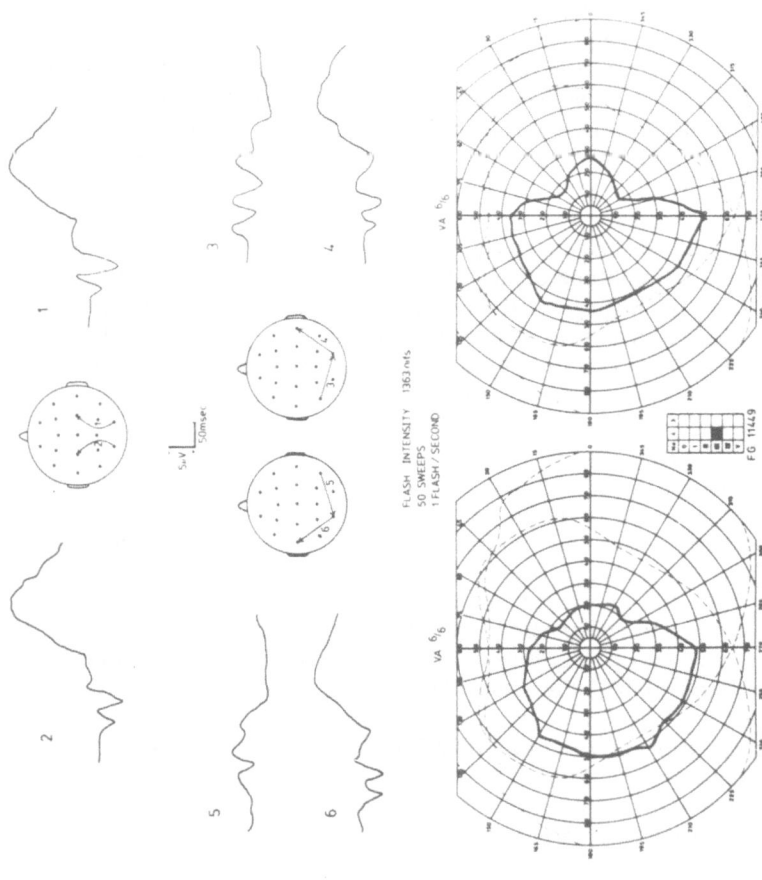

Fig. 8. Patient with a right homonymous hemianopia (and macular sparing) as shown in the field plots following brain stem vascular disturbance. Binocular flash stimulation showed the major positive component of the visual evoked cortical potential P2, at 120 milliseconds. The amplitude being 10 uVs on the right (Channel 1) and 5 uVs on the left (Channel 2). Phase reversal was seen more clearly to the right occiput than to the left (Channels 5 and 6).

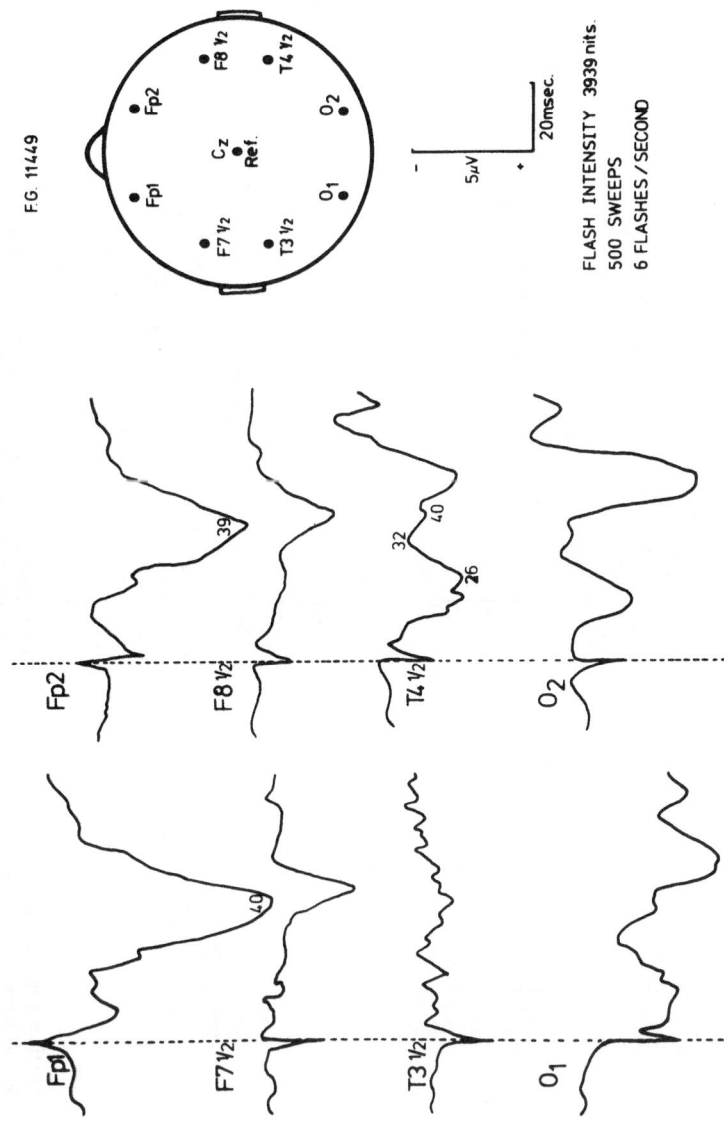

Fig. 9. VESP technique used on the same patient with right homonymous hemianopia following brain stem vascular disturbance. A clear VESP complex is seen on the right at $T4\frac{1}{2}$ (P26, N32, P40) but such a complex is absent on the left ($T3\frac{1}{2}$). It is interesting to note that the ERG from the left eye (Fp1) is of higher amplitude than that from the right eye (Fp2).

61

62

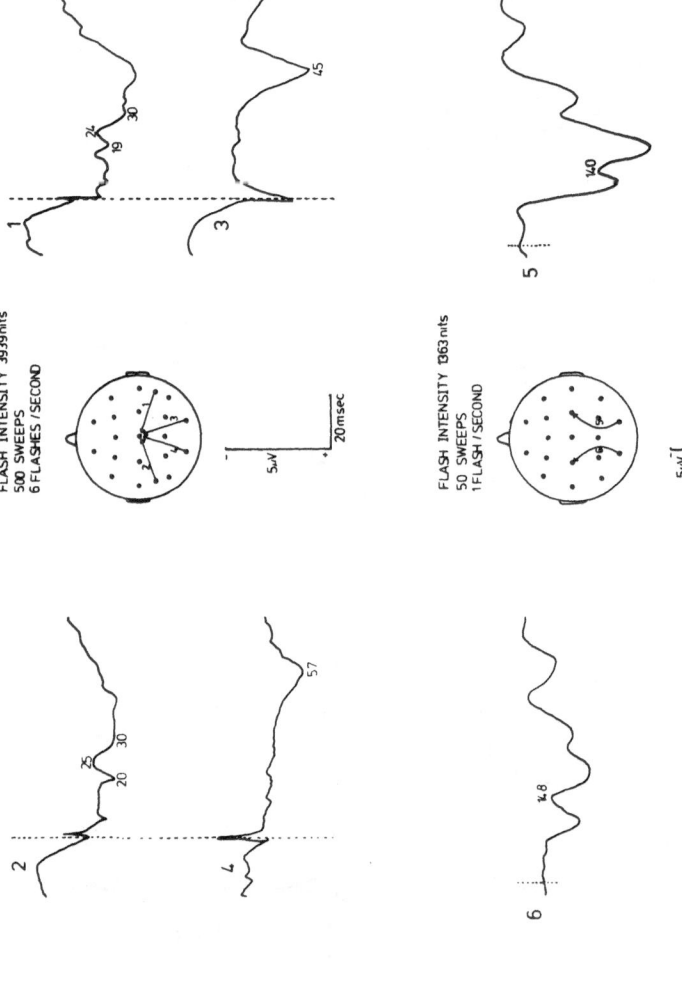

Fig. 10. Patient with cortical abnormality. The VESP is clearly preserved bilaterally. (Channels 1 and 2). The P1 component of the VECP is delayed and reduced on the left (Channel 4) compared with the P1 component of the right (Channel 3). The VECP on the left (Channel 6) is markedly reduced in amplitude and slightly delayed, compared with the VECP on the right (Channel 6), during binocular stimulation.

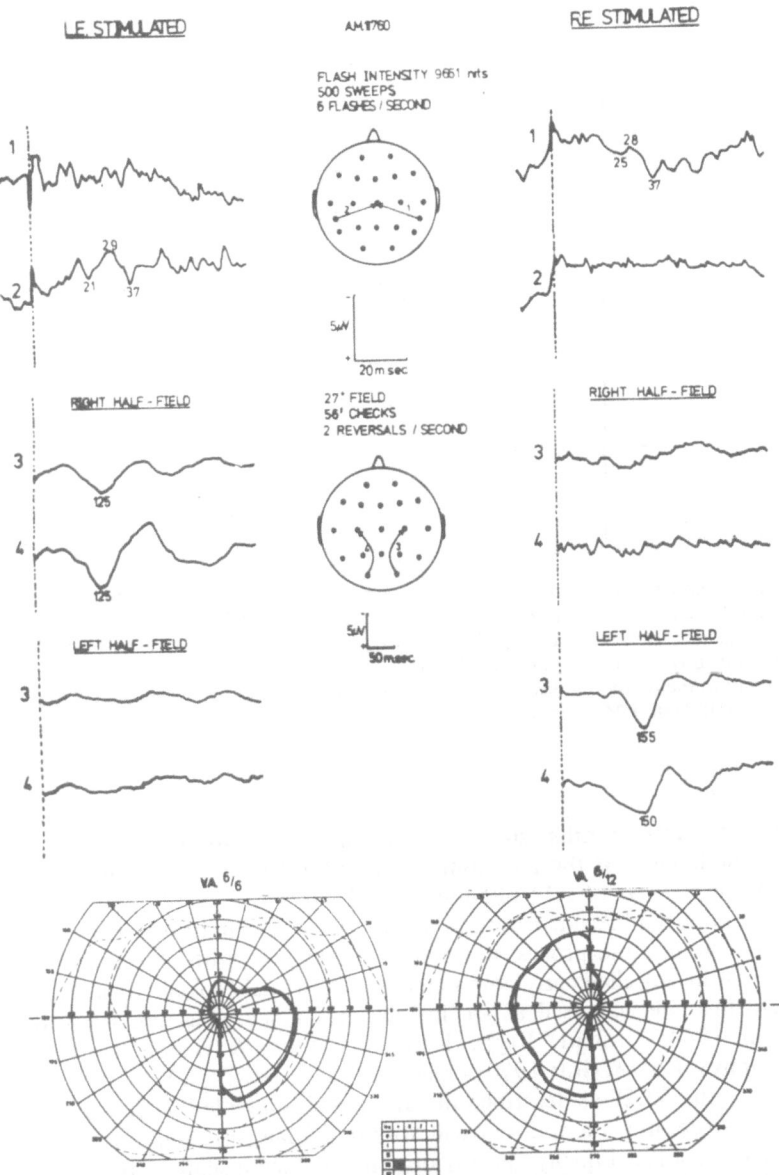

Fig. 11. Patient with pituitary adenoma producing chiasmal compression and associated bitemporal hemianopia. The VESP technique on monocular stimulation of the right eye showed a P25, N28, P37 complex on the right (Channel 1) but absence of any response on the left (Channel 2). On monocular stimulation of the left eye, no response was seen on the right (Channel 1) but a P21, N29, P37 complex as seen on the left (Channel 2). Half-field pattern reversal stimulation shows absence of response when the right half-field of the right eye was stimulated but a major positive component at 150– 155 milliseconds when the left half-field was stimulated. When the right half-field of the left eye was stimulated a major positive was seen at 125 milliseconds but was absent on left half-field stimulation. The field plots are shown at the bottom of the figure.

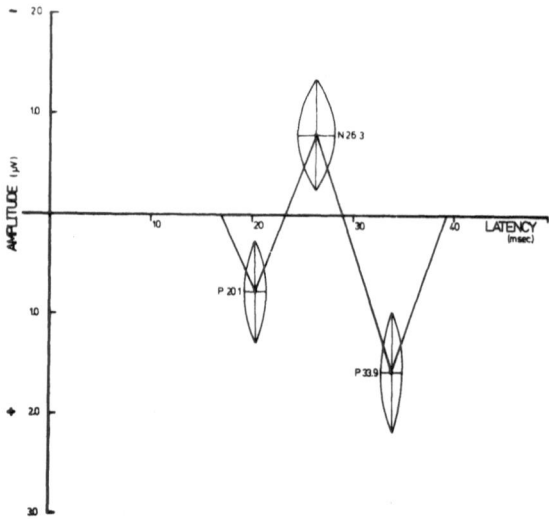

Fig. 12. Graphical representation of the mean VESP in normal subjects (N = 30). The mean difference in amplitude and latency of the VESP between recording on two occasions on nine subjects are shown as elipsoids. It is clearly seen that the mean amplitude differences are considerably greater than the mean latency differences of all three components of the complex. The mean latency variations are 1.11, 1.88, and 1.11 for the P20, N26, P34 wave respectively.

reliability over months, shows remarkably little variation in latency (Fig. 12). The latency of the P34 component is the least variable, only varying in latency by a mean of 1.11 of a millisecond.

The topographical distribution of the component indicates that is maximal around the mastoid process and indeed it may constitute the explanation for some of the so-called early components of the visual evoked cortical potential where this site was used as an 'inactive' reference. (Ciganek 1961; Kooi & Bagchi 1964; Gastaut, Regis, Lyagoubi, Memo & Simon 1967; Allison Matsumiya, Goff & Goff 1977; Cracco & Cracco 1978).

Since the VESP as described in this paper is unrelated to the amplitude of the electroretinogram and its oscillatory potentials, it is unlikely that it arises from this source. Equally since it does not reduce ipsilateral to an occluded eye it is unlikely to arise from an optic nerve site and must be post-chiasmal. The findings from patients support the suggestion that the origin of the signal is post-chiasmal and the finding of reduced cortical potentials co-existing with preserved sub-cortical potentials would indicate that the signal is not of cortical origin. In this connection it should be noted that Corletto et al. reported in 1967 preservation of an early N23, P28 millisecond wave following an occipital lobectomy.

The most likely explanation is that this potential arises from a thalamic or optic radiation site and such an origin would be entirely consistent with all our findings. It is possible that this technique may supplement the electroretinogram and the visually evoked cortical potential in ophthalmic electro-diagnosis of lesions of the visual pathway.

ACKNOWLEDGEMENTS

We are most grateful to Mr Bernard Williams and Dr Milne Anderson of the Midland Centre for Neurosurgery for allowing us to study their patients.

REFERENCES

Allison, T., Matsumiya, Y., Goff, G.D. & Goff, W.R. The scalp topography of the human visual evoked potentials. Electroenceph. clin. Neurophysiol. 42: 185–197 (1977).

Ciganek, L. The EEG response (Evoked Potential) to light stimulus in man. Electroenceph. clin. Neurophysiol. 13: 165–172 (1961).

Cobb, W.A. & Morton, H.B. The human retinogram in response to high intensity flashes. Electroenceph. clin. Neurophysiol. 4: 547–556 (1952).

Cobb, W.A. & Dawson, G.D. The latency and form in man of the occipital potentials evoked by bright flashes. J. Physiol. 152: 108–121 (1960).

Corletto, F., Gentilomo, A., Rasadini, A., Rossi, G.F. & Zattoni, J. Visual evoked potentials as recorded from the scalp and from the visual cortex before and after surgical removal of the occipital pole in man. Electroenceph. clin. Neurophysiol. 22: 378–380 (1967).

Cracco, R.Q. & Cracco, J.B. Visual evoked potentials in man: early oscillatory potentials. Electroenceph. clin. Neurophysiol. 45: 731–739 (1978).

Desmedt, J.E. (Ed.) Visual evoked potentials in man: new developments. Clarendon Press, Oxford (1977).

Gastaut, H., Regis, H., Lyagoubi, S., Memo, T. & Simon, L. Comparison of the potentials recorded from the occipital, temporal and central regions of the human scalp, evoked by visual, auditory and somator-sensory stimuli. Electroenceph. clin. Neurophysiol. 26: 19–28 (1967).

Harding, G.F.A. Inaugral Lecture. 'A Mirror for the Brain'. University of Aston in Birmingham (1979).

Kooi, D.A. & Bagchi, B.K. Observations on the early components of the visual evoked response and occipital rhythms. Electroenceph. clin. Neurophysiol. 17: 638–643 (1964).

Van Hasselt, P. A short latency visual evoked potential recorded from the human mastoid process and auricle. Electroenceph. clin. Neurophysiol. 33: 517–519 (1972).

Authors' address:
Clinical Neurophysiology Unit
Dept. of Ophthalmic Optics
University of Aston in Birmingham
Birmingham, England

VISUAL POTENTIALS EVOKED BY PATTERN STIMULATION WITH DIFFERENT SPATIAL FREQUENCIES IN RETROBULBAR NEURITIS

V. PORCIATTI & G.P. VON BERGER

(*Livorno, Italy*)

ABSTRACT

Numerous studies on psychophysical reaction times in man in response to pattern stimulation demonstrate a progressive increase in the latency of the response when the spatial frequency of the stimulus is increased. A similar behaviour has been recently observed with the use of evoked potentials. In this particular study the Authors demonstrate that the increase in the latency manifested by increasing the spatial frequency may be observed in the transient responses but not in those steady-state responses of relatively high temporal frequencies. This leads to the hypothesis of the progressive selection of smaller receptive fields mainly within the X-system. Keeping in mind that at the level of the retinal ganglion cells there is a progressive increase in the dimensions of the receptive fields, the Authors demonstrate that retrobulbar neuritis (either axial or peripheral) may be detected by changing the spatial frequency of the stimulus.

INTRODUCTION

Many Authors (Kaswan 1965; Breitmeyer 1975; Vassilev 1976; Lupp 1976; Parker 1977; Jones 1978) have demonstrated that the increase of spatial frequency of an onset-presented grating stimulus evokes an increase both in psychophysical reaction times and in the latency of visual potentials. Some of them believe that this behaviour is due to a progressive transition from Y system with fast conduction to X system with lower conduction; others think that this behaviour could happen also within each system, keeping in mind that at the retinal ganglion cell level both systems show ranges of conduction velocities partially overlapped. (Saito 1970; Fukada 1971; Cleland 1971). In order to verify the relative share of X and Y systems we have studied the latency of both transient and steady-state responses evoked by a checkerboard-reversal stimulation of different spatial frequencies in normal subjects. Further, considering that the retinal spatial distribution of X system is mostly central and that of Y system is mostly peripheral (Cleland 1971, 1972; Ikeda 1972; Cleland 1973), we have applied the same experimental conditions to patients affected by unilateral neuritis either axial or peripheral.

METHODS

We have employed a high contrast check-reversal stimulus with fundamental spatial frequencies ranging from 0.4 cycles/degree to 35 cycles/degree (the check sizes ranged from 1.2' to 111') and with temporal frequencies ranging from 1 Hz (for the transient response) to 8–16 Hz (for the steady-state response). Such stimulation seems very apt to our purposes for the following reasons: 1) it evokes high amplitude responses which allow the study of patients with low visual acuity, 2) the transient response shows a time-to-peak of its main positive component markedly constant either in the same subject or in a group of subjects with similar age, 3) the steady-state response, in a non-linear system as the visual one, may yield further information beside transient responses, and may also be usefully studied by Fourier analysis.

RESULTS AND DISCUSSION

Normal subjects

The transient response as a function of spatial frequency is shown in Fig. 1.

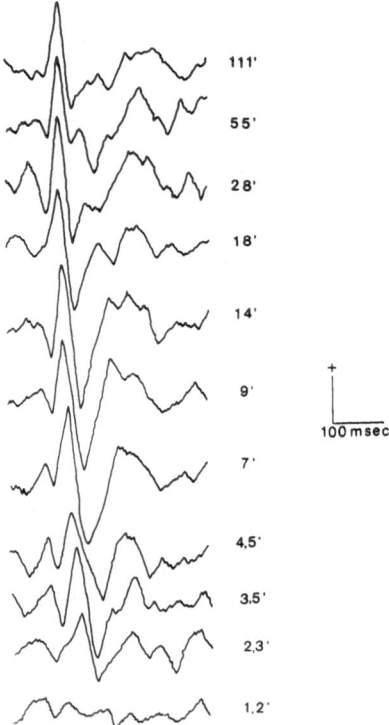

Fig. 1. Normal subject. Transient responses to a 1 Hz check-reversal stimulation of different angular size. Calibration is 4 uV for the first 6 tracings and 2 uV for the last 5 tracings.

From this figure we can mention two main behaviours: 1) the response follows checks of decreasing angular size until 2.3 minutes of arc; 2) the latency gradually increases with the rise of spatial frequency. This behaviour is strikingly shown in Fig. 2: the P_2 wave latency has a practically constant

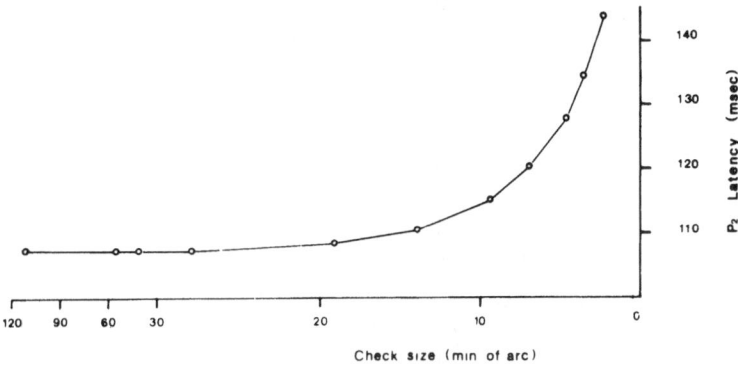

Fig. 2. Normal subject. Latency of transient response as a function of check size. For further details see text.

value of about 108 msec. for check-sizes ranging from 120 to 20 minutes and then gradually increases with the rise of spatial frequency reaching the value of 147 msec. for check sizes of 2.3 minutes. With smaller checks the response becomes undetectable. The behaviour of the steady-state response is shown in Fig. 3, where two main considerations are evident: 1) the response is detectable until 3.5 minute checks, so that it shows a higher spatial discrimination threshold in comparison with the transient response, 2) the phase of the response does not change across the full range of spatial frequencies. The apparant latency of the steady-state response, as evaluated by the slope of the phase versus temporal frequency function, is about 110 msec.; this value is quite similar to the latency of the transient response in the range of lower spatial frequencies. Comparing the transient and the steady-state behaviour (Fig. 4), we may point out: 1) the transient response follows higher spatial frequencies, 2) the latency of the transient response increases in the range 20–2.3 minutes, meanwhile the steady-state latency does not change with spatial frequency and shows a value of about 110 msec. This value is similar to that of the transient response in the range 120–20 minutes. The increase of latency with spatial frequency could be explained as follows: considering that at the retinal ganglion cell level the conduction velocities are correlated with the amplitude of receptive fields, namely to smaller receptive fields correspond axons with lower conduction (Wiesel 1960; Stone 1965; Enroth-Cugell 1966; Stone 1971; Ikeda 1972; Fischer 1973; Cleland 1973), it could be possible that the increase of spatial frequencies select smaller and smaller receptive fields with lower conduction velocities. The increase of latency could be related to a gradual transition from the fast Y system to the slower X system. However, considering that

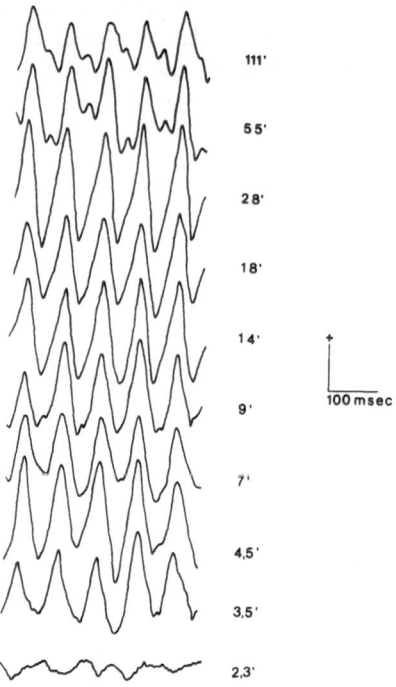

Fig. 3. Normal subject. Steady-state responses to a 12.5 Hz check-reversal stimulation of different angular size. Calibration is 4 uV for the first 7 tracings and 2 uV for the last 3 tracings.

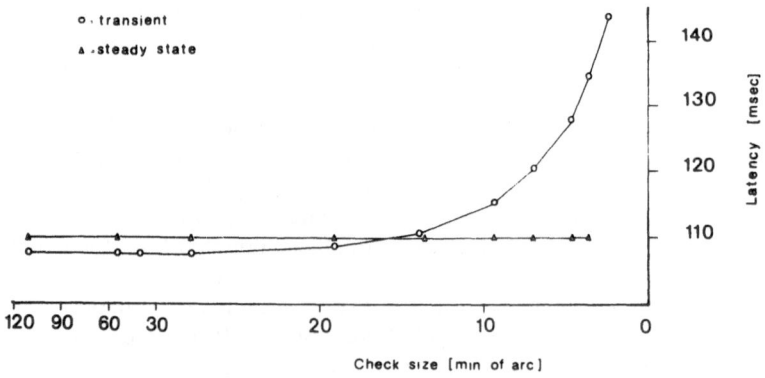

Fig. 4. Normal subject. Latency of transient (circles) and steady-state (triangles) responses as a function of check-size. For further details see text.

70

the two systems have conduction velocities partially overlapped, the variations in latency could occur in either system. In fact, in the transient response, both systems may contribute to the evoked response. However, as at lower spatial frequencies the X system is probably not activated because of its smaller receptive fields, the Y system could be the most involved in the response. This opinion matches with our experimental data which show the lower latencies for the lower spatial frequencies. The constant value of the response latency in the range 120–20 minutes could be related to the low sensitivity of the Y system to the spatial structure of the stimulus.

In the steady-state response of relatively high temporal frequency (12.5 Hz), we tried to penalize the sustained X system in favour of the transient Y system. Since the latency of the steady-state response is similar to the minimum constant value detected in the transient response, it follows that at lower spatial frequencies the Y system seems to be the most involved. On the contrary, at the higher spatial frequencies, followed only by the transient response, only the X system seems to be involved. At middle spatial frequencies, in the range 20–3.5 minutes, the increase in latency of the transient response seems to be correlated to the selection of smaller and smaller receptive fields mainly within the X system.

Patients affected by retrobulbar neuritis

We have selected two cases of unilateral retrobulbar neuritis: the first one mainly axial, the second one mainly peripheral as is shown by clinical examinations (Fig. 5 and 6). Both cases showed a marked Pulfrich stereophenomenon. In the axial neuritis the response of the affected eye in comparison with the contralateral shows a delay detectable only in the transient response at the higher spatial frequencies (Fig. 7).

In the mainly peripheral neuritis (Fig. 8), the transient response of the affected eye, compared with the contralateral, shows a delay both at low spatial frequencies and at high ones. The delay is more evident at lower frequencies. In the steady-state response, the delay of the affected eye is detectable only at low spatial frequencies and its value is smaller than that evaluated in the transient response.

The results obtained in patients affected by retrobulbar neuritis confirm our remarks in normal subjects. In addition, the different behaviour of transient and steady-state evoked responses allows us to foresee an interesting use of this research in clinical applications, mainly in cases with a lower symptomatology.

71

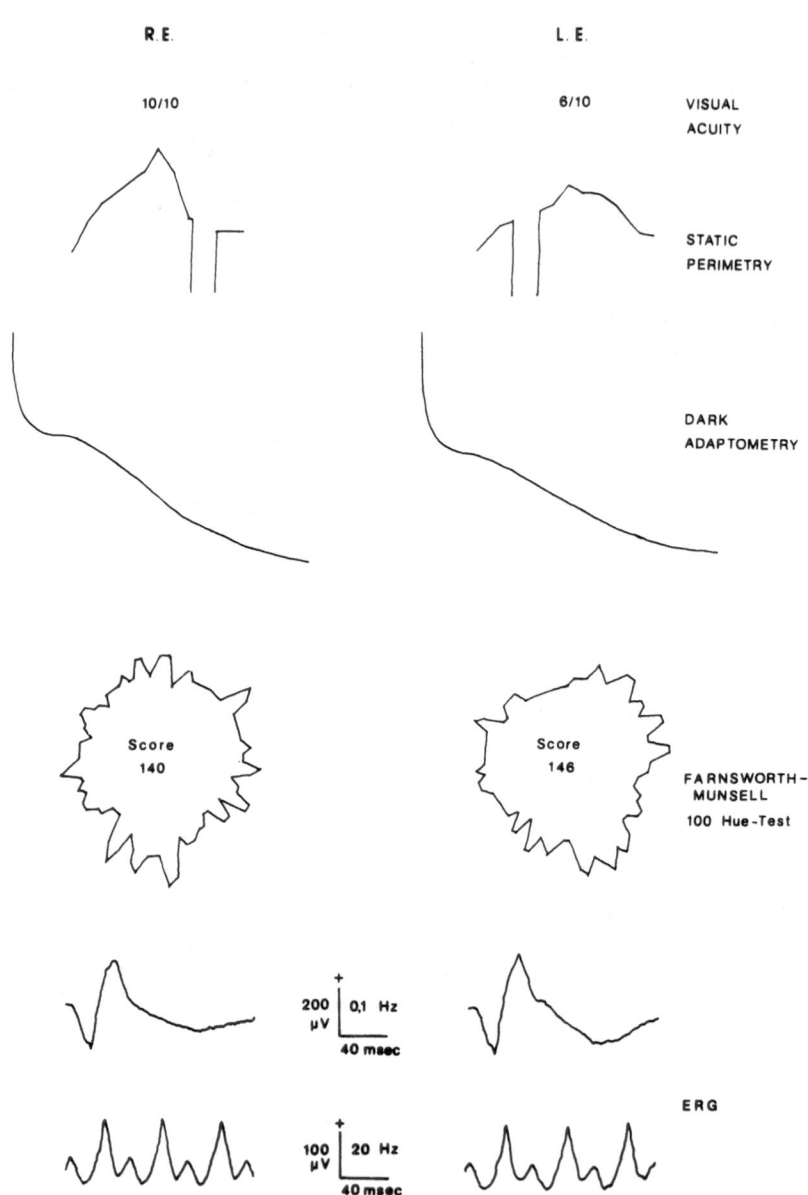

Fig. 5. Axial neuritis. Functionsl findings.

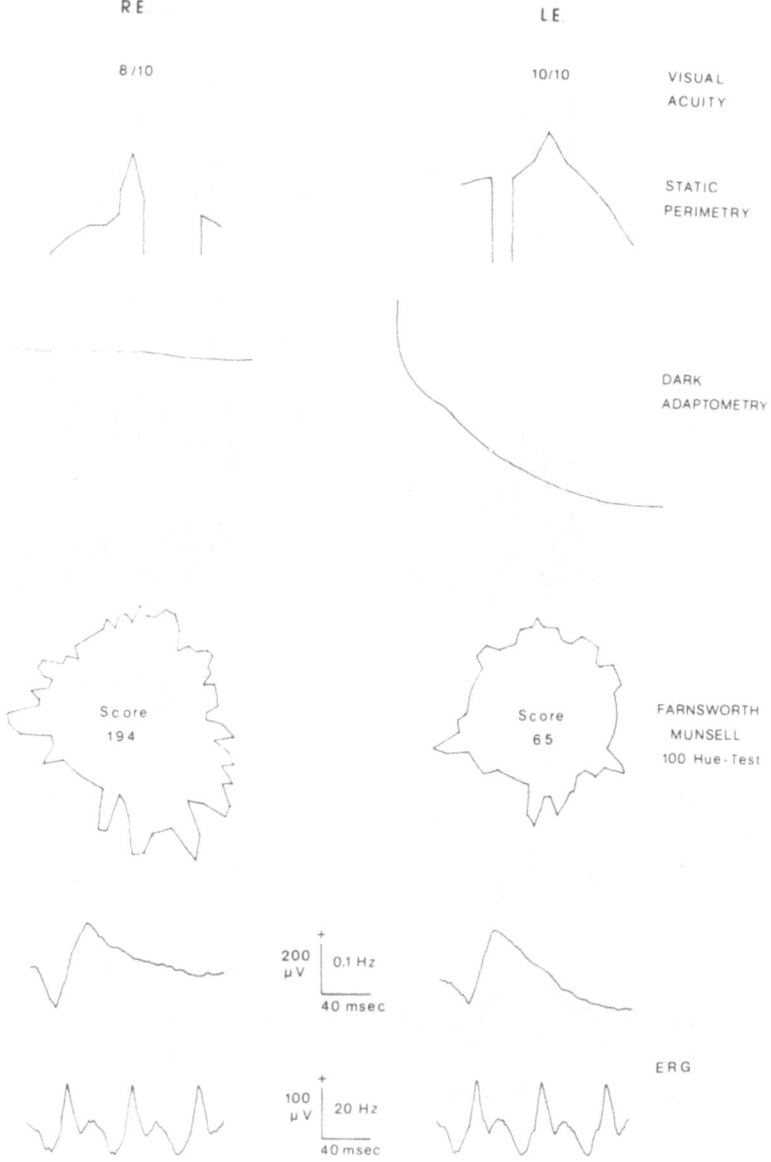

RE   LE

8/10   10/10   VISUAL
                                         ACUITY

                                         STATIC
                                         PERIMETRY

                                         DARK
                                         ADAPTOMETRY

Score   Score   FARNSWORTH
194   65   MUNSELL
                                         100 Hue-Test

200   0.1 Hz
μV
       40 msec

                                         ERG

100   20 Hz
μV
       40 msec

Fig. 6. **Mainly peripheral neuritis. Functional findings.**

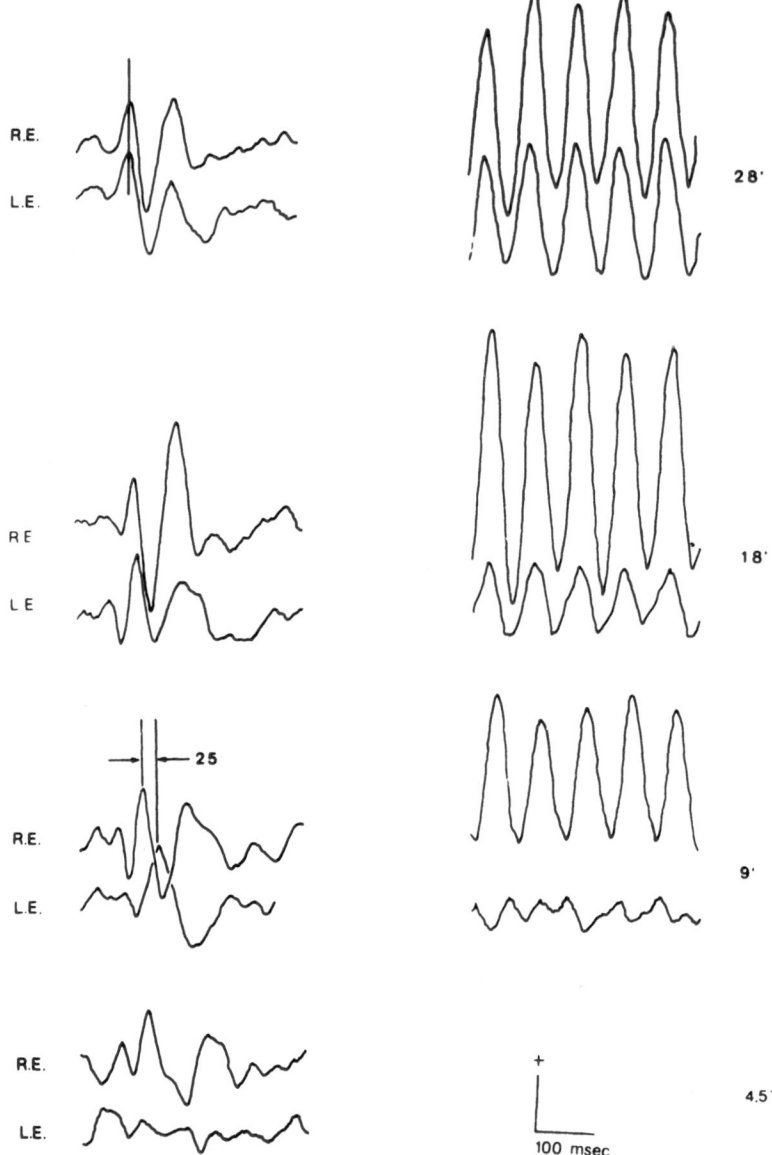

Fig. 7. Axial neuritis. Transient and steady-state responses to checks of different angular size. The affected left eye shows a marked delay only in the transient response to smaller checks. Calibration is 4 μV.

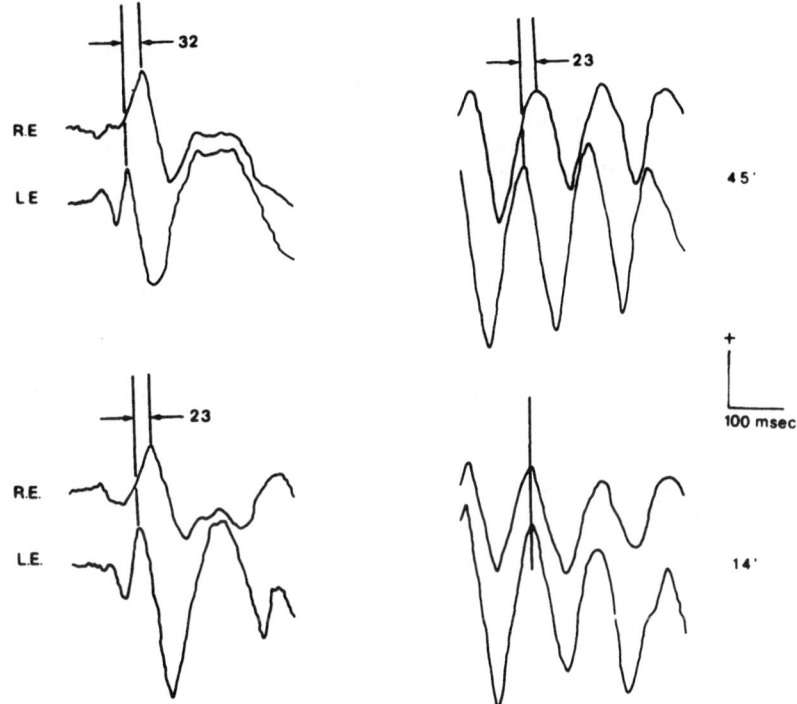

Fig. 8. Mainly peripheral neuritis. Transient and steady-state responses to checks of different angular size. In the transient response the delay of the affected right eye is more evident to large checks. In the steady-state response the delay is evident only to large checks. Calibration is 4 μV.

REFERENCES

Breitmeyer, B.G. Simple reaction time as a measure of the temporal response properties of transient and sustained channels. Vision. Res. 15: 1411–1412 (1975).

Cleland, B.G., Dubin, M.W. & Levick W.R. Sustained and transient neurones in the cat's retina and lateral geniculate nucleus. J. Physiol. (Lond.) 217: 473–496 (1971).

Cleland, B.G. & Levick W.R. Physiology of cat retinal ganglion cells. Invest. Ophthalmol. Vis. Sci. 11: 285–290 (1972).

Cleland, B.G. & Levick W.R. Properties of sustained and transient ganglion cells in the cat retina. J. Physiol. (Lond.) 228: 649–680 (1973).

Enroth-Cugell, C. & Robson J.G. The contrast sensitivity of retinal ganglion cells of the cat. J. Physiol. (Lond.) 187: 517–552 (1966).

Fisher, B. Overlap of receptive field centers and representation of the visual field in the cat's optic tract. Vision. Res. 13: 2113–2120 (1973).

Fukada, Y. Receptive field organisation of cat optic nerve fibres with special reference to conduction velocity. Vision. Res. 11: 209–226 (1971).

Fukada, Y & Saito H.A. The relationship between response characteristic to flicker stimulation and receptive field organisation in the cat's optic nerve fibres. Vision. Res. 11: 227–240 (1971).

Ikeda, H. & Wright, M.J. Differential effects of refractive errors and receptive field organisation of central and peripheral ganglion cells. Vision. Res. 12: 1465–1476 (1972).

Jones, R. & Keck, M.J. Visual evoked response as a function of grating spatial frequency. Invest. Ophthalmol. Vis. Sci. 17: 652–659 (1978).

Kaswan, J. & Young, S. Effects of luminance exposure duration and task complexity on reaction time. J. Exp. Psychol. 69: 393–400 (1965).

Lupp, V., Hauske G. & Wolf, W. Perceptual latencies to sinusoidal gratings. Vision. Res. 16: 969–972 (1976).

Parker, D.M. & Salzen, E.A. Latency changes in the human evoked response to sinusoidal gratings. Vision. Res. 17: 1201–1204 (1977).

Saito, H., Shimahara, T. & Fukada, Y. Four types of responses to light and dark spot stimuli in the cat optic nerve. Tokyo J. Exp. Med. 102: 127–133 (1970).

Stone, J. A quantitative analysis of the distribution of ganglion cells in the cat's retina. J. Comp. Neurol. 124: 337–352 (1965).

Stone, J. & Hollander, H. Optic nerve axon diameters measured in the cat retina. Some functional considerations. Exp. Brain Res. 13: 498–503 (1971).

Vassilev, A. & Mitov, D. Perception times and spatial frequency. Vision. Res. 16: 89–92 (1976).

Wiesel, T.N. Receptive fields of ganglion cells in cat's retina. J. Physiol. (Lond.) 153: 583–594 (1960).

Authors' address:
Laboratorio di Fisiopatologia Oculare
Divisione Oculistica
Spedali Riuniti
57100 Livorno, Italy

PART TWO

VISUAL PATHWAYS: CLINICAL ASPECTS

PATTERN EVOKED POTENTIAL LATENCY AND CONTRAST SENSITIVITY IN GLAUCOMA AND OCULAR HYPERTENSION

S. SOKOL, A. DOMAR, A. MOSKOWITZ & B. SCHWARTZ

(Boston, U.S.A.)

ABSTRACT

The latency of the first major positive component (P_1) of the pattern reversal visually evoked potential (VEP) and constrast sensitivity, using the Arden grating plates, were measured in 3 groups of age matched subjects. One group consisted of 14 normal subjects (mean age 66 yrs.) with no ocular disease; a second group contained 21 patients (mean age 58 yrs.) with ocular hypertension; and a thrid group contained 20 patients (mean age 66 yrs.) with glaucoma. Analysis of the Arden grating scores revealed no significant differences between the 3 groups. These findings indicate that the Arden gratings have limited usefulness in the detection of glaucoma, at least in older patient populations. On the other hand, the VEP data showed that the mean P_1 latency for the glaucomatous eyes was significantly longer than the P_1 latency for the normals and ocular hypertensives. Further, there was no significant difference in mean P_1 latency between the normals and ocular hypertensives.

INTRODUCTION

The latency of the pattern reversal visually evoked potential (VEP) and sensitivity to changes in contrast of sine wave gratings of differing spatial frequencies are now widely used to detect optic nerve pathology. Initially, abnormal prolongation of the VEP latency was thought to be pathognomonic for demyelinating disease (Halliday, McDonald & Mushin 1973). Abnormal VEP latencies have now been reported in ischemic optic neuropathy, Leber's hereditary optic neuropathy, compressive lesions of the anterior visual pathways and glaucoma (Sokol 1980). Further, abnormal contrast sensitivity has been found in amblyopia (Hess & Howell, 1977), optic neuritis (Arden & Gucukoglu 1978) and glaucoma (Arden & Jacobson 1978; Atkin, Bodis-Wollner, Wolkstein, Moss & Podos 1979).

The purpose of the present experiment was to study changes in the latency of the pattern reversal visually evoked potential (VEP) and contrast sensitivity to sine wave gratings in glaucoma and ocular hypertension. To date, we know of no comparison between the VEP and contrast sensitivity in the same group of age matched normals, glaucoma patients and ocular hypertensives, nor has the fact that many patients have miotic pupils due to ocular medication been taken into account when VEP latencies have been evaluated (Huber & Wagner 1978). Our psychophysical measure of optic nerve function was the Arden Grating Test and our electrophysiological measure was the latency of the first major positive component (P_1) of the pattern reversal VEP.

METHODS

Subjects

Three groups of age matched subjects were included in the present study: 20 glaucoma patients (mean age: 66 years), 21 patients with ocular hypertension (mean age: 58 years), and 14 normals (mean age: 66 years). The glaucoma patients' field defects as measured with the Goldmann perimeter included peripheral nasal step (9 eyes), arcuate scotoma (5 eyes), nasal step and arcuate scotoma (4 eyes), paracentral scotoma (7 eyes), and one quadrant loss (5 eyes). The glaucoma patients had visual acuities of 6/12 or better. All of the patients with ocular hypertension had intraocular pressures of 21 mmHg or higher on repeated testing, symmetric cupping and pallor of the optic discs, normal visual fields, open angles, and visual acuities of 6/12 or better. All of the normal subjects underwent complete ophthalmic examinations and were included in the study only if there was no ocular pathology, visual fields using the Goldmann perimeter were normal, and intraocular pressures were less than 21 mmHg on two occasions. All normal subjects had acuities of 6/9 or better.

Arden grating plates. The test consists of 7 plates: a screening plate (plate 1) and 6 diagnostic plates (#2–7). At a testing distance of 50 cm, the spatial frequency of the 6 diagnostic plates ranges from 0.4 to 6.4 cycles/degree in increments of 1 octave. The contrast of each plate changes from the top to the bottom of the plate and covers a range of approximately 1.75 log units. The observer's task is to view each plate as the tester slowly uncovers it and report when the grating bars are first seen. A score of 1 to 20 is assigned for each plate based on when the observer first sees the grating.

The grating test was administered to all subjects by the same tester according to the instructions which are supplied with the plates; all subjects and patients were tested monocularly. The luminance of the plates was 1.56 log cd/m². The grating score obtained from the fellow eye of glaucoma patients with uniocular field defects were not included in the analysis of the data.

Visual evoked potentials. Pattern reversal VEPs were recorded from the same patients who were tested with the Arden Grating Plates. Each subject sat 1 meter from a TV monitor which generated a checkerboard pattern stimulus. The mean luminance of the screen was 1.90 log cd/m², field size was 14.5

degrees by 18 degrees and the contrast was 0.84. Each check subtended 48 minutes of arc. The VEP was recorded from a gold cup electrode 1 cm anterior to the inion on the midline and referenced to the earlobe; the other earlobe was ground. Signals were led into a Grass P511 preamplifier with band pass settings of 1 and 35 Hz. The amplified signals were averaged by a Nicolet Med-80 minicomputer and stored on a floppy diskette for later retrieval and measurement of peak latencies. The first major positive component (P_1) was measured with a software program which allowed the operator to place a cursor at a point on the VEP waveform which was displayed on an oscilloscope screen; the resolution of this program was accurate to wihtin 400 micro-seconds.

RESULTS

Arden grating test. For plates that were seen with each eye separately, the mean score of the right and left eye was calculated (Ederer, 1973). These data were analyzed with a one-way analysis of variance according to ocular status matched for age (Edwards, 1962). We did not use Arden's method of scoring 25 for each plate which was not seen, because this would violate the assumptions underlying the analysis of variance. Accordingly, data from any subject who did not see any one of the seven plates were excluded from the analysis of variance; responses to individual plates were categorized as either 'seen' or 'not seen' and analyzed with a Chi Square test.

The mean scores for the glaucoma patients, ocular hypertensives and normals for each plate is shown in Fig. 1. The F-ratios for plates 2, 3, 5, 6 and 7 showed no significant differences among the 3 groups. Only plate 4 revealed a significant F-ratio ($F = 3.25$, $p < 0.05$). Further analysis of plate 4 with paired t-tests showed no difference between the normals and ocular

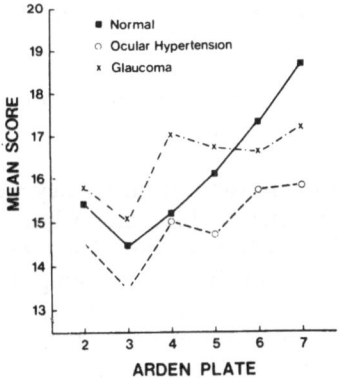

Fig. 1. Mean Scores on Arden Grating Test for each plate for age matched normals, ocular hypertensives and glaucoma patients. Only plate 4 was significant, with glaucoma patients showing significantly higher scores.

81

hypertensives, and significantly higher scores or lower sensitivity ($p < 0.05$) for the glaucoma patients.

Fig. 2 shows the percentage of each of the 3 groups who saw or did not see plate 6 or 7 with either eye. The number of patients who did not see

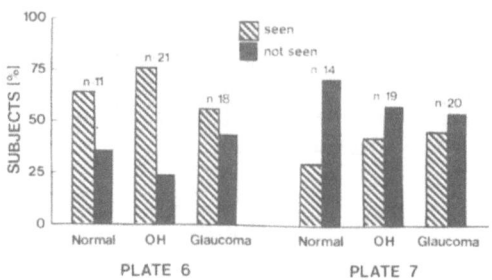

Fig. 2. Histogram showing the proportion of age matched normals, ocular hypertensives (OH) and glaucoma patients who saw or did not see plate 6 and 7 with both eyes. Not included in the histogram are data from three normals and two glaucoma patients who saw plate 6 with only one eye and two ocular hypertensives who saw plate 7 with only one eye (Sokol, Domar & Moskowitz 1980).

plates 2–5 was too small to include in the analysis. χ^2 analysis of the data showed no significant difference among the 3 groups: $\chi^2 = 1.88$ for plate 6 and $\chi^2 = 1.01$ for plate 7.

Visual evoked potential. In a related study we have found, not surprisingly, that pupil size affects the latency of P_1. As seen in Fig. 3, a decrease in pupil diameter results in a prolongation of P_1, most likely because of the decrease in retinal illuminance. For example, an increase of nearly 20 msec. occurs when the pupil diameter is reduced from 9 to 1 mm. On this basis, it becomes important to control for pupil size, particularly in view of the fact that many glaucoma patients use medication which constricts the pupil. For example, Fig. 4 shows the distribution of pupil diameters of the glaucoma patients, normals and ocular hypertensives. Statistical analysis of pupil diameter showed that, as a group, the glaucoma patients had significantly smaller pupils ($p < 0.001$) than normals and ocular hypertensives (who had equal mean pupil diameters).

In order to increase the precision of the latency measurement and remove pupil size as a source of potential bias, an analysis of covariance was used (Edwards, 1962). Briefly, analysis of covariance provides an indirect statistical control for pupil size by first determining the relationship between pupil size and latency and then adjusting the mean latencies from each group so that any bias due to pupil size is eliminated. As seen in Fig. 5, analysis of covariance revealed that after adjustment for the differences in pupil diameter the mean P_1 latency from the normals and ocular hypertensives was equal and the mean P_1 latency obtained from the glaucoma patients was significantly longer than either the normals' or ocular hypertensives'.

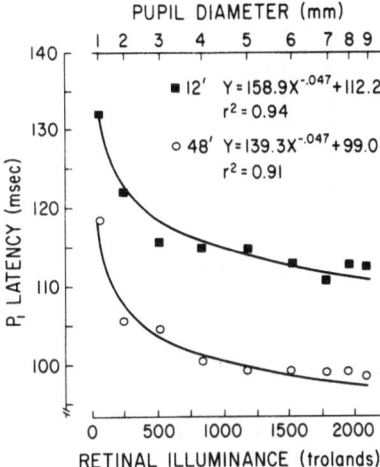

Fig. 3. P$_1$ latency in a normal subject for 12 and 48 minute checks as a function of pupil diameter (upper scale). The subject's eye was dilated with 2.5% phenylephrine and artificial pupils ranging in diameter from 1 to 9 mm in 1 mm steps were used. Also, shown on the lower scale is the effective retinal illuminance for each pupil diameter, which takes the Stiles-Crawford effect into account (Le Grand, 1968). The data were best fit by a hyperbola with an equation of the form $Y = aX^{-b} + c$. Values for a, b and c and for r^2, the coefficient of determination, are given in the figure.

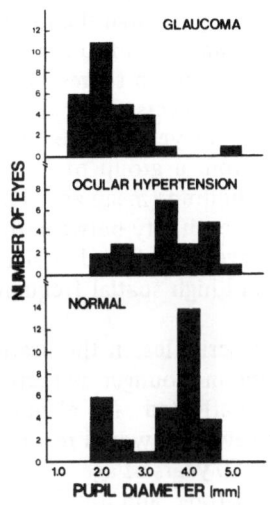

Fig. 4. Histogram showing distribution of pupil diameter for the three groups.

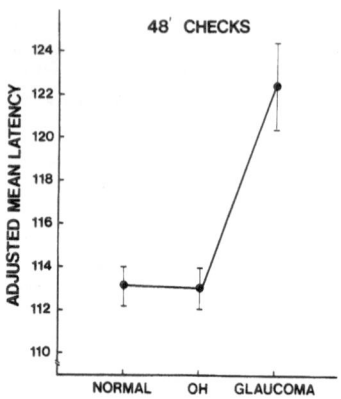

Fig. 5. Adjusted mean latency of P_1 for normals, ocular hypertensives and glaucoma patients. Vertical lines indicate ± 1 standard error.

DISCUSSION

The results obtained with the Arden grating test demonstrate that a large number of false-positives occur in older subjects. Thus, the Arden grating test may be inaccurate as an indicator of glaucoma, at least in older patients. For example, had we used Arden's method of scoring 25 for 'not seen', there would have been a false positive rate of 37% on plate 6 and 71% on plate 7.

The most likely explanation for the inability of older normals to see plate 6 and 7 is the decrease in contrast sensitivity with age. Skalka (1980) found that the mean total Arden scores for normal subjects between 50 and 60 years of age were 19 points higher than the mean scores for subjects between 10 and 20 years of age. We have also found a significant age effect with the Arden plates. Fig. 6 shows the mean scores obtained on each plate for three groups of visually normal subjects. The scores obtained for a group of 14 older adults (mean age: 66 years) were significantly higher ($p < 0.001$) than the scores obtained from a group of 24 young adults (mean age: 28 years) and a group of 26 children (mean age: 12 years). There was no significant difference in contrast sensitivity between the young adults and children. Derefeldt et al. (1979) have also found a significant decrease in contrast sensitivity in the middle and high spatial frequency regions in subjects older than 60.

Our results do not necessarily lessen the usefulness of the Arden plates in the detection of glaucoma in younger patients nor do they indicate that contrast sensitivity is unaffected in glaucoma (Atkin, Bodis-Wollner, Wolkstein & 7 1979). However, we would recommend that the plates be used judiciously in patients over 50 years of age.

The VEP results demonstrate abnormal prolongation of P_1 in patients with glaucoma. Further, these results indicate that pupil size must be carefully controlled, either statistically, as we have done, or experimentally by

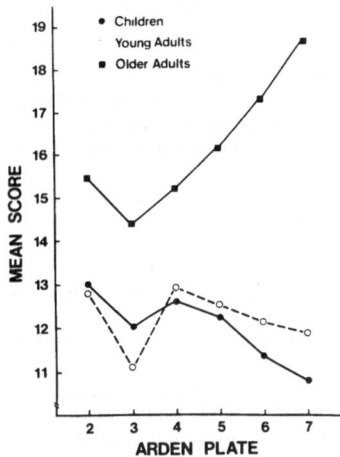

Fig. 6. Mean scores on Arden Grating Test for each plate for 3 groups of visually normal subjects. The mean scores for the group of older adults were significantly higher (sensitivity lower) than the scores for either the yound adults or children.

using an artificial pupil of constant diameter. While the mean latency for the glaucoma group was significantly longer than the mean for either the normals or the ocular hypertensives we cannot say how many individual galucoma patients were abnormal on the basis of the commonly used criterion of 2.0 standard deviations longer than the mean.

Further studies with constant pupil size are necessary before it can be determined if the percentage of glaucoma patients with abnormal prolongation of VEP latency is as high as that found in patients with optic neuritis (90%) or a definite diagnosis of multiple sclerosis (80–90%). Huber et al. (1978) report that 74% of their glaucomatous patients had peak latencies greater than twice the standard deviation of their control group. However, it should be noted that while they report that their glaucoma patients had miotic pupils they did not give any specific information regarding the pupil size differences in their groups.

The VEP probably adds little to the diagnosis of glaucoma because other less sophisticated techniques such as measurement of intraocular pressure, visual fields and ophthalmoscopic examination of the optic disc are available. However, whether the VEP will be of any value in the early detection of glaucomatous damage, that is, prior to the onset of visual field defects or the appearance of abnormal cupping and pallor of the optic disc, remains to be determined.

ACKNOWLEDGEMENT

This work was supported by research grant EY00926 from the National Eye Institute.

85

REFERENCES

Arden, G.B. & Gucukoglu, A.G. Grating test of contrast sensitivity in patients with retrobulbar neuritis. Arch. Ophthal. 96: 1626–1629 (1978).

Arden, G.B. & Jacobson, J.J. A simple grating test for contrast sensitivity: preliminary results indicate value in screening for glaucoma. Invest. Ophthalmol. Vis. Sci. 17: 23–32 (1978).

Atkin, A., Bodis-Wollner, I., Wolkstein, M., Moss, A. & Podos, S.M. Abnormalities of central contrast sensitivity in glaucoma. Am. J. Ophthalmol. 88: 205–211 (1979).

Derefeldt, G., Lennerstrand, G. & Lundh, B. Age variations in normal human contrast sensitivity. Acta. Ophthal. 57: 679–690 (1979).

Ederer, F. Shall we count numbers of eyes or numbers of subjects? Arch. Ophthal. 89: 1 (1973).

Edwards, A.L. Experimental Design in Psychological Research. Holt, Rinehart and Winston, New York. (1962).

Halliday, A.M., McDonald, W.I. & Mushin, E. Visual evoked response in diagnosis of multiple sclerosis. Br. Med. J. 4: 661–664 (1973).

Hess, R.F. & Howell, E.R. The threshold contrast sensitivity function in strabismic amblyopia: evidence for a two type classification. Vision. Res. 17: 1049–1055 (1977).

Huber, C. & Wagner, T. Electrophysiological evidence for glaucomatous lesions in the optic nerve. Ophthal. Res. 10: 22–29 (1978).

Le Grand, Y. Light, Colour and Vision (2nd ed.). Translated by R.W.G. Hunt, J.W.T. Walsh, and F.R.W. Hunt. Chapman and Hall, Ltd., London. 107–108 (1968).

Skalka, H.W. Effect of age on Arden grating acuity. Br. J. Ophthal. 64: 21–23 (1980).

Sokol, S. Visual evoked potentials. In: Electrodiagnosis in clinical neurology (Ed. M.J. Aminoff). Churchill Livingstone, New York 348–369 (1980).

Sokol, S., Domar, A. & Moskowitz, A. Utility of the Arden grating test in glaucoma screening: high false positive rate in normals over 50 years of age. Invest. Ophthalmol. Vis. Sci. 19: 1529–1533 (1980).

Authors' Address:
Department of Ophthalmology
New England Medical Center and
Tufts University School of Medicine
171 Harrison Ave.
Boston, MA 02111, U.S.A.

PATTERN EVOKED CORTICAL POTENTIALS AND AUTOMATED PERIMETRY IN CHRONIC GLAUCOMA

C. HUBER

(*Zurich, Switzerland*)

ABSTRACT

Chronic glaucoma causes visual field defects and in some cases an increase in the latency of pattern evoked visual potentials (P E P). To assess the contribution of field defects to the latency increase in PEP we have reexamined 16 glaucoma patients out of a group of 27 whose PEP had been recorded two years before (Huber and Wagner 1978). PEP measurements and visual fields measured by automated static perimetry (Octopus) where compared. A significant increase in PEP latency could only be demonstrated in the presence of a *relative central scotoma*. The depth of the relative scotoma is related to the increase in latency. Peripheral field defects do not affect the PEP latency as a small central island of vision with normal sensitivity is sufficient to produce a normal PEP. A large visual field with reduced central sensitivity can however result in a large latency increase. Over a period of two years the shape of the individual PEP is constant. The latency increase in glaucoma thus represents a differential diagnosis of increased PEP latency in the context of neurological diseases. PEPs are not an adequate method for the detection of early glaucoma as the sensitivity of the visual field's center can be unaffected for a long time in this disease.

INTRODUCTION

Chronic glaucoma in man produces a localised, slowly progressing destruction of the optic nerve in the region adjacent and posterior to the papilla. Early functional defects are relative scotomatas in the visual field which tend to progress toward the visual field center in the course of the disease. Visual evoked potentials have been recorded in glaucoma with the hope that an objective perimetry (Müller, Haase & Henning 1975; Cappin & Nissim 1975) or an electrophysiological measure of the neural lesion might be possible (Bartl, Benedikt, Hiti & Mandl 1975). The fact that pattern evoked responses can show pathological changes in glaucoma even when the central part of the visual field and the visual acuity are intact (Huber & Wagner 1978; Cappin & Nissim 1975) seems surprising, because the pattern evoked responses have been shown to depend only on the function of the central part of the retina. Luminance evoked potentials have large summation areas not only under scotopic (Kojima & Zrenner 1977) but also under photopic conditions (12° Armington 1968; 20° Oguchi & Van Lith 1974: 10° Henkes & Van Lith 1969). Pattern evoked responses, however, are more dependant on the foveal function. The size of the retinal area sufficient to elicit normal pattern evoked potentials depends on the check or bar size used (Abe & Iwata 1976; May, Forbes & Piantanida 1971; Van der Tweel 1979). The critical area is smaller than the 10 to 20° given for the luminance responses and can be limited to the inner 3 to 5° of the retina. In glaucoma, Ermers et al. (1974) have shown in some patients that a reduction of light sensitivity by 0.5 to 1.0 log unit in the visual field center is sufficient to reduce the amplitude of the pattern evoked potentials compared to a normal fellow eye. Huber et al. (1978) have shown an increase in the latencies of evoked potentials in a glaucoma population. With the advent of automated perimetry systems precise question oriented static perimetry is now possible in most adult patients. To evaluate the influence of glaucomatous field defects on pattern evoked potentials we have reexamined the group of glaucoma patients seen in 1977 (Huber & Wagner 1978), 2 years later, by measuring pattern evoked potentials (PEP) and by automated static perimetry.

MATERIALS AND METHODS

Twenty-seven glaucoma eyes in 16 patients could be re-examined out of the original group of 39 eyes in 27 patients. Only patients with a visual acuity of 0.4 or better were included, as an optical reduction of visual acuity to that level in healthy eyes does not result in an increase of PEP latency with the 38' large check size used (Huber & Wagner 1978).

PEP pattern stimulation. Reversing checkerboard patterns with check sizes of 38' 19' and 9' were generated with the Medelec pattern generator on a television screen covering a field of $10° \times 14°$ (Arden & Faulkner 1977; Arden, Faulkner & Mair 1977). The pattern contrast was 50% and the pattern reversal rate 1 or 2 Hz. The average luminance on the screen is $90 \, cd/m^2$. The EEG was recorded from a midline electrode placed 5 cm above the inion referred to the ear. The latency is measured from the time of pattern reversal to the apex of the first positive peak at about 100 msec. If the signals were small the normal number of averaged sweeps (n = 128) was doubled or tripled to define more clearly the apex of the waveform (Fig. 3).

Static perimetry. The static visual fields were measured with the Octopus system developed by Fankhauser and his colleagues (Octopus Interzeag AG, CH-8952 Schlieren, Switzerland). Both Octopus-programs 31 and 21 were used on each eye. The resulting topographical resolution is 6° up to 30° eccentricity and 15° in the outer periphery. The resolution in sensitivity is theoretically 1 dB or a tenth of a log unit. To help evaluate pathology we have used the age-matched normal values and standard deviations given in the Octopus visual field atlas (Zühlke 1978). In the illustrations a sensitivity profile in the 0°/180° axis is drawn under a normal band with a width of 2 SD (Fig. 3, 6).

RESULTS

Change of PEP configuration over time

Small changes in measured latency should be considered irrelevant due to the inherent difficulty in determining the apex of a not too sharp wave. In a well controlled glaucoma case (Fig. 1), without any latency increase

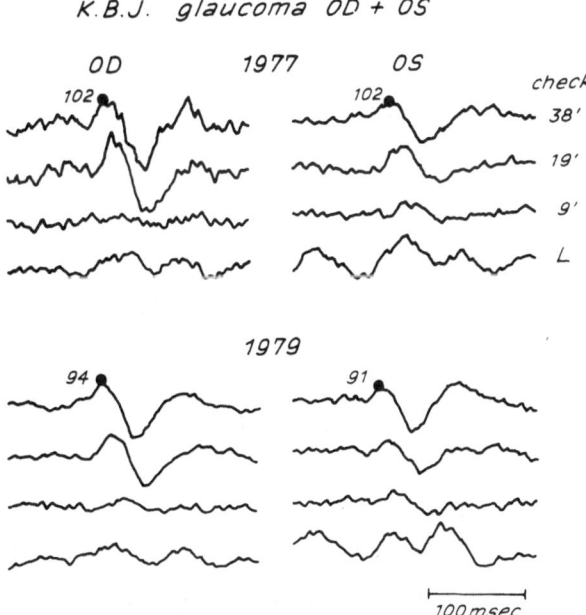

Fig. 1. Pattern evoked potentials in a glaucoma patient measured with an interval of two years. Visual acuity 1977 and 1979 1.0 both eyes. The form of the evoked potentials induced by the different check sizes (38, 19 and 9′) does not change over two years. The earlier latencies measured in 1979 are probably due to a different noise level. The time resolution of the digital averager (1 msec) is not the limiting factor for precise latency measurements. The choice of the maximum peak is difficult when noise ripples are added to the evoked potential curve.

the shape of different PEPs is unchanged after an interval of two years. The earlier latency measured in 1979 is due to a different amount of noise level. The width of the recorded wave makes the precise measurement of an apex difficult. This is in part due to an artefact pointed out by Van Lith et al. (1979). As the pattern reversal is not synchronized to the frame rate of the TV monitor, to avoid 50 Hz visual and electrical interference, there is an inherent variability in the interval between trigger and pattern reversal in the center of the TV screen. This variability leads, after averaging, to a broadening of the recorded curves so that the resolution of the averager in time, of

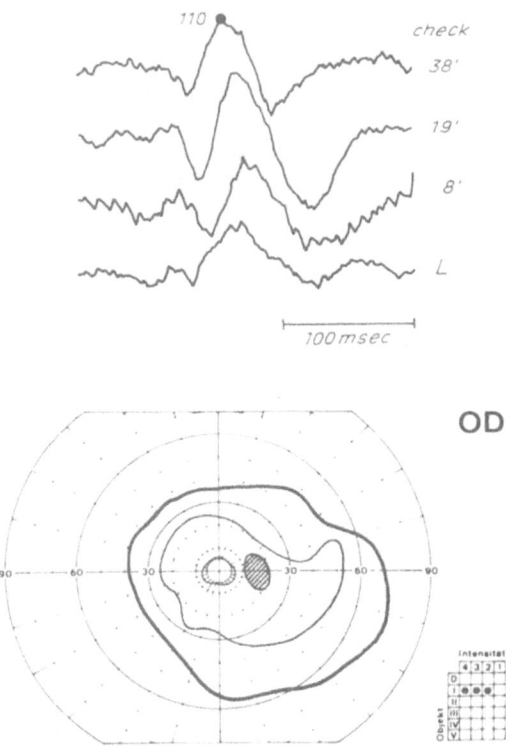

Fig. 2. Normal pattern evoked potentials to different check sizes in a glaucoma patient with only slight peripheral field defects in Goldmann perimetry as measured in 1977. The latency is measured in the evoked potential to the larger 38′ pattern. With those larger patterns the latency is not affected by a reduction in visual acuity down to a visual acuity of 0.3.

1 msec, is much better than the ability of the examiner to localise the maximum of the PEP wave. Under identical recording conditions the shape of the individual PEP does not change over a period of two years even if the latency increases by as much as 30 msec (Fig. 2, 3).

The latencies measured under identical conditions in the same glaucoma eyes two years apart are plotted as histograms in Fig. 4. Assuming an upper limit of normal latency (mean ± SD) of 115 msec (Huber & Wagner 1978) there are 11 eyes in 1977 and 13 in 1979 with latencies in the pathological range. Seven eyes show an increase of over 10 msec in latency over a period of two years. The large spread of latencies in a glaucoma population described in 1977 is confirmed.

A relation between subjective reduction in light sensitivity and pattern evoked potential latency could only be found for the single spot measured in the center of the visual field. If one takes into account the sensitivity loss as near as 6° away from the fixation point the subjective data can be quite reduced without a pathological increase in latency. A plot of the sensitivity in the visual field center against PEP latency however shows a progressive decrease in light sensitivity with increasing PEP latency (Fig. 5). The fact that the delay in the evoked potentials is mainly due to the very center of the visual field is illustrated in two extreme cases (Fig. 6 and 3). In Fig. 6 more than 6° in size. Points measured with an eccentricity of 3° are in the normal range but with an eccentricity of 6° are already pathological. The PEP latency is only increased to the upper limit of our normal range in spite the visual field is constricted to a small central island of less than 12° but of the obliteration of the greatest part of the visual field. In Fig. 3, on the contrary, the size of the visual field is intact. The sensitivity is reduced in the whole field but the reason for the large delay in PEP latency is that the sensitivity in the centre of the visual field is reduced by nearly 2 log units.

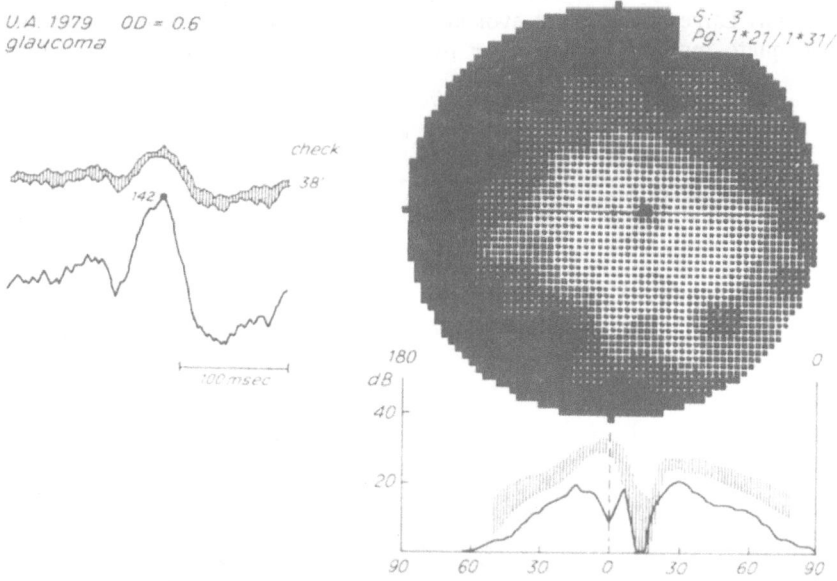

Fig. 3. Delayed pattern evoked potential in the same eye as in Fig. 2 two years later. The upper broader band on the left is a superposition of 3 averaged potentials, the lower curve is the sum of 3 identical evoked potentials. The form of the evoked potential is identical to the upper curve in Fig. 2 but the latency is increased by 32 msec. The Octopus perimetry shows a decrease in sensitivity over the whole visual field. The lower curve under the visual field is a sensitivity profile in the 0/180° meridan under a band showing the normal sensitivity in the corresponding age group (the width of the band is 2 SD).

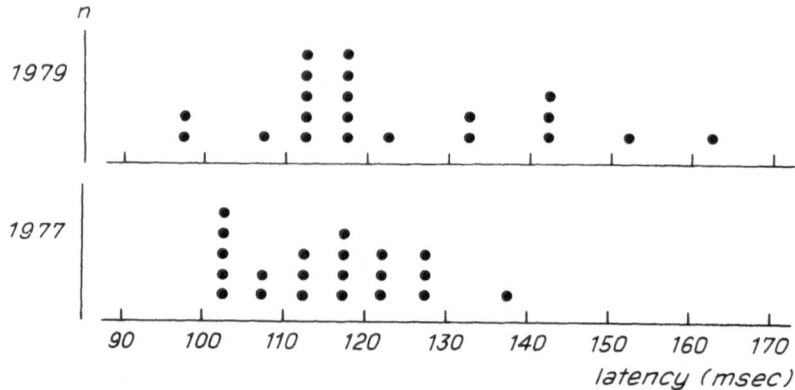

Fig. 4. Latency histogram of pattern evoked visual potentials in 21 glaucoma eyes after an interval of 2 years. The latencies are grouped in classes of 5 msec. The normal mean latency is 102 msec ± 6 msec. In 1977 11 eyes have a latency above 115 msec in 1979 13 eyes. The visual acuity is in all cases above 0.3.

DISCUSSION

In glaucoma a delay in pattern evoked potential seems to be clinically measurable only when the disease affects the sensitivity of the visual field center. Large field pattern evoked potential methods will probably not be an adequate method to detect or follow early glaucomatous changes. In our

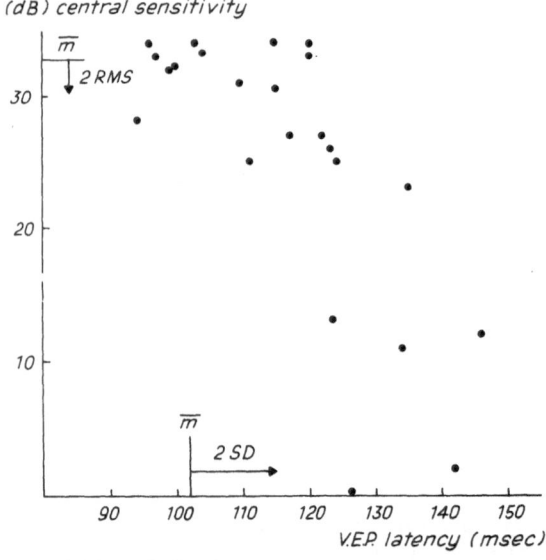

Fig. 5. Subjective sensitivity of the fovea in 23 glaucoma eyes as a function of the latency in the visual evoked potential (VEP). The mean value and SD of a normal population are indicated on both axes. There is a progressive decrease of sensitivity in the visual field center as the latency of the evoked potentials increases. The visual acuity is in all cases above 0.3. The stimulus for the evoked responses is a reversing checkerboard pattern of 38' size for the single checks.

92

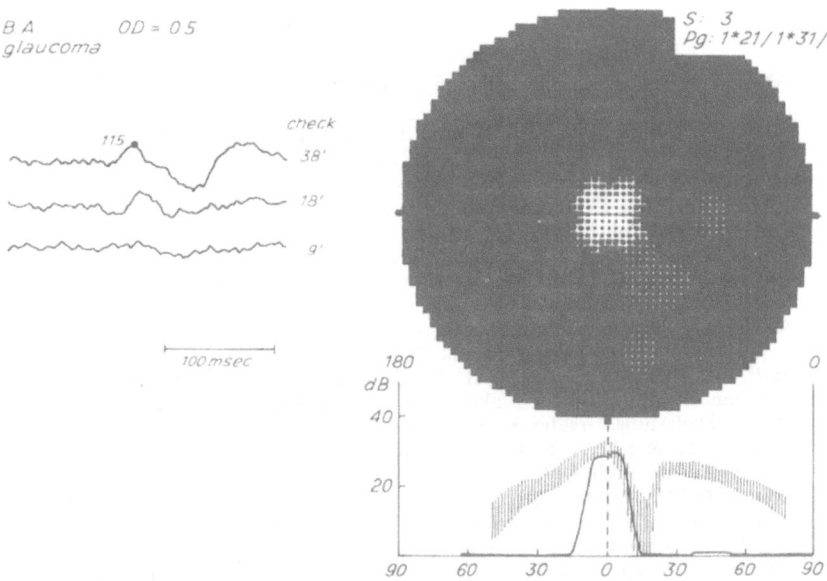

Fig. 6. Pattern evoked potential and Octopus visual field in an advanced glaucoma case. The latency of the evoked potential is only increased to the limit between norm and pathology (115 msec). The sensitivity of the visual field center is still normal in spite of an extreme constriction of the visual field.

experience the subjective information given by the automated perimetry is more relevant and sensitive than the objective measure of PEP latency. The possibility of very large latency increments present in glaucoma eyes with a good visual acuity must be kept in mind in the differential diagnosis of neurological diseases. To miss the diagnosis of a glaucoma should not happen to an ophthalmologist but might easily happen if the patient is seen by a neurologist alone. Subjectively the patient, whose visual field and PEP are shown in Fig. 3, may not realize that anything is wrong with her eye. The fact that the PEP latency can increase with time in glaucoma and that it is quantitatively related to the sensitivity reduction in the visual field center speaks for a direct relation to the optic nerve lesion. Theoretically the methods could be made more sensitive to earlier glaucomatous change by using stimulus patterns nearer to the threshold of perception. The size of the squares or the contrast could be reduced. The population examined is however quite old (Huber & Wagner 1978) and some of the patients have a beginning of cataract. This is not a problem with large check sizes as the evoked potential is then not very sensitive to either contrast or defocussing. In this group of patients finer stimuli would only have detected the slight, glaucoma independent, reductions of visual acuities.

ACKNOWLEDGEMENTS

This work was supported by a grant from the Swiss National Funds Nr. 3.020.73.

93

REFERENCES

Abe, H. & Iwata, K. Checkerboard pattern reversal VER in the assessment of glaucomatous field defects. Acta Soc. Ophthal. Jap. 80: 829–841 (1976).

Arden, G.B. & Faulkner, D.J. A versatile pattern generator for neuro-ophthalmological and paediatric EP and psychophysical tests, using standard television techniques compatible with boradcast colour programs. In: Experimental and clinical amblyopia. 13th ISCERG Symposium (Ed. E. Auerbach) Junk, The Hague. (Doc. Ophthal. Proc. Series Vol. 11). 49–55 (1977).

Arden, G.B., Faulkner, D.J. & Mair, C. A versatile television pattern generator for visual evoked potentials. In: Visual evoked potentials in man: new developments (ed. J.E. Desmedt) Clarendon Press, Oxford. 90–109 (1977).

Armington, J.C. The electroretinogram, the visual evoked potential and the area luminance relation. Vision Res. 8: 263–276 (1968).

Bartl, G., Benedikt, O., Hiti, H. & Mandl, H. Das elektrophysiologische Verhalten gesunder und glaukomkranker menschlichen Augen bei durzeitiger intraokularer Druckbelastung. Graefes Arch. Ophthal. 195: 201–206 (1975).

Cappin, J.M. & Nissim, S. Visual evoked responses in the assessment of field defects in glaucoma. Arch. Ophthal. 93: 9 18 (1975).

Ermers, H.J.M., de Heer, L.J. & Van Lith, G.M.H. VECP's in patient with galucoma. In: 11th ISCERG Symposium (Ed. E. Dodt & J.T. Pearlman). Junk, The Hague. (Doc. Ophthal. Proc. Series Vol. 4). 387–393 (1974).

Huber, C. & Wagner, T. Electrophysiological evidence for glaucomatous lesions in the optic nerve. Ophthal. Res. 10: 22–29 (1978).

Henkes, H. & Van Lith, G.M.H. Evaluation and clinical application of macular responses in ERG and VER. J. Chiba Med. Soc. 45: 481–535 (1969).

Kojima, M. & Zrenner, E. Local and spatial distribution of photopic and scotopic responses in the visual field as reflected in the visually evoked potential. In: 14th ISCERG Symposium (Ed. Th. Lawwill) Junk, The Hague. (Doc. Ophthal. Proc. Series Vol. 13). 31–40 (1977).

Van Lith, G.H.M., Henkes, H.E., & Van Marle, G.W. Projector or TV as a pattern stimulator? In: 16th ISCEV Symposium (Ed. Y. Tazawa). Jap. J. of Ophthal: 210–206 (1979).

May, J.G., Forbes, W.B. & Piantanida, T.P. The visual evoked response obtained with an alternating barred pattern: Rate spatial frequency and wave length. Electroenceph. clin. Neurophysiol. 30: 222–228 (1971).

Müller, W., Haase, E. & Henning, G. Vergleichende Untersuchungen von subjektiv und objektiv ermittelten Gesichtsfeldern. Graefes Arch. Ophthal. 194: 143–152 (1975).

Oguchi, Y. & Van Lith, G.H.M. Contribution of the central and the peripheral part of the retina to the VECP under photopic conditions. In: 11 ISCERG Symposium (Ed. E. Dodt & J.T. Pearlman). Junk, The Hague. (Doc. Ophthal. Proc. Series Vol. 4), 261–268 (1974).

Van der Tweel, L.H. Pattern evoked potentials facts and considerations. In: 16th ISCEV Symposium (Ed. Y. Tazawa). Jap. J. Ophthal: 201–206 (1979).

Zühlke, G. Visual field atlas 2nd Edition. Interzeag AG, Riebbachstr. 5, CH-8952 Schlieren, Switzerland (1978).

Authors address:
C. Huber
University Eye Clinic
Rämistrasse 100
CH-8091 Zurich
Switzerland

THE TRANSIENT PATTERN ONSET VEP IN GLAUCOMA

N.R. GALLOWAY & C. BARBER

(*Nottingham, England*)

ABSTRACT

Alternate upper and lower half field stimuli with 30 minute checks were applied to each eye of a series of nine normals and twelve patients suffering from field defects due to chronic simple galucoma. The responses from the glaucoma patients tended to be markedly abnormal but they could not be related to the visual field defect.

INTRODUCTION

Testing visual fields is a routine part of the management of chronic simple glaucoma, and the decision for surgery may sometimes depend on the detection of progressive field loss. It seems possible that the visually evoked potential could be developed as an objective test of field loss and some attempts have already been made to achieve this using the steady state VEP (Cappin & Nissim 1975; Abe & Iwata 1976). The effect of raised intraocular pressure on the VEP has also been assessed in normal (Bartl, Benedikt, Hiti & Mandl 1975) and glaucomatous eyes (Ermers, De Heer & Van Lith 1974). In its early stages the visual defect in glaucoma tends to be asymmetrically positioned in upper and lower half fields, sometimes involving largely the upper half field. For this reason it was felt that more information might be obtained if upper and lower half fields were stimulated separately in these patients.

METHOD

A projection television system was used to produce upper and lower half pattern onset 30 minute check stimuli. The stimulus was presented alternately to upper and lower half fields with the subject fixing centrally. The size of the stimulus was varied in separate runs from a maximum of ten degrees down to six degrees in two degree steps, the smaller horizontal strips being progressively further away from fixation. The horizontal width of all

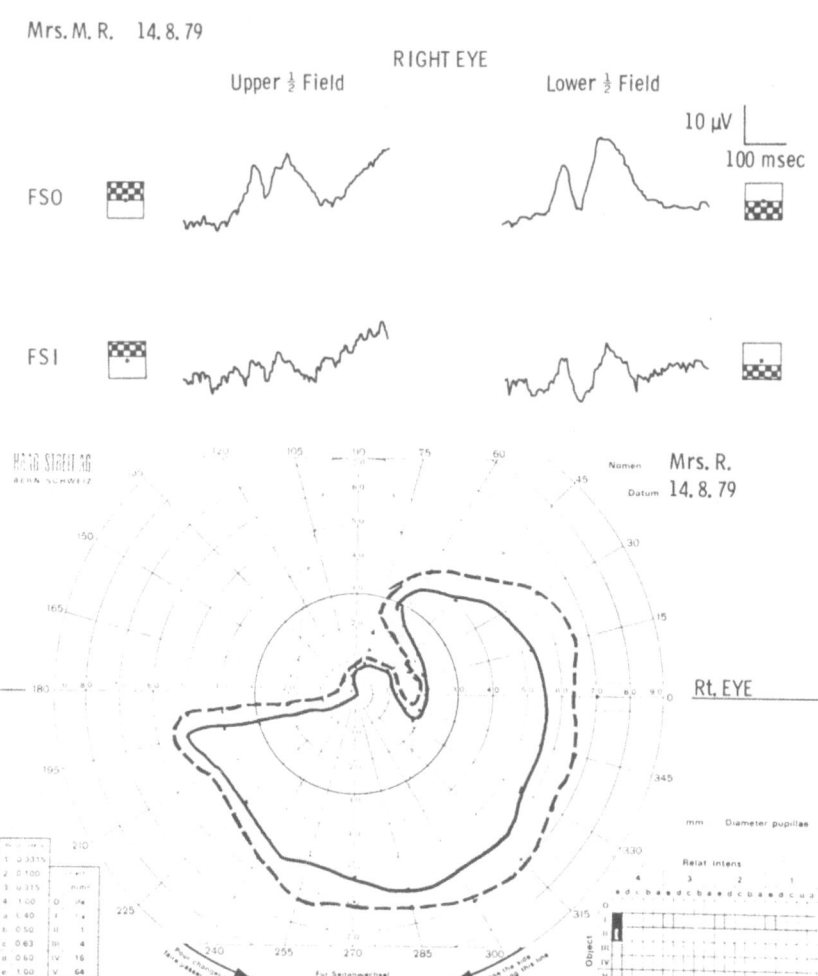

Fig. 1. The response from the right eye of a patient with early constriction of the visual field.

FSO – Stimulus 20° wide, 10° vertically through fixation.
FSI – Stimulus 20° wide, 8° vertically, 2° above fixation.

the stimuli was 20°. The smallest was therefore a horizontal strip 29° wide and 6° vertically being offset 4° from fixation. In practice this stimulus did not give reliable responses, and in most cases the VEP was too small to record. These results have therefore been omitted from the paper. In Figs. 1, 2 and 3, FSO refers to the stimulus which subtended 10° in a vertical direction, either below or above fixation. The letters FSI refer to the stimulus which subtended 8° vertically and was offset 2° from fixation.

Silver-silver chloride electrodes were attached to the scalp at 2.5 cm above

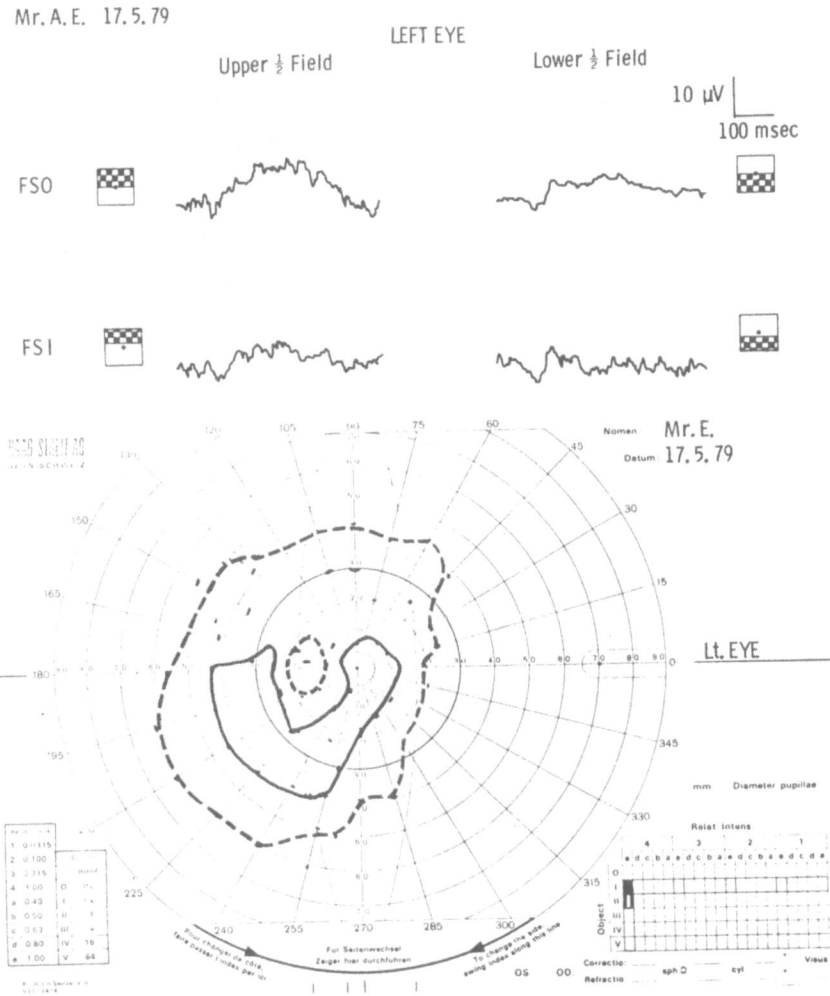

Fig. 2. Small response from an eye with grossly constricted field and visual acuity of 6/18.

the inion and forehead and ears were used as earth points. All leads were connected to a preamplifier and averaging was then carried out using a Nicolet computer. The average of 256 sweeps each of one second was recorded from each eye. The patients' visual fields were tested with a Goldmann perimeter. Each patient was tested on two separate occasions with an intervening interval of about two months.

MATERIAL

The nine normal subjects were confirmed to be free of eye disease or injury

97

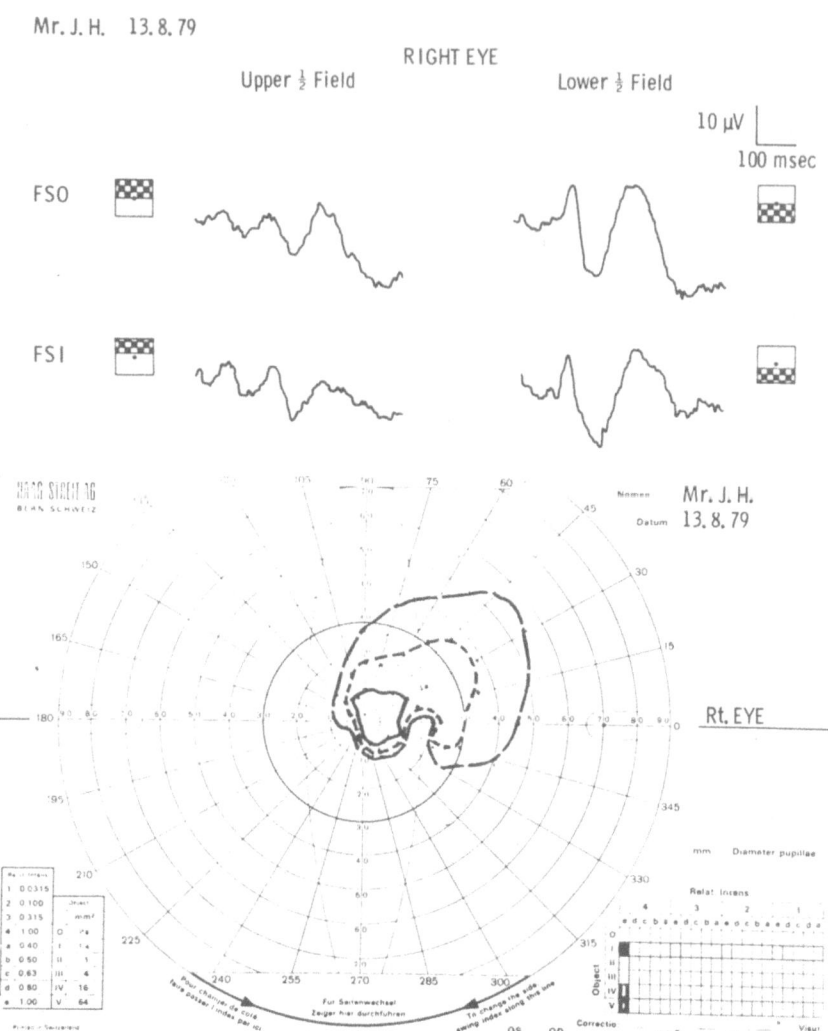

Mr. J. H.   13. 8. 79

RIGHT EYE

Upper ½ Field   Lower ½ Field

10 µV

100 msec

FSO

FSI

HAAG STREIT 1G
BERN SCHWEIZ

Mr. J. H.
Datum 13. 8. 79

Rt. EYE

mm   Diameter pupillae

Relat Intens

Fig. 3. Good response from a patient with a severely constricted field but a visual acuity of 6/9.

and had normal fields. The twelve patients were all confirmed cases of chronic simple galucoma with field defects in one or both eyes.

RESULTS

In general the normal results showed a gradual reduction in size of response as the stimulus was applied to a more peripheral part of the visual field. The responses form the lower half of the field were larger than those from the upper half. Intersubject variation was considerable.

Table 1.

Patient		Visual acuity	Field	V.E.R.
D.P.	R	CF	Central loss	Absent response
	L	6/12	Central loss	Absent response
C.A.M.	R	6/5	Grossly constricted	Absent response
	L	6/5	Grossly constricted	Absent response
G.B.	R	6/18	Moderately constricted	Good responses
	L	6/9	Moderately constricted	from lower half
A.E.	R	6/18	Moderately constricted	Small response
	L	CF	Moderately constricted	Absent response
A.Y.	R	6/18	Full field	Small response
	L	6/12	Grossly constricted	Good response
J.H.	R	6/9	Grossly constricted	Good response
	L	6/12	Slightly constricted	Good response
C.C.	R	6/36	Grossly constricted	Absent response
	L	6/24	Grossly constricted	Absent response
J.G.	R	6/6	Full field	Good response
	L	6/6	Upper half loss	Slightly reduced
C.H.	R	6/6	Upper half loss	Good response
	L	6/6	Upper half loss	Good response
M.R.	R	6/12	Upper half loss	Good response
	L	6/9	Full field	Good response
F.W.F.	R	6/6	Upper half loss	Reduced response
	L	6/9	Full field	Reduced response
A.S.			No follow-ups	

Table 1 shows the results obtained from eleven patients with chronic simple glaucoma. One patient was excluded because he failed to keep his follow up appointment and his results could not therefore be repeated. All the other cases had repeatable results, the waveform and amplitude being very similar on each of the two occasions that they were tested. The considerable intersubject variation made it difficult to make reliable physical measurements on the traces and this applied to the results from normal subjects as well as from patients.

Table 2 shows that the degree of field loss bears a relationship to the amplitude of the transient VEP.

Fig. 1 shows the response of the right eye of a patient with early constriction of the visual field and Fig. 2 shows a small response from an eye with a grossly restricted field and a visual acuity of 6/18. Fig. 3 in contrast shows a good response from a patient with a severe field defect and a visual acuity of 6/9 FSO: Stimulus subtending 10° vertically to fixation. FSI: Stimulus subtending 8° vertically but offset 2° from fixation.

DISCUSSION

The larger response normally obtained from lower half field stimuli is well recognised. This was also present in the glaucomatous patients sometimes

Table 2

Type of field defect	No of eyes	VEP
Central loss	2	Absent in both
Grossly constricted	6	Absent in four out of six good response in two eyes
Moderately constricted	4	Absent in one our of four
Upper half loss	5	Good response in all
Slightly constricted	1	Good response
Normal field	4	Two good, two reduced

even when the defect was in the lower part of the field. In general the more severely constricted fields produced small or absent VEPs; in one case with severely constricted fields the VEP was absent even with a visual acuity as good as 6/5 in each eye. Although results were recorded using different sizes of target, in most instances the more peripheral stimulus simply produced slightly smaller results than the larger 10° stimulus. We were not able to show that the use of a slightly peripheral stimulus gave any extra information, when trying to detect glaucomatous field defects. It had been hoped that the comparison of responses from upper and lower stimuli aimed at 2–10° from fixation might show up early glaucoma cases. It is well recognised clinically that many glaucoma cases show early loss of visual field in the region above fixation. The most obvious difficulty here is the fact that these perimacular areas of the retina do not contribute greatly to the normal VEP and damage in these areas might not be expected to alter the response. In practice such damage does seem to alter the response but in a rather unpredictable manner. Some of the cases with early visual field defects had quite good responses and these results seem to show that this method of eliciting the VEP is not suitable for detecting early field defects. On the other hand the consistency of results on repeated testing of individual cases suggest that the technique might provide a means of monitoring defects in a patient with advancing disease. It seems probable that a more appropriately designed stimulus and perhaps a different electrode position could give more useful information in the future.

ACKNOWLEDGEMENTS

This study was supported in part by a grant from the Trent Regional Health Authority. We acknowledge with thanks the assistance of Mrs. S. Khan.

REFERENCES

Abe, H. & Iwata, K. Chequerboard pattern reversal VER in the assessment of glaucomatous field defects. Acta Soc. Japan 80: 829–841 (1976).
Bartl, G., Benedikt, O., Hiti, H. & Mandl, H. The electrophysiological behaviour of normal and glaucomatous eyes with short term intraocular pressure elevation. Albrecht v. Graefes Arch. Klin. exp. ophthal. 195: 201–206 (1975).

100

Cappin, J.M. & Nissim, S. Visually evoked response in assessment of field defects in glaucoma. Arch. Ophthal. 93: 9–18 (1975).

Ermers, H.J., De Heer, L.J. & Van Lith, G.H.M. VECPs in patients with glaucoma. In: 11th ISCERG Symposium (Ed. E. Dodt & J.T. Pearlman) Junk, The Hague. (Doc. Ophthal. Proc. Series Vol. 4) 387–393 (1974).

Authors' address:
Queens Medical Centre
Nottingham NG1 5DN
England

OPTIC PATHWAY ACTION POTENTIALS AND INTRAOCULAR PRESSURE (IOP) RISE

A clinical and experimental study

A. NEETENS, Y. HENDRATA & J. VAN ROMPAEY

(Antwerp, Belgium)

ABSTRACT

Before the occurrence of visual field losses, the visual evoked potential (VEP) in patients with open angle glaucomatous disease (OAG) may be disturbed. In OAG-patients pharmacological lowering of systemic blood pressure can result in a decrease of the VEP amplitude. Prior systemic lowering of IOP, however, does not always result in improvement of the VEP response.

Inadequate capillary perfusion under conditions of elevated IOP threatens axonal function of the optic pathway. Conditions of diseased vessel wall also threaten axonal function. Experimental animal models confirm these clinical findings. Repeated IOP increases cause permanent lowering of action potentials, released only by increasing the systemic blood pressure.

INTRODUCTION

In disseminated as well as in selective optic pathway damage, regardless of the etiology, visual evoked potential (VEP) changes do not seem to be specific (Neetens, Hendrata & Van Rompaey 1979a). In patients with open angle glaucoma (OAG), for example, both wave-shape and latency following flash reversal pattern stimulation may be altered, but the changes observed are typically similar to those detected in patients with demyelinating diseases (Neetens, Hendrata, Van Rompaey 1979b). The VEP, however, can provide subclinical information on the functional integrity of the optic pathway in many neuro-ophthalmological conditions (Neetens, Hendrata, Van Rompaey, Rubbens & Verschueren 1979).

Because of the importance of an objective diagnostic tool for determining subclinical damage, as in patients wtih elevated intraocular pressure (IOP) but without detectable peripheral visual field losses, further investigation of the VEP under this clinical condition seemed indicated. We therefore examined the VEP in OAG patients. For a more direct electrophysiological assessment of optic nerve involvement under conditions of increased intraocular pressure, an experimental study was also performed in the cat.

PART I. CLINICAL STUDY

METHODS AND MATERIALS

Stimulus

A photostimulator S.I.L.T. (Ahrend-Van Gogh), used without having the patients previously dark adapted, provided flash stimulation. For pattern stimulation a digitimer pattern reversal type D112 provided a chequer-board reversal screen (32 × 32 cm) with black and white squares (2 × 2 cm). Alternation of the checks was sinusoidal (half maximum luminance), and the total number of alternating stimuli presented at 1/s was 100.

The fixation point, subtending 1'30″, was placed on the display screen at the height of the patient's eye. The patient was seated comfortably upright at a 70 cm viewing distance from the screen, wearing appropriate correction for near. Muscular strain and activity were monitored as myogenic acitivty especially at the neck may significantly alter the wave-shape of the VEP response. The right and the left eyes were examined separately. Both the stimulator and the patient were in an electrically shielded room. Some patients were tested under the influence of a myotic collyrium.

Amplification and recording

An active midline electrode, 2 cm above the inion, and one reference earlobe clip electrode were used with a multichannel amplifying recorder (Ahrend-Van Gogh). Placement of the active electrode was carefully noted.

Features which facilitated our averaging techniques include: automatic scaling and centering on the cathode ray tube (CRT) display screen, digital display of the relevant data, the possibility of photographing the screen with a Polaroid camera, and the possibility of displaying either the averaged results or the buffer contents (response to the latest accepted stimulus).

Subjects

The patients who participated in this study included: 10 established cases (5 male and 5 female) of OAG ranging from 48 to 63 years of age, 5 newly diagnosed probable OAG cases in the 50 year old age group and an additional 4 probable OAG cases with small unilateral field defects, 17 cases of narrow angle glaucoma and 6 cases of secondary eye ball contusion resulting in temporary IOP elevation.

RESULTS

Previous studies (Neetens, Hendrata and Van Rompaey 1979b) describe the results obtained in 13 young healthy individuals to establish normal values (see Table 1). We shall only mention that a typical normal VEP in our laboratory contains six waves, three positive (P) and three negative (N) deflections. We take into consideration only N_1 and P_1 because the remaining waves are frequently equivocal (Fig. 1). The amplitude and latency obtained

104

Table 1

Disease	Latency (m sec)				Amplitude (μV)			
	Flash		Pattern		Flash		Pattern	
	X̄	s.d.	X̄	s.d.	X̄	s.d.	X̄	s.d.
Control cases (13)	108.9	15.7	102.0	5.3	14.4	6.0	9.3	2.0
OAG (10 cases)	95	19	109.0	34	8.6	2.3	7.7	3

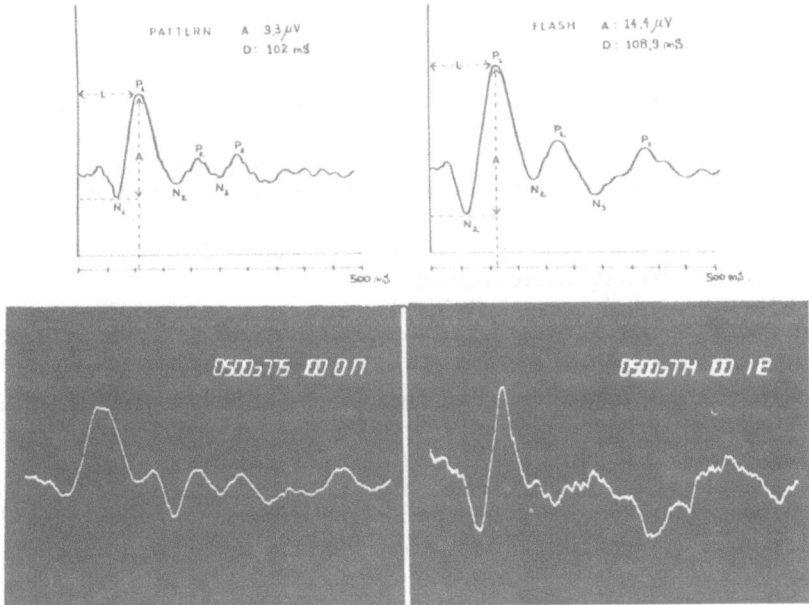

Fig. 1. Typical VEP response to pattern (left) and to flash (right) stimulation obtained under our recording conditions in a normal observer.

in the 10 OAG cases also are presented in Table 1. Latency is especially increased in cases wtih nasal visual field defects but amplitude is always low and waveshape disturbed, already with beginning Bjerrum-zone involvement. In OAG a decrease of IOP does not improve the VEP response. In the narrow angle glaucoma cases with sudden closure of angle (17 cases), after medical treatment (5 cases) or surgery (12 cases) the VEP remained slightly disturbed, especially in wave-shape.

In cases of secondary eyeball-contusion resulting in elevation of intra-ocular pressure (IOP) of relatively short duration (2 to 4 weeks), the VEP responses are disturbed. However, normalisation of IOP normalised the amplitude in 4 cases of a total of 6 patients.

Also tested were 5 newly diagnosed probable OAG patients with elevated daytime IOP who had never been treated. They attended the outpatient

Table 2

Patient		mm Hg IOP (apl.)		OAPm-difference		VEP	
age	sex	RE	LE	RE	LE	RE	LE
47	f	23	24	+ 5	+ 2	N	N
46	m	22	25	− 7	− 10	wl	wl
49	m	30	23	− 9	+ 6	a	N
48	f	28	24	− 5	− 3	wl	wl
50	f	25	30	+ 1	− 4	a	al

N = normal; w = wave-shape; a = amplitude; l = latency
w, a, l: disturbed VEP (pattern reversal)

department for presbyopia problems, unaware of a possible eye disease. In this group of 5 patients only questionable field-defects were detected by Goldmann-perimetry. We observed 4 additional patients with unilateral but small field defects under similar conditions. Our findings from these nine patients are shown in Tables 2 and 3. Also presented in Tables 2 and 3 are the results of ophthalmo-dynamometry (ophthalmic artery pressure: OAP) and systemic blood pressure examinations.

The theoretical mean ophthalmic artery pressure (OAPm) for the measured intraocular pressure and mean systemic blood pressure was calculated and compared to the actual OAPm. If the excess value is higher (+) a better capillary perfusion may be expected. If the difference is negative, considering the actual OAPm, it is accepted that the capillary disk perfusion is inadequate to supply the nerve tissue (Delaunois 1978).

It appears from Tables 2 and 3 that, regardless of the initial IOP, those eyes with a positive excess value (better capillary perfusion), have better VEP responses. These clinical data suggest that the first objective subclinical symptom of increased IOP may be a disturbed VEP and that a higher capillary blood perfusion pressure protects against axonal damage, since in the latter event VEPs are nearly normal. In glaucoma cases, a change in wave-shape and a decrease in the amplitude of the VEP exists even before any important visual field defects appear (Fig. 2). The patient with IOP rise should be examined under conditions of high IOP and after IOP lowering treatment. If the initial IOP is to be considered within normal limits, the investigation may be done after provocative tests (water-drinking test). We are convinced that some OAG patients tolerate higher intraocular pressures without functional impairment because their optic nerve axons remain better oxygenated, with adequate capillary perfusion

PART II. EXPERIMENTAL ANIMAL STUDY

The results from our clinical study suggested an experimental study in the cat of the action potentials (ap) of the optic nerve under varying conditions of intraocular pressure (Po) and systemic blood pressure (Neetens, Hendrata & Van Rompaey 1980).

Table 3

Patient		mm Hg IOP (apl.)		Vis. field		OAPm-difference		VEP	
age	sex	RE	LE	RE	LE	RE	LE	RE	LE
63	m	26	43	N	u.B.	− 5	− 16	wl	wal
58	f	22	32	N	n.q.	0	− 12	Nw?	wal
60	m	21	28	N	n.q. + B	− 4	− 6	al	wal
52	m	25	22	rel u.B.	N	− 7	− 2	wa	al

N = normal; u.B. = Bjerrum; n.q. = nasal quadrant; n.q. + B = nasal quadrant and relative upper Bjerrum. w, a, l: cfr. Table 2.

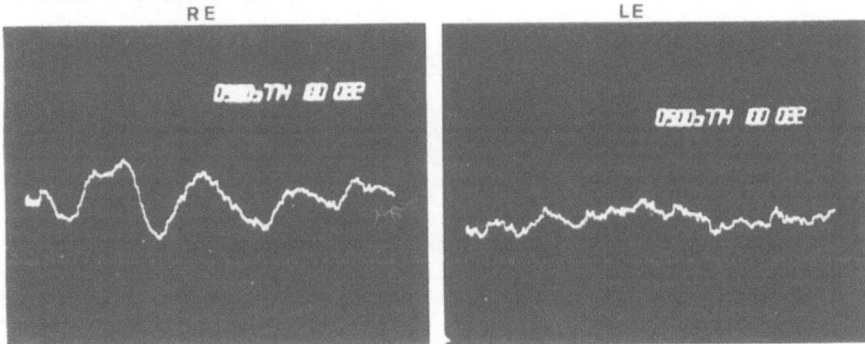

Fig. 2. Pattern reversal VEP in a 58 year old femal OAG patient (upper traces). The response in the left eye was disturbed both in amplitude and latency, OAPm differences were noted with a left eye value of − 12.

MATERIALS AND METHODS

Experiments were performed on cats with an average weight of 2,500 gr., i.v. anaesthetized with sodium-pentobarbital (30 mg/kg). The tracheotomized animal is connected to an artificial respirator (Palmer-pump) in order to maintain blood g/ass levels at PaO_2 105 mm Hg (s.d. = ± 10), and $PaCO_2$, 36 mmHg (s.d. = ± 4). The femoral artery and vein are prepared and catheterised, the catheters being perfused with heparinised saline (5,000 u.i./ ml).

The intraocular (Po) pressures are recorded by direct cannulation of the anterior chamber. Both systemic mean arterial (PAm) and intraocular (Po) pressures are recorded with a Beckman Dynograph. Anterior chamber (AC), femoral artery and vein-cannulae are connected each by three position-stopcocks with high precision Hamilton syringes to apply i.v. injections or to permit changes of small, well determined amounts of aqueous humor from the AC or blood from the artery.

Systemic arterial blood pressure was altered pharmacologically after i.v. injection of noradrenaline (10 μg/kg) or isopropylnoradrenaline (isoproterenol) (10 μg/kg). The optic nerve is placed on a bipolar electrode

107

(Delaunois 1978) eliminating interference, and coupled to the Beckman Dynograph to register the optic nerve action-potentials (ap).

Light flash stimulation (1/sec) of the retina is accomplished with a 2.4 W-bulb, fed at 1.3 V and switched off and on with a Grass stimulator at 1 hz, 150 ms, through a reed-relay. The eye is not previously dark-adapted.

The mean normal value of the optic nerve action potentials from 22 animals is 35 uV (s.d. = ± 6 μV) for Po oscillating between 12.8 and 37 mm Hg and PAm between 45.3 and 51.1 mmHg.

RESULTS

The results are presented in Fig. 3, 4 and 5. With PAm unchanged, increased

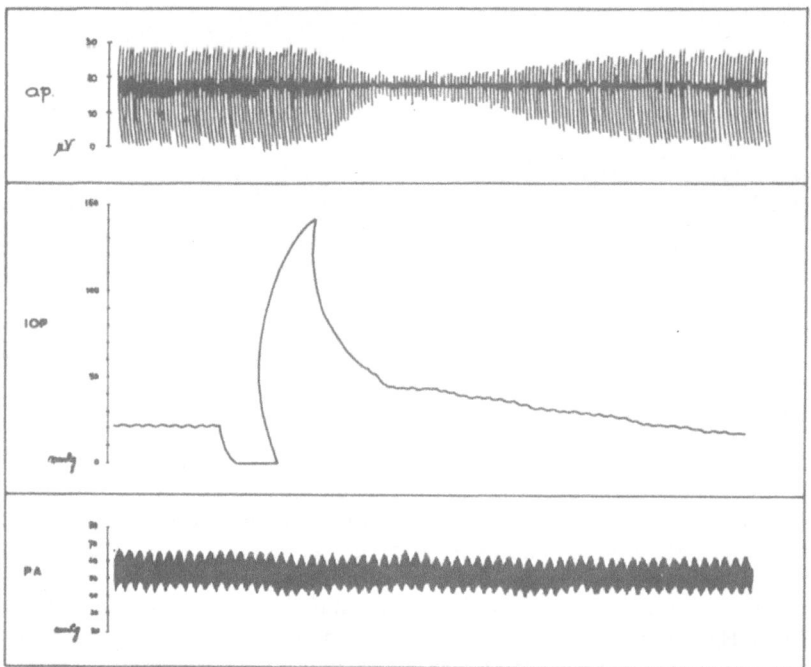

Fig. 3. Increased Po with PAm unchanged. Note action potential decrease.

Po lowers the action potentials of the optic nerve. The action potentials remain unchanged until a high Po (mean value 43 mmHg, (s.d. = ± 9) is applied. Then suddenly they decrease and, with further increases in Po, remain present but at extremely low values. If Po is lower than the original normal value the action potentials will not increase in amplitude but stabilize at values identical to the initial ones. By increasing PAm the action potentials improve rapidly, already from 70–80 mmHg PAm.

If PAm is high, as a rule Po-rise needs to be higher to lower the action

108

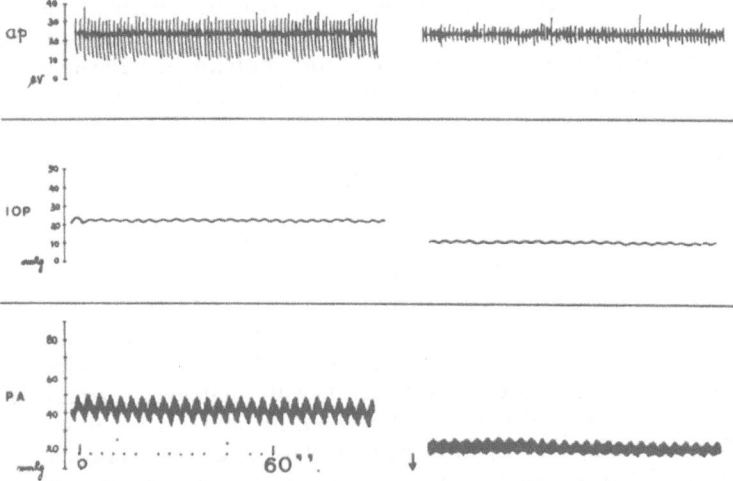

Fig. 4. Lowering of PAm even with lowering Po results in action potential decrease (withdrawal of blood and aqueous).

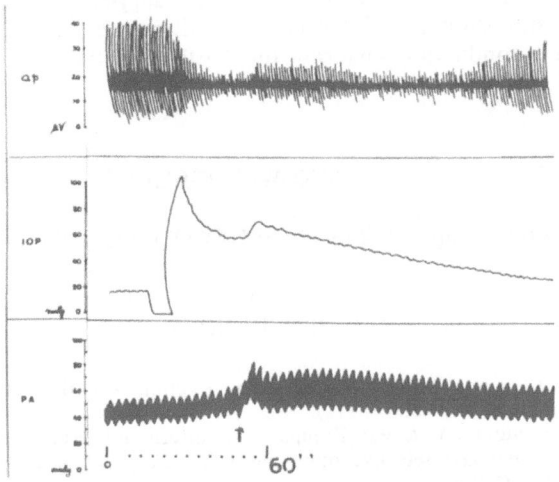

Fig. 5. The decrease of action potential caused by increased Po improves with rise of PAm, even if simultaneously Po also rises (arrow: i.v. injection of 10 μg Noradrenaline).

potentials. When PAm falls a slight Po-rise is followed by an important, sometimes sudden, decrease of action potential. Repeated increases with subsequent lowering of Po, lower the action potentials more and more after each rise, and they never recover to the original amplitude. Lowering the Po to the baseline does not result in increase of action potentials as long as the original PAm is maintained. If we increase PAm we observe an improvement of the action potentials, even if Po rises simultaneously. In summary, an experimental animal model to study optic pathway action potentials demonstrates that high Po and lowered PAm cause inadequate capillary flow and oxygenation, which result in an action potential decrease. Raising PAm protects against the effects of a rise of Po, but a decrease of Po in conditions of lowered PAm does not imporve action potentials. Repeated increases of Po cause a lowering of action potentials, only released by increasing PAm.

CONCLUSIONS

The clinical correlation of the action potentials of the optic nerve, the VEP, may be considered as the earliest objective parameter of functional damage, and may already be disturbed before any visual field loss.

Rise of intraocular pressure is only one of the mechanisms to threaten capillary perfusion, other mechanisms include hemodynamic crises and pathological tissue-spaces. In patients with deficient capillary perfusion, repeated increase of IOP may be necessary and sufficient to result in a definitive capillary collapse. In patients with a diseased vascular system and (or) low PAm, if capillary perfusion is not adequate, there will very easily occur a subsequent capillary closure, with a corresponding decrease in visual function and visual field loss.

These clinical and experimental results suggest that critical capillary closure-pressure should be determined. Furthermore, because critical closure may induce conduction changes the VEP of patients with elevated and normalised IOP should be evaluated.

ACKNOWLEDGEMENT

This research was supported by Grant NFWO 3.0001.79.

REFERENCES

Delaunois, A.L. Easy recording of extra-cellular action-potentials. Med. and Biol. Eng. and Comput. 16: 219–220 (1978).
Neetens, A., Hendrata, Y. & Van Rompaey, J. Pattern and flash visual evoked response in disseminated and selective optic pathway damage. Trans. Ophthal. Soc. U.K. 99: 103–110 (1979a).
Neetens, A., Hendrata Y. & Van Rompaey, J. Pattern and flash visual evoked response in multiple sclerosis. J. Neurol. 220: 113–124 (1979b).
Neetens, A., Hendrata, Y., Van Rompaey, J., Rubbens, M.C. & Verschueren, C. VER and subslinical optic pathway damage. Bull. Soc. Belg. Ophth. 185: 83–98 (1979).
Neetens, A., Hendrata, Y. & Van Rompaey, J. Experimental animal study of the effects of intraocular pressure and systemic blood pressure on optic pathway action potentials. Exp. Eye Res. in press (1980).

Authors' address:
Dept. of Ophthalmology
University of Antwerp
Antwerp, Belgium

TEMPORAL BEHAVIOUR OF VEPs IN OPTIC DISC EDEMAS

M. ANASTASI, M. LAURICELLA & F. PONTE

(*Palermo, Italy*)

ABSTRACT

The Authors studied VEPs' temporal behaviour in papillitis, anterior ischemic optic neuropathy and choked disc in order to distinguish these diseases in a later stage. A comparison between the electro-functional and clinical data has been done. These three forms sometimes difficult to distinguish from the clinical point of view, present typical electrophysiological features, in the early stage as well as in the later stage, so that the VEPs seem to be a good tool for retrospective diagnosis.

INTRODUCTION

The VEPs' behaviour in the optic disc neuritis course is well known. The evoked responses undergo an alteration which remains for a long time even after the recovery of all the visual functions (de Haas 1972; Spekreijse & Van der Tweel 1974; Van Lith & Mak 1974; Oguchi 1979). Less attention has been dedicated to the VEPs' temporal behaviour in anterior ischemic optic neuropathy (A.I.O.N.) and the choked disc. Therefore, we felt that it would be interesting to follow a long term comparative study of the VEPs in such forms of optic disc edemas in order to distinguish in these three diseases, if possible, tardy electro-functional stigmata.

MATERIALS AND METHOD

We examined 22 patients of both sexes, between 25 and 65 years of age, where 12 were affected by papillitis, 6 by anterior ischemic optic neuropathy (A.I.O.N.) and 4 by choked disc.

The research was done only with patients with papillitis and A.I.O.N. where the time between the beginning of the symptomatology and the examination was no longer than 5 days, and with patients affected by choked disc with a visual acuity not below 7/10 and with initial damages of the visual field. In all subjects the electro-functional examinations were done in the acute stage of the disease and repeated from 8 to 12 months later in a control stage. In the patients with choked disc the control examinations were done after surgical or medical reduction of endocranial hypertension. All subjects were studied both from the clinical and functional point of view. In all, the visual acuity and visual field was checked. The normal VEP values were calculated on a population of 30 healthy subjects of both sexes between 30 and 60 years of age.

VEPs were obtained in mesopic adaptation with an averaging of responses to two kinds of visual stimuli: white flashes of 0.3 Joules elicited once per second and sinusoidal light with frequencies between 9 and 50 Hz. The active electrode was a needle inserted into the skin 2.5 cm above the inion. The reference electrode was a silver plate fixed to the ear lobe. The ground electrode was a needle inserted in frontal midline skin. All the electro-functional examinations were done on subjects with midriasis maxima obtained by using 1% tropicamide. Bioelectrical responses were modulated with OTE Biomedica Mod. 1076 Pre-amplifiers, sent to an OTE Biomedica Mod. 1172 Neuro-averager and written by a plotter OTE Biomedica Mod. 1013. Continuous monitoring was insured by Tektronix Type 502A dual-beam oscilloscope.

The stimuli for transient VEPs were obtained from a stroboscope OTE Biomedica Mod. SL1B with light intensity between 0.3 and 1.6 Joule/flash; the stimuli for steady-state VEPs were obtained by means of an indirect illumination with fluorescent tubes of a diffusing sphere. The mean luminance was $50 \, cd/m^2$, modulation depth was 85%.

The latency of the transient VEP response was measured from the beginning of the record, triggered by the flash, to the peak of the highest positive deflection of the primary response. The latency of steady-state VEP was calculated as phase lag (π).

RESULTS

Fig. 1 shows the clinical and bioelectrical picture, in the acute stage and one year later, of a 48 year old woman affected by papillitis in O.S.; in the acute stage there is papilloedema, visual acuity is 1/50 with an absolute central scotoma in the visual field. VEPs to single flashes are normal in amplitude but pathological in latency. Flicker VEPs are pathological both in amplitude and latency.

The visual acuity at the control stage one year later is restored to 10/10. The central scotoma has disappeared, the optic disc is still slightly blurred, but VEPs show a similar response to the foregoing examination. All parameters in O.D. have always been normal. This model of evolution of the disease is not constant in all patients examined as we found in the control stage a large variability of the visual acuity, visual field and optic disc appearance whereas VEPs both in the acute stage and in the later control stages have not shown important changes and remained pathological at all stimulus parameters including frequency.

Fig. 2 shows the clinical and bioelectrical pictures in the acute stage and 10 months later, of an A.I.O.N. in a woman 56 years of age. The immediate decay of the visual functions without changes after some time is obvious. The flash VEPs have quite an abnormal amplitude with a normal latency as the flicker VEPs show a rapid extinction of the responses with the increase of stimuli frequency. This behaviour continues 10 months later. The group studied follows this model even though with a large variability of visual field pictures.

Fig. 3 shows the clinical picture of a 34 year old man affected by bilateral choked disc due to intracranial hypertension. He has a good visual acuity, a widening of the blind spot in the visual field, VEPs which are normal in the beginning of the disease (A) and normal visual acuity, normal visual field and normal VEPs one year later (B). At a first examination (A) the surface of the disc is elevated above the plane of the retina and disc margins are blurred with a slight venous engorgement. At the second examination there is still a little blurring of the disc margins while the other parameters are normal. Such a clinical and electro-functional finding is constant in all patients with a choked disc even though with a great morphological variability in visual field alterations.

We made a distinction between single flash VEPs and flicker VEPs for a global analysis of our data. The VEPs' amplitude calculated on the highest positive deflection of the primary response is drawn in Fig. 4. We have plotted the results obtained at the initial stage of the three diseases (A) and at the later stages (B) in relation with normal values (dashed area). The papillitis shows average values in the normal range with a large variation. The average amplitude in the A.I.O.N. is quite subnormal with a large variation too. The amplitude in choked disc shows values in the normal range.

In the later control (B) the range of amplitudes of papillitis and choked disc does not show important variations compared to the initial control (A) and the average values are in the normal range. On the contrary, in A.I.O.N., the amplitudes of the later control (B) are below normal values.

More concentrated data can be found in the latency graph (Fig. 5). The latency in papillitis is abnormal in the acute stage (A) as well as in the later control (B) with a little tendency towards normality. The average latency in the other diseases is normal in both stages.

Fig. 6 shows the amplitude values of steady-state VEPs in the studied diseases in relation with the normal range (dashed area). The results, as is evident from the graph, are arranged in three well distinct levels in the initial stage (A) as well as in the later stage (B). The average values of amplitude in choked disc are normal, in papillitis they are always subnormal but rarely extinct, in A.I.O.N. they are seriously altered with early extinction.

Fig. 7 reports the phase lag behaviour in papillitis and choked disc at the initial (A) and later stages (B) (dashed area indicates normal range). A differentiation between these two forms is evident because in choked disc the average phase lag is normal, while in papillitis it is altered in medium and in high frequency regions (A and B). We found a large variation of the data in abnormal area in the high frequency range. The results in A.I.O.N. are not reported because of early extinction of the responses. It was possible to calculate the phase lag only in two subjects with low stimulation frequency and in the later control stage; the values obtained were normal.

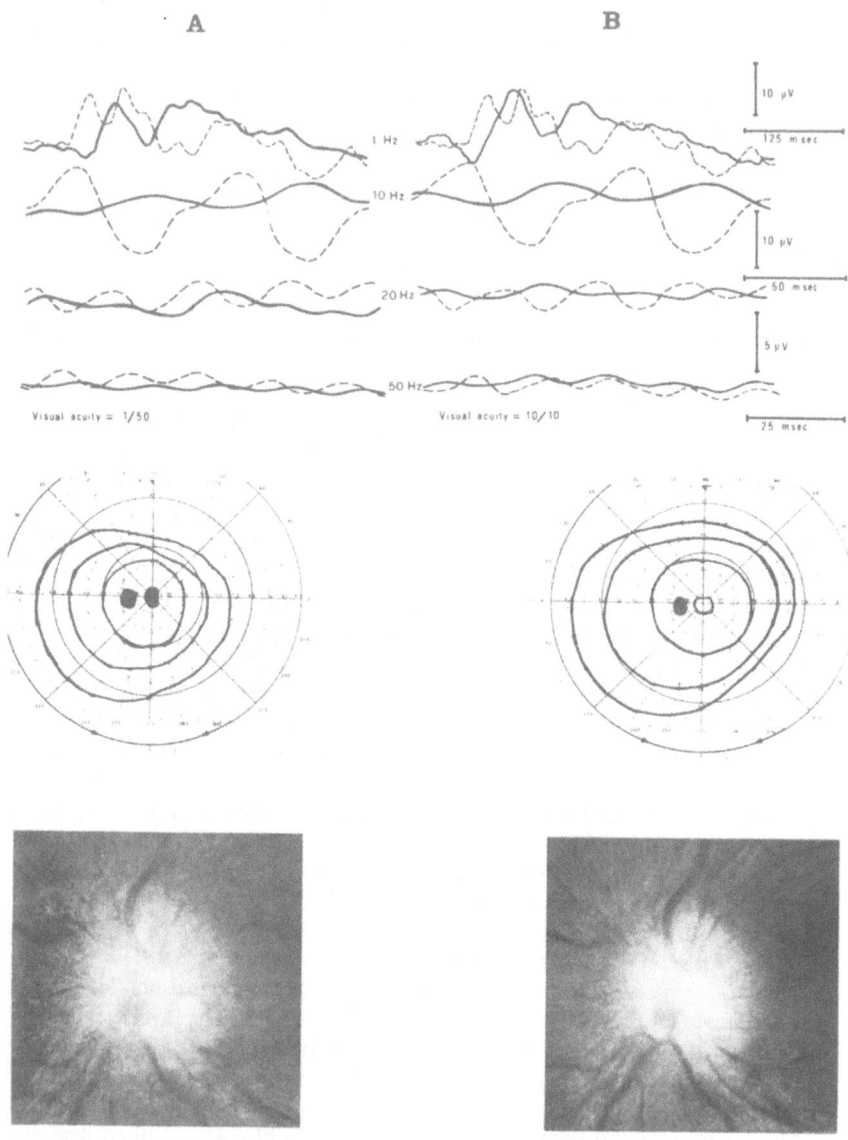

Fig. 1. Clinical and electrophysiological behaviour in papillitis in the acute stage (A) and one year later (B). Improvement of visual acuity and visual field. In the acute stage there is a papilloedema. The optic disc is still blurred at the control stage. Single flash VEPs are normal in amplitude but abnormal in latency; flicker VEPs are abnormal both in amplitude and in latency. Similar responses are also in the later control. (Dashed line: normal VEPs).

114

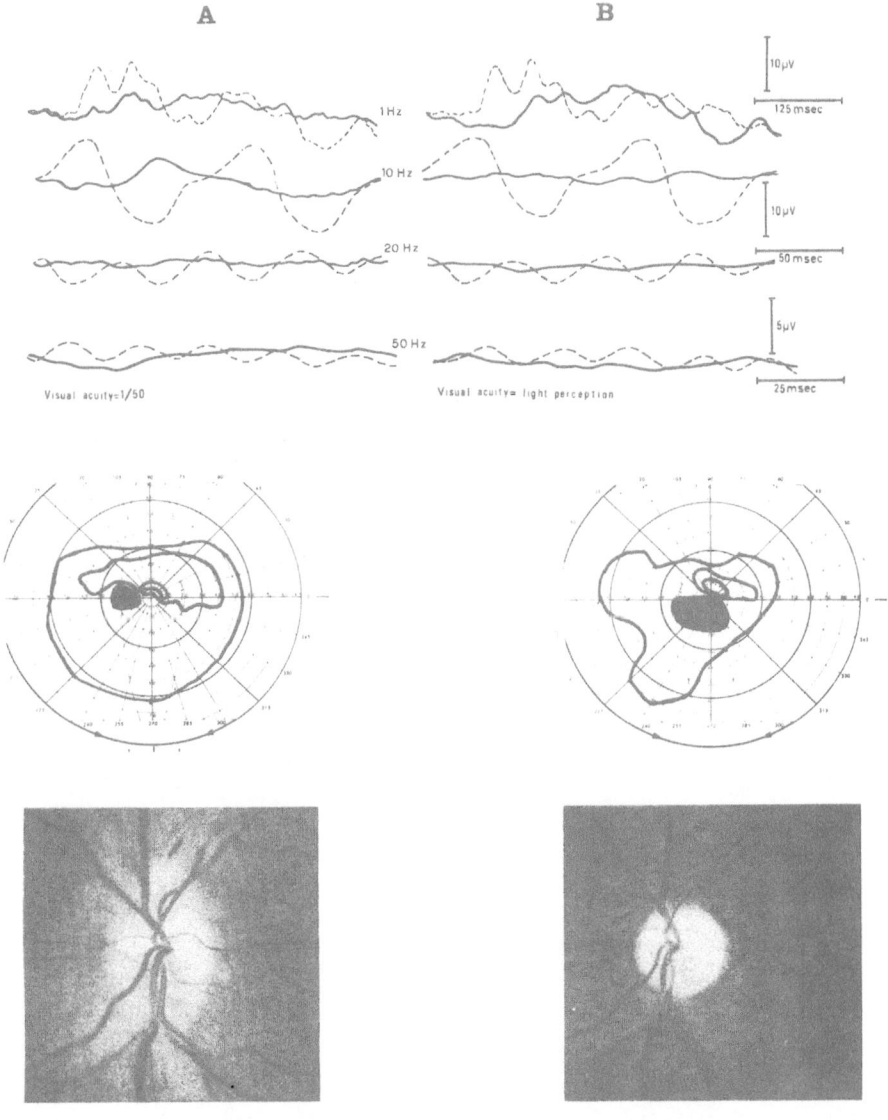

Fig. 2. Clinical and electrophysiological behaviour in anterior ischemic optic neuropathy (A.I.O.N.) in the acute stage (A) and ten months later (B). Immediate decay of the visual function. In the acute stage there is an ischemic papilloedema which develops in optic atrophy. Single flash VEPs have abnormal amplitude with a normal latency and the flicker VEPs show a rapid extinction of the responses with increasing stimulus frequency. Similar behaviour is also in the later control. (Dashed line: normal VEPs).

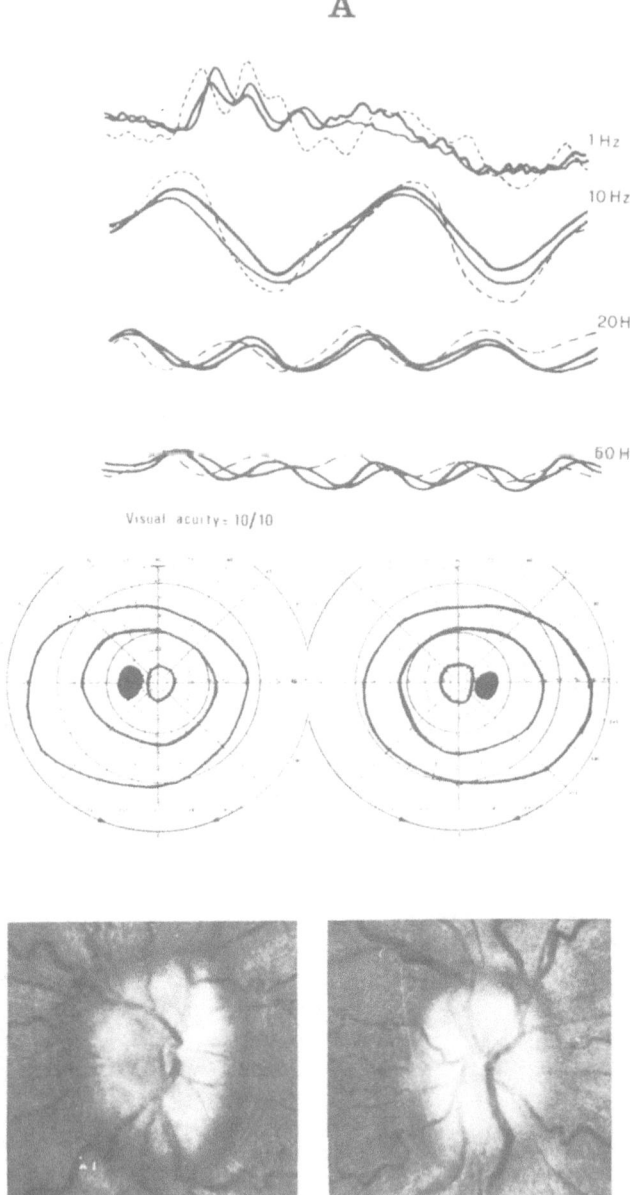

Fig. 3. Clinical and electrophysiological features in choked disc at the beginning of the disease (A) and one year later (B). Good bilateral visual acuity, widening of the blind spot in the visual field, typical picture of the choked disc in the beginning (A)

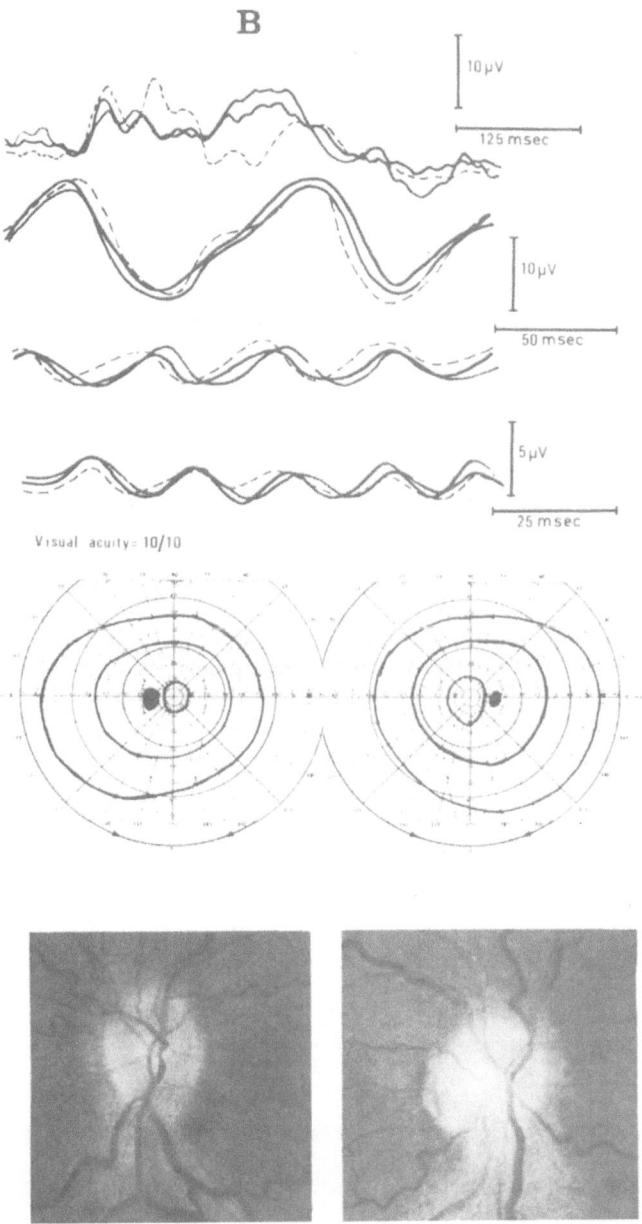

B

10 µV

125 msec

10 µV

50 msec

5 µV

25 msec

Visual acuity = 10/10

and improvement of the visual field feature with a slight persistent blurring of the optic disc one year later (B). VEPs are normal both in the early and later controls. (Dashed line: normal VEPs).

117

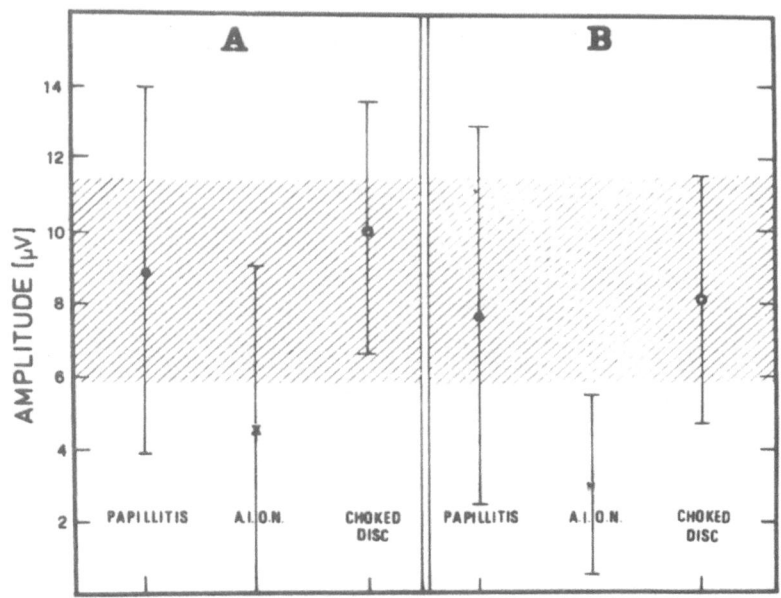

Fig. 4. Amplitude distribution of single flash VEPs in papillitis (●), anterior ischemic optic neuropathy (X) and choked disc (o) at the early (A) and later control stages (B). Normal range is included in dashed area. Vertical bars are the standard deviations (± 1).

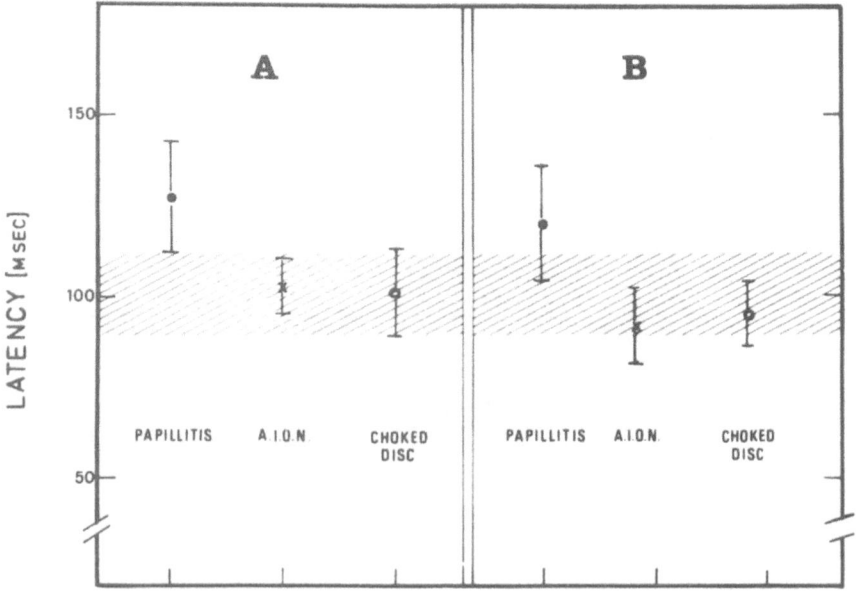

Fig. 5. Latency distribution of single flash VEPs in the considered diseases. See also Fig. 4.

118

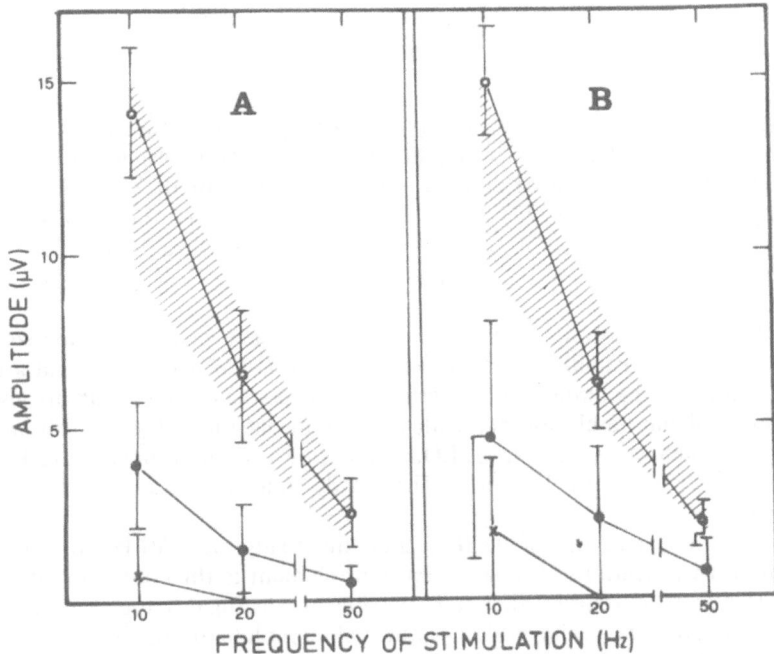

Fig. 6. Amplitude distribution of steady-state VEPs. See also Fig. 4.

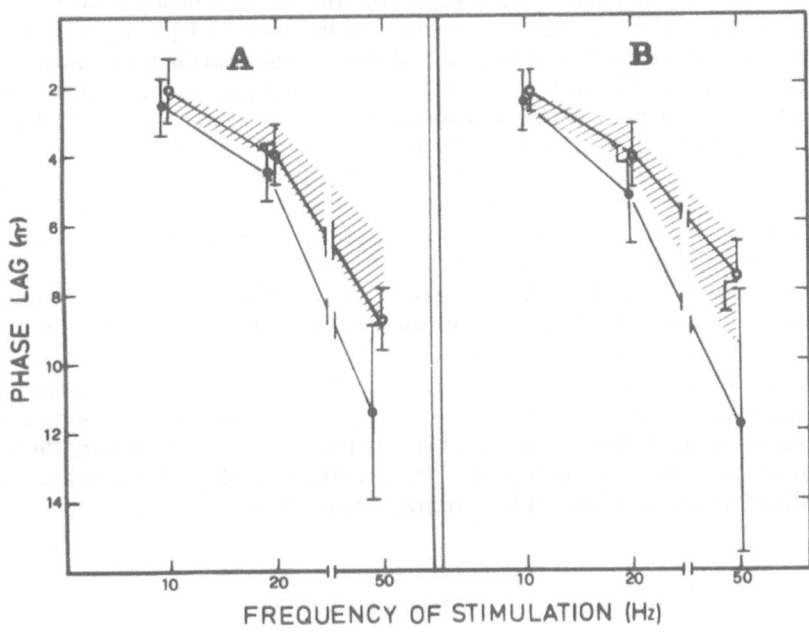

Fig. 7. Phase lag (π) distribution of steady-state VEPs. The data of A.I.O.N. are not plotted because of rapid extinction of the responses. See also Fig. 4.

DISCUSSION

The most important points of our results agree with the observations of other authors about the variability of clinical data (visual acuity, visual field, fundus appearance) and the temporal behaviour of VEPs in papillitis (Barber & Galloway 1977). With regard to VEPs in the other two forms we do not have the possibility of any comparison because studies that have been done at present are still at the incipient stage (Babel & Korol 1975; Wilson 1978).

The considerations drawn from our experience can be summarized in several points. Papillitis is characterized by an abnormal latency and a large variability of the amplitude of flash VEPs. The steady-state VEPs are always subnormal but rarely extinct with a pathological phase lag in medium and high frequency regions. In A.I.O.N. the single flash responses are low in amplitude with normal latency. The steady-state responses fade away very quickly.

In choked disc the single flash and the steady state VEPs do not show significant alterations. The last important element is the constancy of VEPs' behaviour with time so that it is possible to distinguish the three diseases in a later stage when the clinical picture is incomplete or not clear.

An interpretation of such electro-functional features can be provided by the pathophysiology of these three types of diseases.

In papillitis the lowering of the amplitude and the abnormal latency of VEPs can be related to a demyelinization process which persists for a long time. Moreover it is likely that some of the increased latency is generated at the cortical level; the question of the retinal contribution remains open (McDonald 1977). This contrasts with the pathophysiology of the A.I.O.N. where an axonal ischemic degeneration, which causes an important decrease in amplitude with a normal conduction velocity in surviving fibers, is present.

The basic alteration in choked disc seems to be connected to a block of axonal flow, reversible (at least at the beginning) and with minimal changes in blood supply (Moro 1979). This explains the lack of changes of VEPs and the absence of bioelectrical sequences after recovery.

In conclusion, these three edematous forms of the optic disc, well distinct from the pathophysiological point of view, can present no significant differences among themselves in acute stage as well as when the symptomatology is no longer evolutive. In fact the anamnesis is often vague, the optic disc appearance is always difficult to assess and psychophysical results (visual acuity, visual field) may not provide clarification. On the contrary the VEPs seem to reflect accurately the three pathophysiological mechanisms and therefore are a useful tool for a retrospective diagnosis of these diseases.

ACKNOWLEDGEMENT

This work has been supported by a grant (No. 78.02236.04) from the Consiglio Nazionale delle Ricerche, Roma (Italy).

REFERENCES

Babel, J. & Korol, S. Exploration electrophysiologique des affections vasculaires du nerf optique. In: Proc. Symp. Int. Vascular diseases of optic nerve (Ed. F. Moro). Piccin, Padova. 193–207 (1975).

Barber, C. & Galloway, N.R. The visually evoked response and psychophysical testing in optic neuritis. In: 14th ISCERG Symposium (Ed. Th. Lawwill). Junk, The Hague. (Doc. Ophthal. Proc. Series Vol. 13). 79–86 (1977).

Haas, J.P. de. An electro-ophthalmological study of affections of the optic pathway. (Thesis). Junk, The Hague (1972).

Lith, G.H.M. van & Mak, G.T.M. A quantitative evaluation of the VECP in optic neuritis. In: 11th ISCERG Symposium (Ed. E. Dodt & J.T. Pearlman). Junk, The Hague. (Doc. Ophthal. Proc. Series Vol. 4). 375–386 (1974).

McDonald, W.I. Pathophysiology of conduction in central nerve fibres. In: Visual evoked potentials in man: new developments. (Ed. J.E. Desmedt). Clarendon Press, Oxford. 427–437 (1977).

Moro, F. Otticopatie edematose. In: Le Otticopatie (Ed. F. Moro & M. Maione). Maccari, Parma. 405–433 (1979).

Oguchi, J. The VECP in optic neuritis. In: 16th ISCEV Symposium (Ed. Y. Tazawa). Jap. J. Ophthal. 20: 299–305 (1979).

Spekreijse, H. & Tweel, L.H. van der. Stimulus and visual evoked potentials. In: 11th ISCERG Symposium (Ed. E. Dodt & J.T. Pearlman). Junk, The Hague. (Doc. Ophthal. Proc. Series Vol. 4). 269–284 (1974).

Wilson, W.B. Ischemic visual evoked response. In: Am. J. Ophthal. 86. 530–533 (1978).

Authors' address:
University Eye Clinic
Via Liborio Giuffré, 13
I-90127 Palermo
Italy

THE VISUAL EVOKED POTENTIAL
IN ISCHAEMIC OPTIC NEUROPATHY

G.E. HOLDER

(*London, England*)

ABSTRACT

The potentials evoked by pattern reversal (PVEP) and diffuse flash stimulation (FVEP) are described in 11 patients with ischaemic optic neuropathy,
the findings being compared with extensive normal control groups. Two of
these patients had giant cell arteritis confirmed by temporal artery biopsy.

In both patients with temporal arteritis the PVEP from the affected eye
was absent. In the other patients the PVEP from the affected eye invariably
showed a significant amplitude reduction compared with the normal eye. A
significant interocular latency asymmetry was present in the PVEP of only
one of these 9 patients.

Both of the patients with giant cell arteritis had FVEPs of markedly
reduced amplitude from the affected eye associated with a delay in the early
components, the remainder of the waveform being distorted and precluding
accurate quantification of later components including the major positivity.
Five of the other 8 patients in whom the FVEP was examined showed a
significantly reduced FVEP amplitude from the affected eye, this being
accompanied by a significant interocular latency asymmetry in only one
patient. FVEPs were normal in the other three patients.

The use of VEP examination in the diagnosis of ischaemic optic neuropathy is discussed.

INTRODUCTION

The sudden onset of visual deterioration often seen in ischaemic optic
neuropathy can also occur in demyelinating optic nerve lesions and in some
patients differentiation between these two conditions may be difficult on
clinical grounds alone. The early reports of delayed visual evoked potentials
(VEPs) in optic nerve demyelination both in response to diffuse flash
(Richey, Kooi & Tourtelotte 1971) and pattern reversal stimulation
(Halliday, McDonald & Mushin 1972) have since been confirmed by many
authors and the VEP has become the investigation of choice in cases of

suspected demyelination. To date there have been few reports of the VEP in ischaemic optic neuropathy but the findings of Wilson (1978) suggest that differentiation between the ischaemic and the demyelinating lesion may be facilitated by VEP examination.

This report describes the VEP findings in 11 patients with ischaemic optic neuropathy, 9 idiopathic and 2 arteritic (classification according to Boghen & Glaser 1975). The 'arteritic' patients both had giant cell arteritis confirmed on temporal artery biopsy.

PATIENTS AND METHODS

The 11 patients, with brief clinical details, are listed in Table 1. In most cases the diagnosis was made using clinical ophthalmoscopic criteria or confirmed on fluorescein angiography but in some cases the electro-physiological data were instrumental in the final diagnosis. Patient 2 spoke no English and visual acuity assessment was not considered reliable. There was, however, a strong suggestion of an inferior altitudinal field defect. Ischaemic damage could be seen at the macula in patient 8. Patients 3, 4, 9 and 10 probably had bilateral lesions; in the other 7 patients the condition was unilateral. Of the patients with bilateral disease a visual field defect was only present in the less severely affected eye of patient 9.

Table 1. Patients

		Age	Sex	V.O.D.	V.O.S.	Fields
Idiopathic						
1	M.C.	30	F	C.F.	6/6	C.S.
2	M.G.	37	F	?	?	? I.A.D.
3	H.K.	49	M	6/24	C.F.	C.S.
4	T.D.	50	M	6/18	6/60	I.A.D.
5	D.C.	56	F	6/18	6/5	S.A.D.
6	F.B.	59	F	6/9	6/9	I.A.D.
7	R.W.	59	F	6/9	6/5	I.A.D.
8	A.R.	71	M	6/18	6/9	P.C.S.
9	E.J.	74	F	6/6	6/12	S.A.D.
Arteritic						
10	A.S.	68	F	6/9	H.M.	
11	L.M.	78	F	6/9	H.M.	

C.S.   = Central scotoma.
P.C.S. = Paracentral scotoma.
I.A.D. = Inferior altitudinal defect.
S.A.D. = Superior altitudinal defect.

Diffuse flash stimulation was not performed in one patient for technical reasons; the other 10 patients all received both diffuse flash and pattern reversal stimulation. Pattern stimulation was provided by a Digitimer moving mirror stimulator routinely situated 80 cm from the patient, subtending a total field of 11° with an individual check size of 26'. Variations in stimulus parameters were occasionally used and will be described where appropriate. Diffuse flash stimulation was provided by a Xenon discharge photostimulator (S.L.E.) situated 30 cm from the open eye. Pattern stimulation was performed with vision corrected, flash stimulation with vision uncorrected. 128 stimulations were normally used but occasionally 256 or even 512 stimulations were necessary. Bipolar recordings were taken with electrodes placed according to the Modified Maudsley system where the occipital electrodes lie 2 cm anterior and 2 cm lateral to the inion (Holder 1978; 1980). In all patients each eye was examined at least twice, the findings being compared with an extensive normal control group, an interocular amplitude asymmetry of greater than 50% or an interocular latency asymmetry of greater than 6 msec being abnormal.

The response latency was taken as the time from the presentation of the stimulus to the peak of the major positive component, normally occurring at some 95 msecs with pattern reversal stimulation and at some 120 msec with diffuse flash stimulation. Response amplitudes were measured from the peak of the major positive component to the peak of the immediately preceding and following negative components. The findings in a given patient were only rated as abnormal if the abnormality found was reproducible. If no consistent abnormality was present the findings were assessed as normal.

RESULTS

The VEP findings are shown in Table 2.

Table 2. VEP abnormalities.

			PVEP		FVEP	
			Amp. ↓	Lat. ↑	Amp. ↓	Lat. ↑
Idiopathic						
1	MC	30	+	—	+	—
2	MG	37	+	—	+	—
3	HK	49	+	—	—	—
4	TD	50	+	+	+	+
5	DC	56	+	—	+	—
6	FB	59	+	—	—	—
7	RW	59	+	—	Not performed	
8	AR	71	+	—	—	—
9	EJ	74	+[a]	—	+	.
Arteritic						
10	AS		Absent		+	+[b]
11	LM		Absent		+	+[b]

[a] Patient 9 had PVEPs from both eyes which were of abnormally low amplitude compared with the normal population; in all other patients there was an interocular asymmetry of amplitude or latency of abnormally large magnitude, the affected or worse affected eye showing the amplitude reduction or latency increase.

[b] The latency increase here refers to the early components; the major positive component was sufficiently poorly formed to preclude accurate quantification.

The 9 patients with non-arteritic lesions all displayed a significant amplitude reduction (+) in the pattern evoked potential (PVEP) when the affected or worse affected eye was stimulated. One patient showed an increased latency (+) compared with the fellow eye and in one further patient (M.C., see below) there was a relative latency delay when a small check pattern was used, but not when the check size was increased. In both patients with giant cell arteritis the PVEP was absent from the (worse) affected eye.

Five of the 8 non-arteritic patients in whom the flash visual evoked potential (FVEP) was examined showed a significant amplitude reduction in the potentials from the affected or worse affected eye, and in one of these 5 there was also a significant interocular latency asymmetry. Three patients had normal FVEPs. Both of the two patients with giant cell arteritis had FVEPs of markedly reduced amplitude in the (worse) affected eye accompanied by delays in the early components. In both cases the waveform was sufficiently distorted to make accurate assessment of the major positive component difficult.

Illustrative examples can be seen in Figs. 1-3. Brief clinical details follow:

Fig. 1. M.C. This 30 year old woman presented with a sudden painless loss

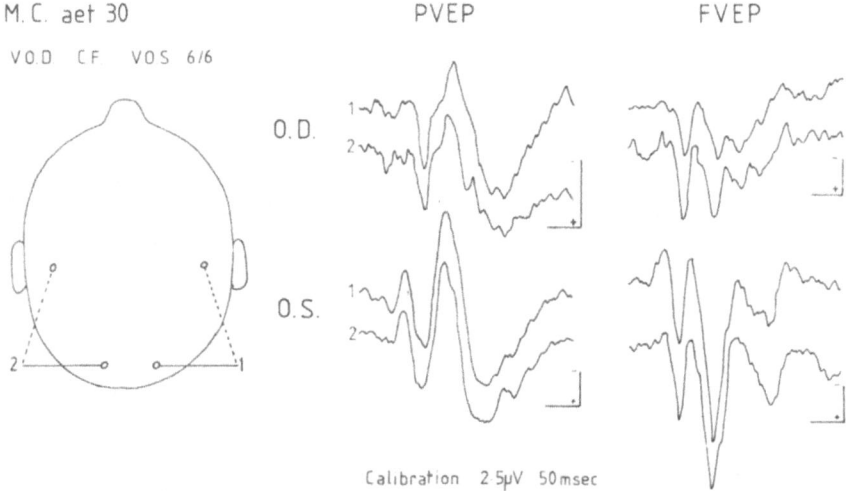

Fig. 1. VEP findings in a 30 year old woman with right ischaemic optic neuropathy (central scotoma). See text for details. Note the differing gains.

of vision in the right eye. There had been two previous minor episodes of 2—10 minutes duration. On examination right visual acuity was reduced to finger counting at one metre; there was a central scotoma. The PVEPs evoked by a 40' check pattern (shown above) are of significantly reduced amplitude from the right eye with no associated latency changes. The FVEPs also show a highly significant amplitude reduction when the right eye is stimulated with no significant interocular latency asymmetry. However, when the 26 minute check pattern was used (results not shown) there was an additional inter-ocular latency asymmetry of some 10 msec in the major positive component of the PVEP, that from the right eye being delayed compared with that from the left.

Fig. 2. D.C. This 56 year old woman developed loss of vision in the right

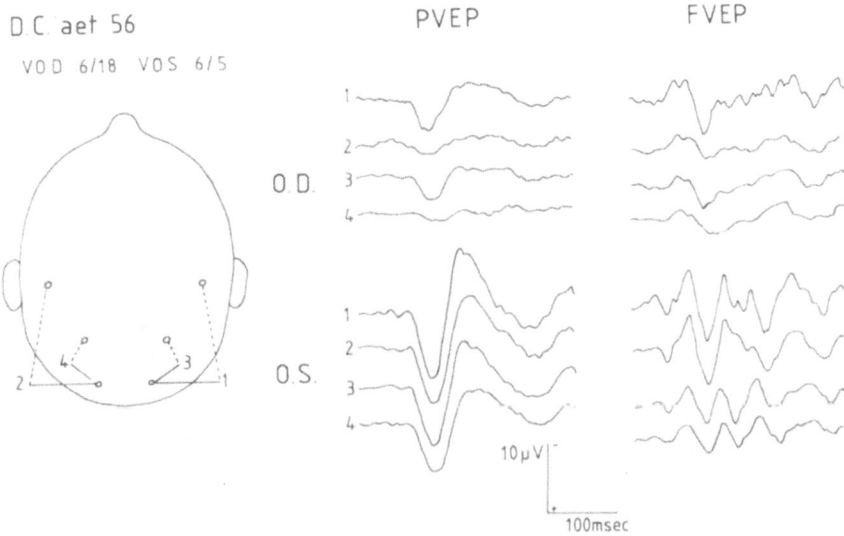

D.C. aet 56

VOD 6/18 VOS 6/5

PVEP

FVEP

O.D.   1 2 3 4

O.S.   1 2 3 4

10µV

100msec

Fig. 2. VEP findings in a 56 year old woman with right ischaemic optic neuropathy (superior altitudinal field defect). See text for details.

eye over about 5 days. There was nothing of relevance in the past history. On examination right visual acuity was 6/18 with a superior altitudinal field defect. There was disc swelling on the right with pallor, some small hemorrhages and axonal debris. The PVEPs from the right eye are of significantly reduced amplitude compared with those from the left, this reduction being particularly well seen in the left hemisphere traces, channels 2 and 4. No significant latency asymmetry is present. The FVEPs from the right eye also show an amplitude reduction, significant in the left hemisphere traces.

Fig. 3. A.S. This 68 year old woman was admitted following two episodes of visual loss. The first affected the right eye and was transient; the second affected the left eye and resulted in persisting deficit. On examination there was bilateral disc swelling with pallor, particularly in the left eye where associated ischaemic changes were seen extending into the peripapillary retina. No ischaemia was apparent on the right. An E.S.R. was not significantly elevated but temporal artery biopsy showed giant cell arteritis. No PVEP is seen when the left eye is stimulated, that from the right being within

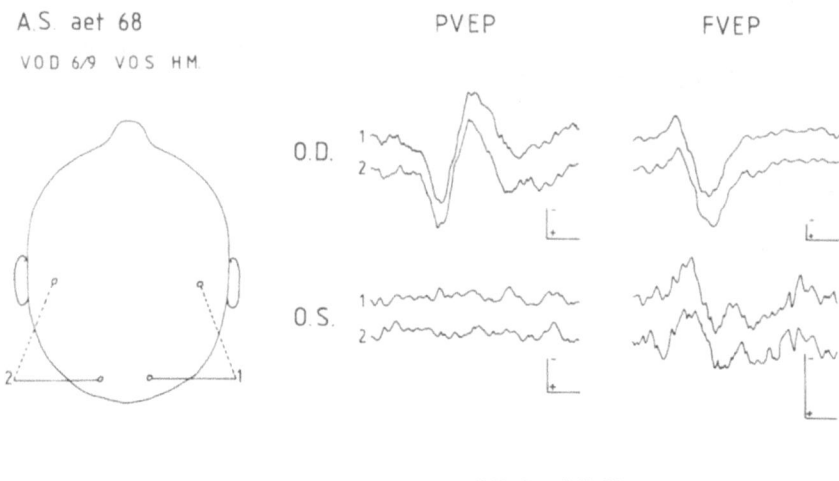

A.S. aet 68

VOD 6/9 VOS HM.

PVEP

FVEP

O.D.

O.S.

Calibration 5uV 50msec

Fig. 3. VEP findings in a 68 year old woman with left ischaemic optic neuropathy secondary to giant cell arteritis. See text for details. Note the differing gains.

normal limits. The FVEPs from the left eye show distortion of the waveform with severely reduced amplitude and delayed early components. Accurate quantification of the major positive component is difficult.

DISCUSSION

The VEP is therefore shown to be of value in the assessment of suspected ischaemic lesions of the anterior visual pathways. The PVEP was abnormal in all 11 patients studied; the FVEP in 70% of the 10 patients in whom this investigation was performed. Wilson (1978) reported that amplitude is the affected variable rather than latency in ischaemic optic neuropathy, and this suggestion is confirmed. However, in the present study this amplitude reduction was usually relative to the fellow eye and was not, as additionally reported by Wilson (1978), relative to the lower limit of normal indicated by the control group.

It is of interest that the two patients with histologically proven giant cell arteritis both had VEPs which were significantly different from the patients without temporal arteritis, particularly in the delayed, distorted responses to flash stimulation. This is in agreement with the findings of Harding et al. (1980) who report that all their patients with ischaemic optic neuropathy who showed a delayed FVEP had temporal arteritis.

The sudden onset of visual loss often seen in ischaemic optic nerve lesions can also occur in optic nerve demyelination and although other factors may indicate the correct diagnosis it seems, as first suggested by Wilson (1978), that VEP examination may supply useful objective evidence to assist the clinician in his decision. In demyelinating optic nerve lesions the latency of the major positive component is increased, often substantially, with or without an associated reduction in amplitude. The clinically uninvolved eye may also show VEP abnormalities, particularly in response to pattern stimulation. In ischaemic optic nerve lesions however, the characteristic finding is that of a reduction in amplitude of the major positive component occasionally accompanied by a minor increase in latency, with stimulation of any clinically uninvolved eye resulting in normal VEPs.

REFERENCES

Boghen, D.R. & Glaser, J.S. Ischaemic optic neuropathy. The clinical profile and natural history. Brain 98: 689–708 (1975).

Halliday, A.M., McDonald, W.I. & Mushin, J. Delayed visual evoked response in optic neuritis. Lancet i: 982–985 (1972).

Harding, G.F.A., Crews, S.J. & Good, P.A. VEP in neuro-ophthalmic disease. In: Evoked Potentials (Ed. C. Barber) MTP Press, Lancaster. 235–241 (1980).

Holder, G.E. The effects of chiasmal compression on the pattern visual evoked potential. Electroenceph. clin. Neurophysiol. 45: 278–280 (1978).

Holder, G.E. Abnormalities of the pattern visual evoked potential in patients with homonymous visual field defects. In: Evoked Potentials (Ed. C. Barber) MTP Press, Lancaster. 285–291 (1980).

Richey, E.T., Kooi, K.A. & Tourtelotte, W.W. Visually evoked responses in multiple sclerosis. J. Neurol. Neurosurg. Psychiat. 34: 275–280 (1971).

Wilson, W.B. Visual evoked response differentiation of ischaemic optic neuritis from the optic neuritis of multiple sclerosis. Am. J. Ophthalmol. 86: 530–535 (1978).

Authors' address:
Department of Clinical Neurophysiology
Brook General Hospital
Shooters Hill Road
London, S.E.18. England

VISUAL PHYSIOLOGIC AND OCULAR EVALUATION IN CAROTID OCCLUSIVE DISEASE

Pre- and post-endarterectomy

J.R. HECKENLIVELY, R.D. YEE, H.R. KRAUSS, D. MARTIN,
R. BUSUTTIL, H. MACHLEDER & J.D. BAKER

(Los Angeles, U.S.A.)

ABSTRACT

Nine patients were evaluated pre- and post-carotid endarterectomy. Each patient received a complete clinical opthalmologic evaluation, Goldmann visual field testing, fundus photography, ophthalmodynamometry, Gee oculopneumoplethysmography, Doppler evaluation of the carotids, color vision testing, visual evoked response (VER) testing, electo-oculography (EOG), macular photostress testing and dark adaptation testing.

Following surgery, there were mild improvements in visual acuity, moderate improvements in visual fields, mild changes in VER, EOG, color vision and photostress recovery time, and improvement in dark adaptation.

INTRODUCTION

Carotid occlusive disease may lead to acute or chronic ocular ischemia; a carotid plaque may be the source of emboli which may travel to the eye or brain, or atheromatous changes may narrow the lumen and produce a chronic ischemic state. Severe carotid occlusive disease may lead to ocular ischemia, with pain and inflammation, or may produce retinal vascular changes, including slowed flow, venous dilatation and tortuosity and intra-retinal hemorrhages (Hedges 1962; Kearns & Hollenhorst 1963). Prolonged severe ischemia may lead to rubeosis iridis with neovascular glaucoma (Kearns 1979). The question we posed in our study is, given that carotid occlusive disease may diminish ocular blood flow, does endarterectomy, with resultant restoration of normal ocular hemodynamics, improve visual function?

MATERIALS AND METHODS

To answer this question we examined the patients of three of us (Drs. Busuttill, Machleder and Baker) scheduled for carotid endarterectomy during the period April, 1979 to January, 1980. We excluded from our study patients with central or branch retinal artery occlusions. Each patient received a complete clinical ophthalmologic examination, including history, refraction, anterior segment inspection at the slit lamp, examination of pupil responses and ocular motility, measurement of intraocular pressure, dilated fundus examination and ophthalmodynamometry. At the time of pre-operative exam, the examiner was not aware of the angiography results. Fundus photos were taken and Goldmann visual fields were performed by a technician who was unaware of the nature of this study or the patients' symptoms. The vascular service independently performed Gee oculopneumo-plethysmography and Doppler examination of the carotids. One of us (Martin) conducted a battery of tests including color perception (tested with the Nagel anomaloscope, Ishihara color plates, AO H-R-R pseudoisochromatic color plates and the Farnsworth-Munsell 100-hue test), VER, EOG, photo-stress recovery time and dark adaptation. The same clinical and laboratory evaluation was performed 6 weeks after endarterectomy.

RESULTS AND DISCUSSION

We studied nine patients. Seven were men and two women. The age range was 53–75, with an average of 62. The presenting symptoms included amaurosis fugax in six, headache in three (one of whom also had amaurosis) and transient ischemic attacks in three (two of whom also had amaurosis). In two of the three patients with headache, the character was severe unilateral retro-orbital pain in one and a chronic unilateral fronto-temporal pain in the other. This pain distribution is characteristic in carotid occlusive disease (Kearns & Hollenhorst 1963).

In this group of patients, concurrent diseases included diabetes in one, hypertension in three and other peripheral vascular disease in four.

Physical examination of the neck revealed carotid bruits in eight patients and diminished carotid pulsation in three.

Visual acuity was good pre-operatively and stable, or improved, post-operatively. Five patients had 20/20 or better vision on the operated side prior to surgery and their vision was unchanged post-operatively. Two patients with 20/25 vision improved to 20/20. Two patients had 20/40 vision pre-operatively; following surgery one improved to 20/20 and one was unchanged.

Visual fields by Goldmann perimetry were normal and unchanged following surgery in three patients. Five patients showed mild to moderate improvements in visual field testing post-endarterectomy.

Fig. 1 displays the pre- and post-operative fields of a 53 year-old woman with a history of episodes of left amaurosis fugax and transient right hemi-paresis, with a left carotid bruit and diminished left carotid pulsation. She underwent a left carotid endarterectomy, since which time she has had no recurrence of symptoms. Pre-operatively her vision was 20/25 in each eye, post-operatively 20/25 on the right and 20/20 on the left. The left field shows a marked expansion in all isopters and the right field reveals a moderate expansion.

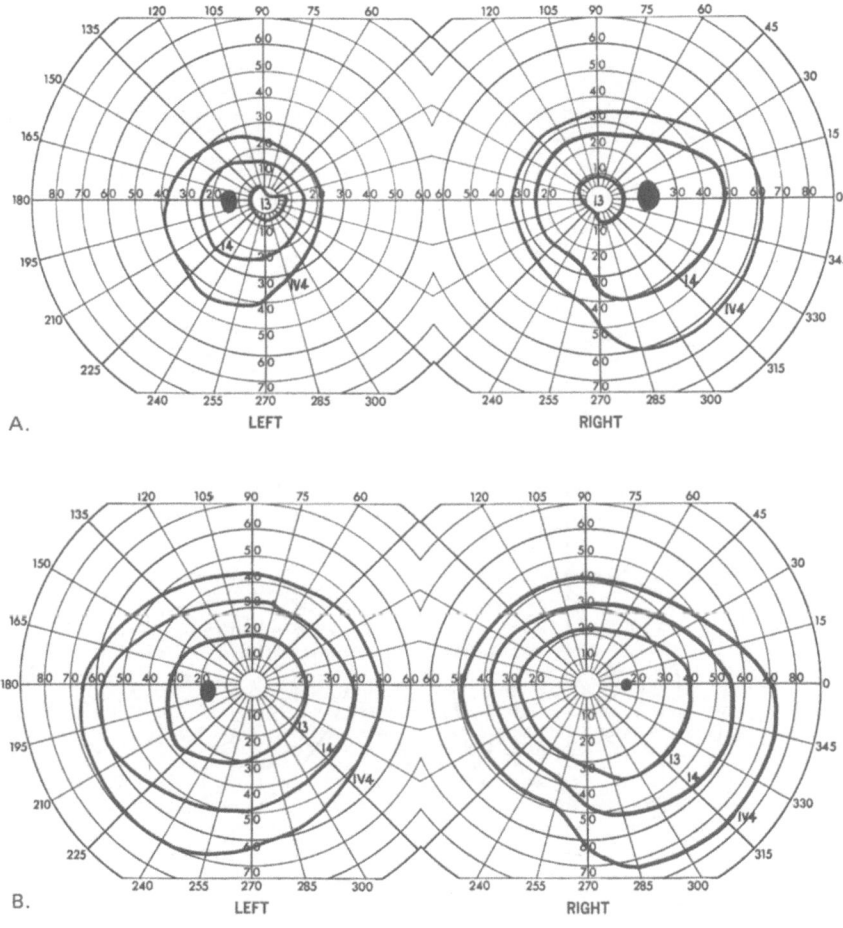

Fig. 1. a) pre-operative (upper), and b) post-operative visual fields in a 53 year-old woman who underwent a left carotid endarterectomy.

Fig. 2 displays the pre- and post-operative fields of a 58 year-old man with a history of left amaurosis fugax with 20/20 vision in each eye pre- and post-operatively, in whom ophthalmodynamometry was 90/40 OD and 50/10 OS and angiography demonstrated mild plaquing of the right carotid and a 90% stenosis of the left internal carotid. There is a moderate improvement in all isopters on the left and a mild improvement on the right. Post-operatively, ophthalmodynamometry was 90/20 OD and 95/20 OS.

In general, comparison of pre- and post-operative fundus photos showed no change, but Fig. 3 shows one case (same patient whose field is seen in Fig. 2) demonstrating a change. Pre-operatively, the disk margin is a bit indistinct and there is some mild capillary dilatation over the disk surface, which may be secondary to ischemia. Post-operatively, the margin is more

133

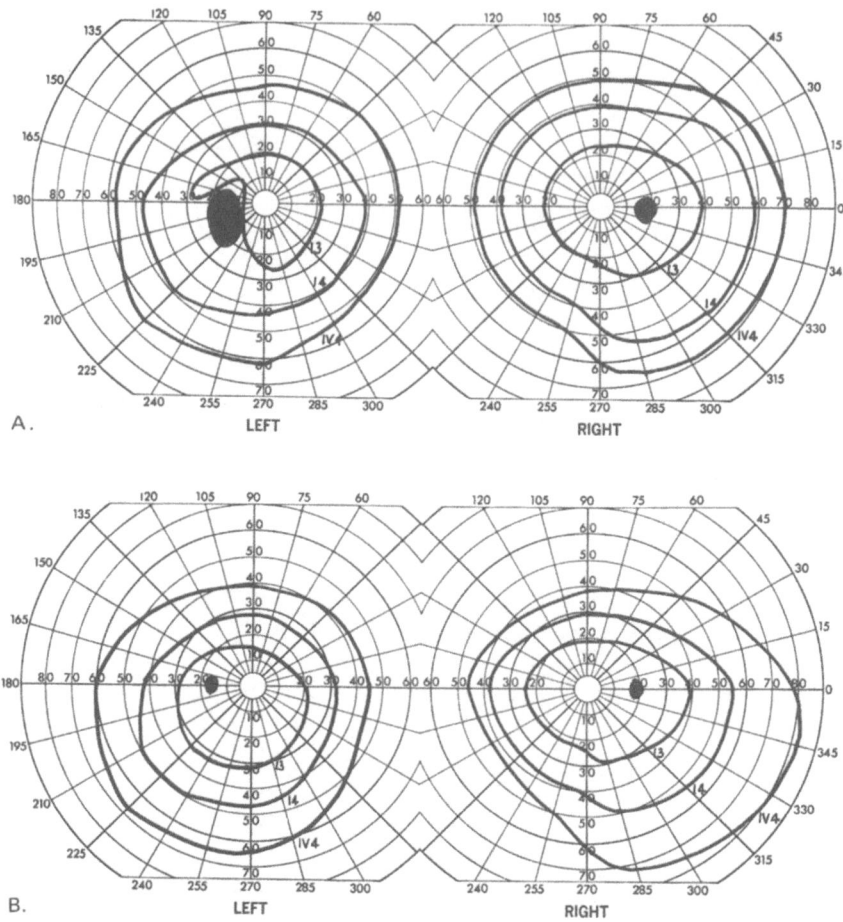

Fig. 2. a) pre-operative (upper), and b) post-operative visual fields in a 58 year-old man who underwent a left carotid endarterectomy.

distinct and the capillary dilatation is not evident. The temporal arteriolar branches demonstrate some widening and less irregularity post-operatively.

An afferent pupillary defect (APD) was present in four patients pre-operatively; this worsened in one patient with pre- and post-operative acuity of 20/40 and moderate worsening of color perception in the same eye. The APD was unchanged in one patient whose vision improved from 20/25 to 20/20. The APD disappeared in two patients in whom the vision improved from 20/25 to 20/20 in one and from 20/40 to 20/20 in the other.

The VER was within our laboratory normal limits, and not significantly changed following surgery, in seven patients. Comparing pre- to post-operative VERs, one patient displayed a shortened implicit time to N2, without a change in time to P2, and another showed a prolonged implicit time to N2 with no change in time to P2.

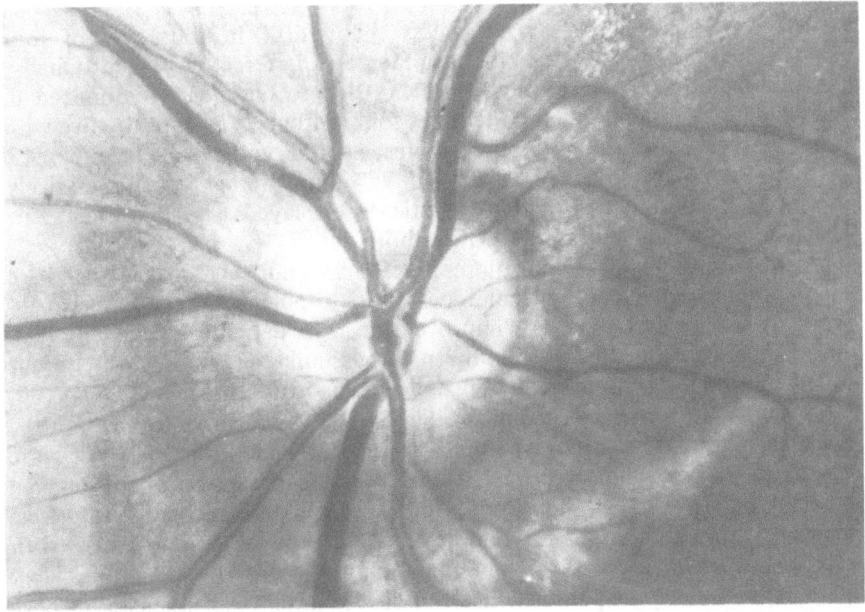

A.

B.

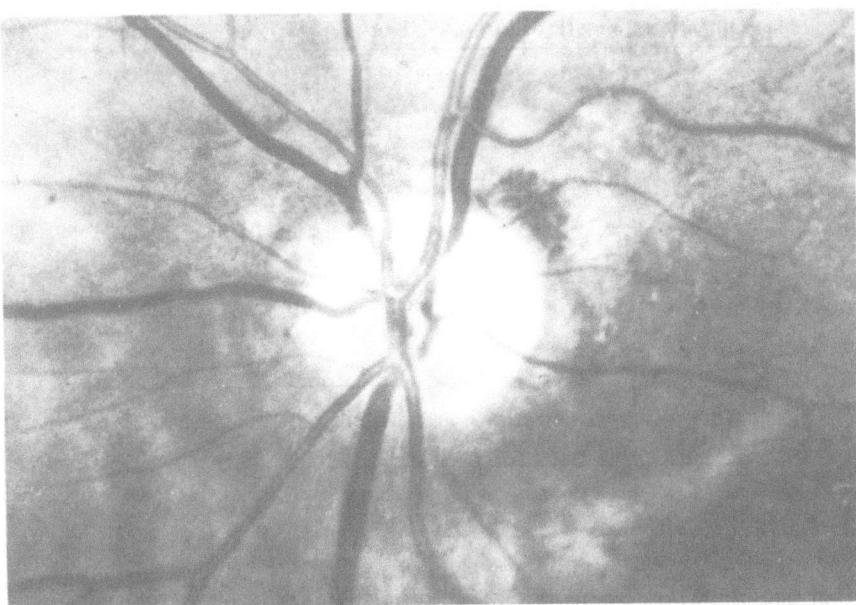

Fig. 3. a) pre-operative (upper), and b) post-operative fundus photos in the same patient as in Fig. 2 (left eye). Temporal arterioles show widening, disk margin is more distinct, and capillary dilatation over disk surface has disappeared.

135

The EOG, pre-operatively, was less than 160% in four eyes of four patients, in each case on the side to undergo endarterectomy. Additionally, the pre-operative EOG was lower on the side to be endarterectomized in five of nine cases and equal in the other four (within ± 10%). In the five with lower EOGs, the difference ranged from 18–40% with an average of 29%. Two patients displayed a greater than 25% improvement post-operatively in the EOG of one eye and two patients displayed a greater than 25% decrease post-operatively in the EOG of both eyes.

As tested by the Nagel anomaloscope, Ishihara and AO H-R-R plates, there was no significant change in color perception. Judging by the Farnsworth-Munsell 100-hue test there was improvement in six patients, a decline in two, and no change in one, but the improvement was mild, and in only one patient was the improvement represented by a decline in error score greater than 100.

A Medin scotometer (Henkind & Siegel 1967) was used to measure the macular photostress recovery time in accordance with the procedure described in a previous report (Heckenlively, Pearlman, Shaver, Brickman & Henkind 1978). Pre-operatively, four of nine patients had photostress recovery times greater than 1 minute; post-operatively three of these with pre-operative times of 5–5½ minutes improved to 1–3 minutes. One patient with a pre-operative time of 1½ minutes was unchanged post-operatively.

Table 1. Dark adaptation (final rod thresholds)

Pt – Endarterectomy (R or L)		Eye	Pre-op	Post-op
CC	L	OD	0.25	0.15
		OS	0.60	0.25
		OU	0.25	0.15
JC	L	OD	0.60	0.35
		OS	1.05	0.65
		OU	0.35	0.35
MW	R	OD	0.90	0.55
		OS	0.50	0.35
		OU	0.50	0.35
EN	L	OD	1.20	0.35
		OS	1.15	0.70
		OU	0.70	0.40

Dark adaptation was carried out with Goldmann-Weekers adaptometer and the final rod threshold was recorded. Table 1 displays the results in four patients who demonstrated improvements of 0.35 log units or more; in all of these cases the improvement was on the operated side. In one case the improvement was bilateral.

The non-invasive studies of carotid function which were performed included ophthalmodynamometry, Gee oculopneumoplethysmography and

Doppler evaluation of carotid flow. Table 2 displays the angiographically demonstrated degree of internal carotid occlusion along with the results of

Table 2. Evaluation of non-invasive pre-operative studies.

Pt	Angiographically documented stenosis			Ophthalmodynamometry		OPPG		Doppler	
	Right	(%)	Left	Right	Left	R	L	R	L
AM	0		90	N*	N	N	N	N	Ab*
KC	0		0	N	N	N	N	N	N
MS	0		30	N	N	N	N	N	Eq*
WR	0		90	90/40	50/10	0.66	0.59	N	Ab
CC	100		80	55/25	105/45	0.57	0.75	Eq	Eq
JC	40–50		90	110/42	92/17	0.72	0.72	Eq	Eq
MW	70		0	60/35	80/40	0.74	0.77	Eq	N
EN	0		30–40	N	N	N	N	N	Eq
IS	30		70	125/45	105/40	0.81	0.78	Eq	N

* N = normal; Eq = Equivocal; Ab = Abnormal.

the non-invasive studies. The results underlined are those which are diagnostic or suspicious of carotid occlusion. The double-underlined result emphasizes a result which is misleading. In ophthalmodynamometry, a difference between the two eyes of greater than 20% in systolic or diastolic pressure is diagnostic and 15–20% is suspicious (Galin, Baras, Cavero & Best 1969). Ophthalmodynamometry was normal pre- and post-operatively in four patients, was diagnostic of carotid occlusive disease in four and suspicious in one, whereas the oculopneumoplethysmography (OPPG) was diagnostic in only two cases. Doppler testing was diagnostic in two, suspicious in five and misleading in one. These results confirm the better accuracy of ophthalmodynamometry reported by others (Sanborn & Miller 1979).

CONCLUSION

We studied nine patients before and after carotid endarterectomy. The most important change post-operatively was an improved sense of well-being in all nine patients and a resolution of presenting symptoms in all nine. In clinical ophthalmologic evaluation, we noted an improvement in visual acuity in some patients, significant improvement in visual field in some and resolution of an afferent pupil defect in two. We found ophthalmo-dynamometry to be superior to Gee oculopneumoplethysmography or Doppler testing in accuracy of diagnosis of carotid occlusive disease. VER, EOG, color testing and the photostress test showed some changes and dark adaptation showed significant improvement in four patients following carotid endarterectomy.

137

REFERENCES

Galin, M.A., Baras, I., Cavero, R. & Best, M. Compression and suction ophthalmodynamometry. Am. J. Ophthalmol. 67: 388–392 (1969).

Heckenlively, J.R., Pearlman, J.T., Shaver, L., Brickman, M. & Henkind, P. Macular recovery from dazzle (photostress) in normal women on birth control pills (BCP). In: 15th ISCEV Symposium (Ed. J. Francois & A. De Rouck) Junk, The Hague. (Doc. Ophthal. Proc. Series, Vol. 15). 313–318 (1978).

Hedges, T.R. Jr. Ophthalmologic findings in internal carotid artery occlusion. Johns Hopkins Med. J. 111: 89–97 (1962).

Henkind, P. & Siegel, I.M. The scotometer. A device for measuring macular recovery time. Am. J. Ophthalmol. 64: 314–315 (1967).

Kearns, T.P. Ophthalmology and the carotid artery. Am. J. Ophthalmol. 88: 714–722 (1979).

Kearns, T.P. & Hollenhorst R.W. Venous-stasis retinopathy of occlusive disease of the carotid artery. Proceedings of the Staff Meetings of the Mayo Clinic. 38: 304–312 (1963).

Sanborn, G.S. & Miller N.R. Evaluation of currently available non-invasive tests of carotid artery disease. Presented at the American Academy of Ophthalmology, San Francisco, Ca., USA, November (1979).

Authors' Address:
Department of Ophthalmology,
Jules Stein Eye Institute,
UCLA School of Medicine,
Los Angeles, CA 90024 U.S.A.

COMPARISON OF VISUAL FIELD EXAMINATION AND VISUAL EVOKED CORTICAL POTENTIALS IN MULTIPLE SCLEROSIS PATIENTS

J.T.W. VAN DALEN & H. SPEKREIJSE

(*Amsterdam, The Netherlands*)

ABSTRACT

Twenty-nine definite patients have been examined by means of visual field examination and visual evoked potentials (VEP). Visual field examination was performed by Friedmann visual field analysis, kinetic perimetry and static perimetry. Visual evoked potentials were obtained by checkerboard stimulation (pattern reversal stimulation on a TV-screen).

In literature VEP techniques are said to be superior to visual field examination in diagnosing lesions of the visual pathways in MS patients. This study shows that in these cases careful visual field examination may be at least as useful as the assessment of VEP. From our 29 patients (58 eyes) a visual field defect was found in 46 eyes, while a VEP latency delay was found in 32 eyes.

INTRODUCTION

Visual evoked cortical potentials (VECP) have become widely accepted in diagnostic schemes for the assessment of multiple sclerosis, especially since the introduction of checkerboard stimulation in the clinic by Halliday and co-workers (Halliday, McDonald & Mushin 1972).

In the situation of checkerboard reversal, the stimulus condition that is most widely used, the major criterion in the VECP is the latency of the first major positive peak. In almost all patients with optic neuritis the peak latency of this component in the pattern reversal response is delayed. However, the VECP delay in multiple sclerosis patients without any visual symptoms or complaints scores a much lower percentage ranging from 61% to 67% as generally reported in literature (Asselman, Chadwick & Marsden 1975; Hennerici, Wenzel & Freud 1977; Duwaer & Spekreijse 1978). It should be noted that this percentage range refers to the whole sample of possible, probable and definite multiple sclerosis patinets; of course higher percentages are reached when only the last two categories are taken into consideration. Visual field (VF) defects in multiple sclerosis patients also have been documented. Although central and paracentral scotomata seem to be rather characteristic, narrow scotomata in the VF 20°–25° from the fixation point have been described as well (Wilson & Reid, 1969; Harms 1976; Foulds, Stewart & McClare 1979). Finally, Hoyt (1972) stresses the close correlation between visible signs of nerve fibre layer defects in the retina and defects in the field of vision.

As more and more examination methods become available for the diagnostic schemes for the assessment of multiple sclerosis, it might be useful to compare two widely used methods: (1) visual field examination and (2) latency estimation of the pattern evoked cortical potentials. Considering the endurance of patients, application of both methods seems only acceptable in clinical routine when they give complementary information.

METHODS

Subjects

Twenty-nine subjects (19 women and 10 men) with well documented histories of multiple sclerosis, classified according to McAlpine et al. (1972) as definite and probable MS patients, were included in the study. All patients unerwent a complete ophthalmological and neurological examination. Seven patients (8 eyes) had a history of at least one attack of optic neuritis; 22 patients had never experienced visual symptoms which could have pointed to involvement of the visual pathways. The 44 eyes from the 22 patients without visual symptoms together with the 6 asymtomatic eyes from the seven patients with optic neuritis form the asymtomatic group referred to further in this paper.

Visual field examination

The visual fields were assessed by means of:
Friedmann visual field analysis
Kinetic perimetry
Static perimetry

Visual evoked cortical potentials

The visual evoked cortical potentials were obtained by checkerboard stimulation generated on a TV-screen. The check sizes used routinely were 20′ and 55′ of visual arc. The pattern reversal frequency was 2 Hz for the transient responses. Eight reversal frequencies between 5.6 Hz and 25 Hz were chosen to estimate the apparent latency from the phase characteristic of the steady-state responses. The VECPs evoked by an appearance-disappearance checkerboard also were determined. As shown in the paper by Riemslag et al. (this volume), this stimulus has a higher detection rate for latency increases than the reversal stimulus, mainly because the small stimulus field (6° by 8°)

used in our study gives, in patients, a more reliable appearance-disappearance response than reversal response.

On the basis of a 3 SD-criterion the latency of the major positive component in the pattern reversal VECP was considered abnormal when the latency of this peak exceeded the value of 126 msec. Note that this latency criterion cannot be transferred to another testing situation. Each clinic has to establish its own normative data since latency varies with many stimulus parameters, including luminance, field size, check size, frame rate of TV-monitor, contrast etc. (Spekreijse, Duwaer & Posthumus Meyes 1979).

Finally, to compare the effectiveness of the VF and VECP latency estimates for MS diagnosis, both tests were performed on the same day for each patient. Thus, the state of the subject may be considered the same during the two tests.

RESULTS

The results for each patient are presented in Fig. 1. Twenty-two patients showed a delayed VECP (in one or both eyes): 21 out of these 22 patients showed an abnormal visual field (in one or both eyes). Seven patients had a normal VECP peak latency; five of these patients had an abnormal VF (in one or both eyes).

Abnormal VECP : 22   Abnormal VF : 21
                        Normal VF   : 1

Normal VECP   : 7   Abnormal VF : 5
                        Normal VF   : 2

Fig. 1. This figure tabulates the VF findings and the pattern VECP latency estimates obtained in the 29 MS patients reported in this study.

	VF norm.	VF abn.
VECP norm.	10	16
VECP abn.	2	30

Fig. 2. In this table the visual fields and VECP latencies are compared for each of the 49 eyes of the MS patients examined.

The VF and latency estimates per eye are tabulated in Fig. 2. In 32 eyes (55%) an abnormal peak latency was found in 46 eyes (79%) an abnormal VF, i.e.:
(a) In 10 eyes VF and VECP latencies were normal.
(b) In 30 eyes abnormal VF and VECP latencies were found.
(c) In 2 eyes with a normal VF the VECP latency was estimated abnormal.

141

(d) In 16 eyes with a normal VECP reversal latency the VF was classified as abnormal.

It may be of interest to consider the 8 eyes with a documented episode of optic neuritis separately six of them showed an abnormal VF and a delayed VECP latency.

On the basis of the above data summary it seems that VF assessment in multiple sclerosis patients is at least as informative as VECP latency determination. The visual fields in the MS patients studied show interesting defects (Fig. 3). Of the 46 eyes with a defective VF only 6 showed a central defect,

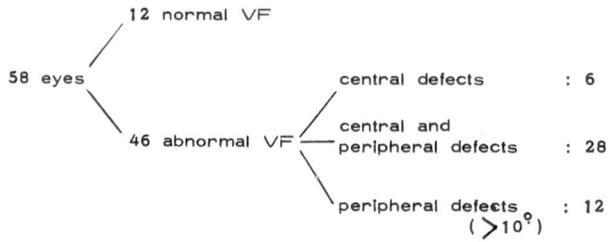

Fig. 3. Overview of the VF examination in 58 eyes.

28 showed both central and peripheral defects, and 12 eyes showed solely a peripheral defect (In this context a peripheral visual field defect is a defect beyond 10° of eccentricity.) It is surprising that 5 of the 12 eyes with solely a VF defect at an eccentricity of more than 10° ofvisual angle, showed also an increased peak latency to a pattern reversal stimulus subtending not more than 6° to 8°.These 5 eyes may be regarded as examples of what Halliday calls the detection of the 'silent lesions' through peak latency estimation. Fig. 4a, b, Fig. 5a, b, c and Fig. 6a, b, c give examples of characteristic field defects as found in two of the multiple sclerosis patients described in the present study. The peripheral defects assessed by means of perimetry turned out to be much more outspoken than expected on the basis of Friedmann's visual field analysis. Friedmann's visual field analysis often did not show any abnormalities in those regions where static perimetry defects were extremely evident.

DISCUSSION AND CONCLUSION

In 6 (out of 8) eyes with a history of optic neuritis an abnormal VECP latency was found, while abnormal VECP latencies were found in 26 (out of 50) asymptomatic eyes. This finding is consistent with previous studies that demonstrated VECP delay in nearly 100% of eyes with a history of optic neuritis, and a far lower percentage (approx. 60%) for visually asumptomatic eyes in the whole sample of possible, probable and definite MS patients (in our sample of visually asymptomatic probable and definite MS patients this percentage is 52%).

In this overall sample the visual fields were found to be abnormal in 46

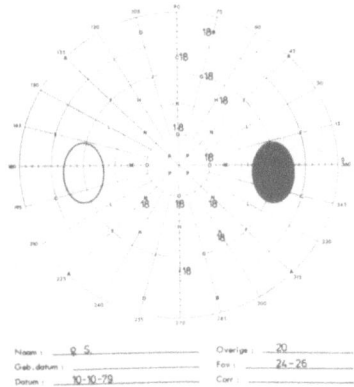

Fig. 4a. The Friedmann visual field analysis of the right asymptomatic eye of a 39 year old female definite MS patient does not show clear defects.

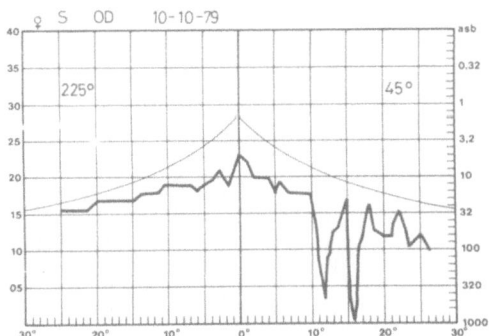

Fig. 4b. Static perimetry (45°−225°) of this eye shows remarkably deep defects at 10°−20° off center. The defects are much more outspoked in the static profile than could be suspected on the basis of the Friedmann visual field analysis. The pattern VECP of this eye also was delayed.

eyes (detection rate of about 80%). This is a higher percentage than usually found in literature. For example Ellenberger and Ziegler (1977) found abnormal VFs in 14% of the eyes in their asymptomatic group. One of the reasons could be that the VFs have to be determined by skilled technicians, otherwise the scattered scotomata, especially in the asymptomatic group, may be overlooked. It is our finding that in this group static perimetry provided a more precise measure of the density of the scotomata than the Friedmann visual field analysis (often these scotomata were quite unexpected on the basis of Friedmann's VFs). No complementary information was gained with kinetic perimetry in the asymptomatic group.

As stated before, of 16 eyes with a normal pattern reversal latency the VF was considered as abnormal whereas the reverse was observed in only 2 eyes. It seems likely that the discrepancy between normal VECP latency and

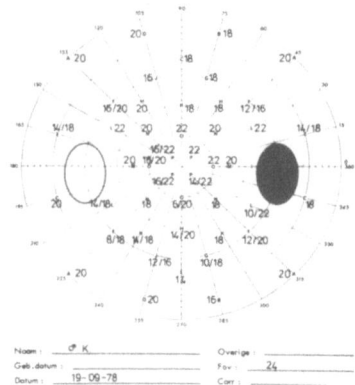

Fig. 5a. Friedmann visual field analysis of the asymptomatic right eye of a 32 year old definite MS patient. Many small defects with extremely strong scatter can be observed. A similar pattern was observed for the other also asymptomatic, eye of this patient.

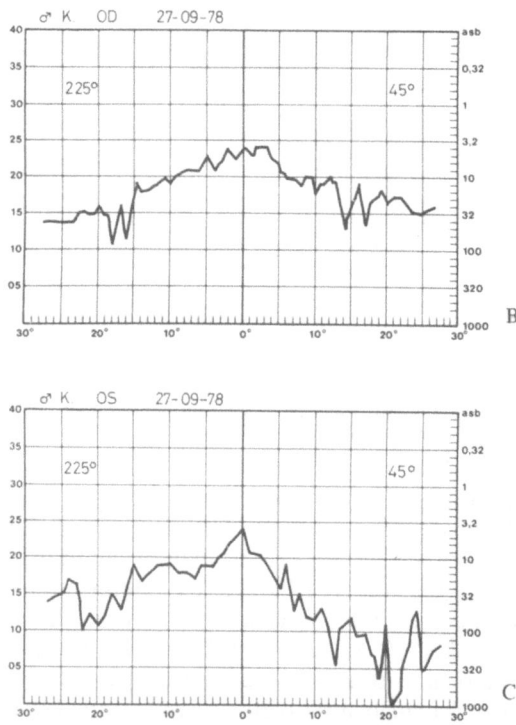

Figs. 5b and 5c. Static perimetry (45°–225°) of the right (Fig. b) and left (Fig. c) eye show marked defects in the peripheral visual field. In these plots scattering is less outspoken than in the Friedmann plots. Note that the pattern VECP latencies of both eyes were normal.

144

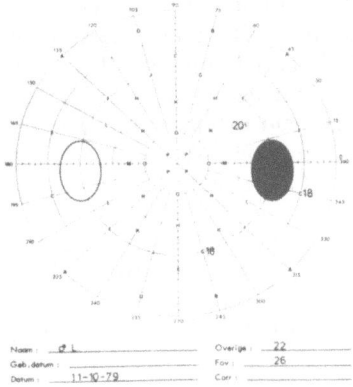

Fig. 6a. Normal Friedmann visual field analysis of the right, asymptomatic, eye of a 22 year old probable MS patient, with a spinal manifestation of MS.

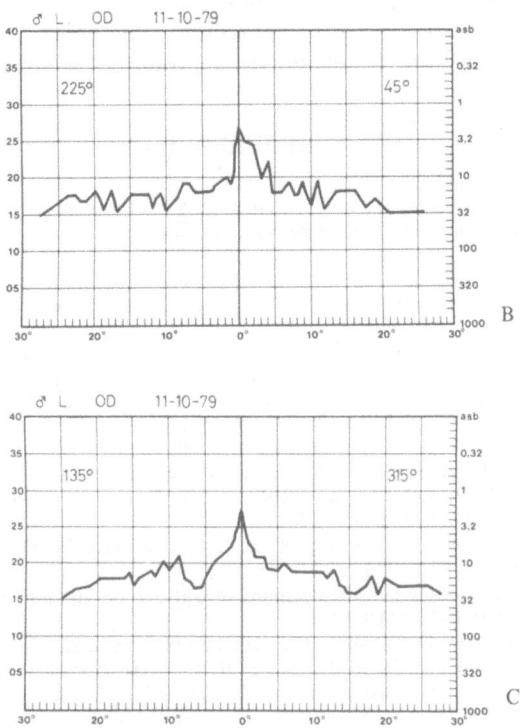

Figs. 6b and 6c. Static perimetry (45°–225° and 135°–315°) of this eye reveals discrete defects 10°–20° off the fixation point. Note that the VECP latency of this eye was found to be normal.

145

abnormal VF can be attributed to the relatively small visual field that is being examined with the pattern reversal stimulus. This suggestion is substantiated by the high correlation of VECP and VF abnormalities when there are both central and peripheral VF defects. It should be noted, however, that for the assessment of MS, visual field defects are even less specific than latency increases of contrast VECPs. This is the major reason why Heron, Regan & Milner (1974) have proposed delay perimetry for diagnostic schemes of MS. Apart from VF and VECP latency tests, colour vision tests (Griffin & Wray, 1978) and grating acuity tests (Regan, Silver & Murray, 1977) also have been described as sensitive candidates for diagnostic schemes of MS. Our present results show that static perimetry as well is a useful method in the assessment of MS as is pattern VECP latency.

ACKNOWLEDGEMENT

We are grateful to Mrs. H. Pijnappel-Groothuyse of the Perimetry Department of the Eye Clinic for the skillful assessment of the visual field plots and Drs. Verduyn Lunel and Riemslag of the Department of Visual System Analysis of the Netherlands Ophthalmic Research Institute for the ophthalmological and EVCP examinations, and to Dr. H. Walbeek of the Alexander van der Leeuw clinic for the neurological examinations.

REFERENCES

Asselman, P., Chadwick, D.W. & Marsden, C.D. Visual evoked responses in the diagnosis and management of patients suspected of multiple sclerosis. Brian 98: 261–282 (1975).

Duwaer, A.L. & Spekreijse, H. Latency of luminance and contrast evoked potentials in multiple sclerosis patients. Electroencephal. clin. Neurophysiol. 45: 244–258 (1978).

Ellenberger, C. Jr. & Ziegler, S.B. Quantitative perimetry and visual evoked potentials in multiple sclerosis. In: International Visual Field Symposium. (Ed. E.L. Greve) Junk, The Hague. (Doc. Ophthal. Proc. Series Vol. 14) 203–212 (1977).

Foulds, W.S., Stewart, J.B. & McClare, E. The diagnosis and prognosis of demyelination in the optic nerve. In: XXII Concilium Ophthalmologicum, Kyoto 1978. K. Shimizu & J.A. Oosterhuis). Excerpta Medica, Amsterdam. 333 (1979).

Griffin, J.F. & Wray, S.H. Acquired color vision defects in retrobulbar neuritis. Am. J. Ophthalmol. 86: 193–201 (1978).

Halliday, A.M., McDonald, W.I. & Mushin, J. Delayed visual evoked responses in optic neuritis. Lancet i: 982–985 (1972).

Harms, H. Role of perimetry in assessment of optic nerve dysfunction. Trans. Ophthal. Soc. U.K. 96: 363–367 (1976).

Hennerici, M., Wenzel, D. & Freud, H.J. The comparison of small rectangle and checkerboard stimulation for the evaluation of delayed visual evoked responses in patients suspected of multiple sclerosis. Brain 100: 119–136 (1977).

Heron, J.R., Regan, D., & Milner, B.A. Delay in visual perception in unilateral optic atrophy after retrobulbar neuritis. Brain 97: 69–78 (1974).

Hoyt, W.F. Funduscopy of the retinal nerve fiber layer in neurosurgical practice. Neurologica Medico-chirurgica 13: 3–12 (1973).

McAlpine, D., Lumsden, C.E., Acheson, E.D. Multiple sclerosis. A reappraisal. Livingstone, Edinborough (1972).

Regan, D., Silver, R. & Murray, J. Visual acuity and contrast sensitivity in multiple sclerosis hidden visual loss. Brain 100: 563–579 (1977).

Spekreijse, H., Duwaer, A.L. & Postumus Meyes, F.E. Contrast evoked potentials and psychophysics in multiple sclerosis patients. In: Human Evoked Potentials (Ed. D. Lehman & E. Callaway) Plenum Publishing Corp., New York. 363–381 (1979).

Wilson, T.M. and Reid, H. Quantitative perimetry in the assessment of optic nerve conduction defects. Trans. Ophthal. Soc. U.K. 89: 67–82 (1969).

Authors' addresses:

J.T.W. van Dalen
University of Amsterdam,
Eye Clinic,
Wilhelmina Gasthuis,
1e Helmersstraat 104,
1054 EG Amsterdam
The Netherlands

and

H. Spekreijse
Netherlands Ophthalmic Research Institute,
Dept. of Visual System Analysis
P.O. Box 6411,
1005 EK Amsterdam.
The Netherlands

147

VER FINDINGS IN RETROBULBAR NEURITIS DUE TO MULTIPLE SCLEROSIS

M. MOSCHOS, G. PALIMERIS, E. PANAGAKIS & H. PAGRATIS

(*Athens, Greece*)

ABSTRACT

In this study the authors analyse the findings of VER in 25 patients suffering from retrobulbar neuritis due to multiple sclerosis.

They stress the diagnostic value of measuring the implicit time of the VER which is greater than in other pathological conditions and they point out that, in these cases, even with eyes that are at least clinically sound, the implicit time, is in a high percentage of cases, greater than normal.

INTRODUCTION

Disturbances of the visual evoked response (VER) in multiple sclerosis and in particular of the implicit time of VER appearance have been the object of studies by numerous investigators during the last decade (Asselman, Chadwick & Marsden 1975; Feinsod & Hoyt 1975; Halliday 1975; 1976; Halliday, McDonald & Mushin 1972; Hennerici, Wenzel & Freud 1974; Korol & Babel 1979; McDonald 1976; Moschos, Palimeris, Panagakis & Pagratis 1979).

A major impetus to these investigations has been given by the pattern stimulator and the registration of VER, by means of which the disturbances of the implicit time become more evident than in VER registration after repetitive flash stimulation.

The present paper, which originated in the Athens University Eye Clinic, represents a study of the implicit time of the VER in retrobulbar neuritis and includes a discussion of the results of this study.

MATERIAL AND METHODS

Our investigation concerns 25 cases with retrobulbar neuritis in various stages, etiologically attributed to multiple sclerosis. Of these cases 10 represent the second or third recurrence of the disease, while in the remaining 15 cases the optic nerve was affected for the first time.

Doc. Ophthal. Proc. Series, Vol. 27, ed. by H. Spekreijse & P.A. Apkarian   149

© *1981 Dr W. Junk Publishers, The Hague/Boston/London*

Visual acuity varied, ranging from 7 to 8/10 in 6 cases, from 4 to 6/10 in 3 cases, from 2 to 3/10 in 10 cases, while in 6 cases it was barely 1/20 to 1/10.

For the registration of the VER an amplifier type NT6 of the British manufacturer MEDELEC was used, which is equipped with an electronic averager. Stimulation of the eye was effected with a pattern stimulator which produces patterns of varying intensity.

In all 25 cases the VER were studied in both the affected and other, clinically at least, sound eye.

RESULTS

In all the cases the VER registered from the affected eye showed marked disturbances of a) the morphology, b) the amplitude, and c) the implicit time of the appearance of the waves, which became increasingly distinct the more the involvement of the optic nerve had progressed and visual acuity had diminished.

Thus, with increasing severity of the disease the wave-shape disturbances correspondingly tend towards diminution of the amplitude of wave III, which in 10 cases with visual acuity from 2 to 3/10 was extremely low, varying between 2 to 4μV, while in the 6 cases with visual acuity from 1/20 to 1/10 it was hardly registered at all. In none of the cases of developing neuritis was the VER completely extinguished.

Regarding the implicit time of appearance of the VER, this amounted in 9 cases to 130–140 ms. In 10 of the remaining 16 cases it varied between 140 to 150 ms. (Fig. 1). In the remaining 6 cases measurement of the implicit

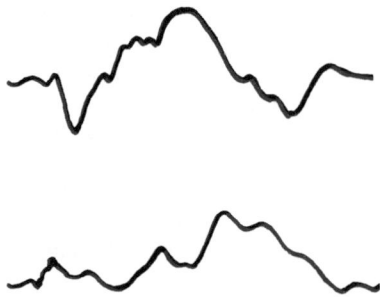

Fig. 1. Pattern responses recorded in the actue phase of optic neuritis in a 24 year-old man. From the left eye, (lower trace) the pattern response is very low and the latent time is delayed. It is interesting that latent time of pattern response from the right eye (upper trace) is also delayed.

time of the waves proved impossible, as these were either of extremely low amplitude or almost extinguished. Given the fact that the normal implicit time of VER appearance is 100 to 110 ms, the increase of the time registered is about 30 to 35% above normal.

After steroid treatment, in the 15 cases in which the disease had affected the nerve for the first time, visual acuity was almost completely restored and the morphology and amplitude of the VER reverted to normal, but the implicit time remained excessive (Fig. 2). In the remaining 10 cases with second or third recurrance the improvement of wave amplitude and

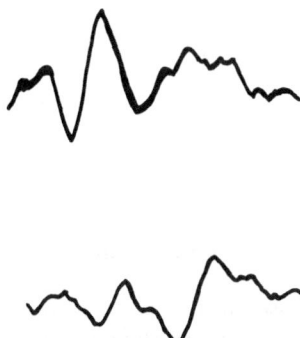

Fig. 2. Pattern responses recorded in the same patient as Fig. 1 two weeks after treatment with corticosteroids. Note the improvement of latency of VER in the right eye (upper trace). The responses from the left eye (lower trace) have recovered in amplitude paralleling the improvement of visual acuity, but the latent time shows no improvement.

morphology of the VER was proportionate to the degree of recovery of visual acuity. On the contrary, the implicit time remained clearly abnormal, although it showed a slight tendency to revert to normal.

Of particular interest is the study of the VER of the other eye, which clinically at least, was sound with visual acuity of 10/10 and unimpaired visual fields. While the morphology and the amplitude of the waves were normal, the implicit time of their appearance in the 17 cases, i.e. in 68%, was abnormal, ranging from 115 to 125 ms (Fig. 1).

DISCUSSION

From the study of our cases it emerges that the implicit time of the appearance of the VER is affected and increases considerably prior to the manifestation of the clinical symptoms or the disturbances of VER morphology and amplitude (Fig. 3). As the disease progresses disturbances of the implicit time become increasingly marked so that in advanced stages the implicit time may show an increase by 30 to 35% above normal, ranging between 130 to 150 ms, while simultaneously a reduction of the wave amplitude may be observed. At this stage there is, of course, from the clinical point of view already a significantly reduced visual acuity and a distinct central scotoma.

A fact worth noting is that, contrary to the observations of Halliday (1976), none of our cases in which the disease was fairly advanced and where visual acuity was even as low as 1/20, showed a complete extinction of the VER. Of particular interest in the cases of unilateral involvement is the

151

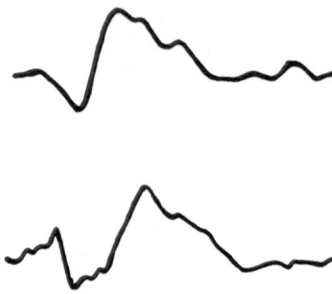

Fig. 3. Pattern responses in a case with multiple sclerosis without visual complaints. Note the delay of the latent time in the left eye (lower trace).

study of the implicit time of the other, clinically and electrophysiologically, sound eye.

In our cases an increase of the implicit time was established in 68%, whereas other investigators, such as Hennerici et al. (1974), Asselman et al. (1975), Halliday (1976) Halliday et al. (1977), Cook & Arden (1977), Chain et al. (1977), Feinsod & Hoyt (1977) and others report increased implicit time in as high as 85 to 93% of the cases.

Finally it is a characteristic aspect that when the crisis of the disease subsides, visual acuity and the amplitude of the VER waves may become normal again, either totally or partially, while the increase of the implicit time remains unaffected by the improvement of the clinical picture.

As an explanation of the fact that the increased implicit time remains undiminished in demyelinating diseases, various opinions have been put forward from time to time (McDonald & Sears 1970; Mastaglia, Black & Cala 1977; Cook & Arden 1977), although none of them offers adequate elucidation of the phenomenon. More recently Korol and Babel (1979) have assumed the possible existence of a system of accelerated transmission of the visual stimulus, which is of extramuscular origin and more vulnerable in multiple sclerosis than the macular bundle. This system would explain the phenomenon that often visual acuity and the amplitude of the VER are normal, while the implicit time of the appearance of the waves of the VER remains abnormal.

REFERENCES

Asselman, P., Chadwick, D.W. & Marsden, C.D. Visual evoked responses in the diagnosis and management of patients suspected of multiple sclerosis. Brian 98: 261–282 (1975).

Chain, F., Mallecourt, J., Leblank, & Lhermit, F. Apport de l'enregistrement des potentiels éviqués visuels au diagnostic de la sclérose en plaques. Révue neurol. (Paris) 113: 81–88 (1977).

Cook, J.H. & Arden, G.B. Unilateral retrobulbar neuritis; A comparison of evoked potentials and psychophysical measurements. In: Visual evoked potentials in man: new developments (Ed. J.E. Desmedt). Claredon Press, Oxford. 450–457 (1977).

Feinsod, M. & Hoyt, W.F. Subclinical optic neuropathy in multiple sclerosis. J. Neurol. Neurosurg. Psychiat. 38: 1109–1114 (1975).

Halliday, A.M., McDonald, W.I. & Mushin, J. Delayed VER in optic neuritis. Lancet 1: 982–985 (1972).

Halliday, A.M. the effect of lesions of the visual pathway and cerebrum on the visual evoked response. In: Evoked Potentials, Handbook of Electroencephalography and Clinical Neurophysiology Vol. 8A (Ed. W.S. Van Leuven, F.H. Lopes da Silva & A. Kamp) 119–129 (1975).

Halliday, A.M. Visually evoked responses in optic nerve diseases. Trans. Ophthal. Soc. U.K. 96: 372 (1976).

Halliday, A.M., McDonald, W.I., Mushin, J. Visual evoked potentials in patients with demyelinating disease. In: Visual evoked potentials in man: new developments (Ed. J.E. Desmedt). Clarendon Press, Oxford. 357–438 (1977).

Hennerici, M., Wenzel, D. & Freud, H.J. The comparison of small side rectangle and checkboard stimulation of the evaluation of delayed VER in patients suspected of multiple sclerosis. Brain 96: 69–78 (1974).

Korol, S. & Babel, J. Les potentiels évoqués visuels et l'ophtalmoscopie à la lumière anerythre dans les formes subcliniques des névrites rétrobulbaires de la sclérose en plaques. J. Fr. Ophtal. 2: 463–470 (1979).

Mastaglia, F.L., Black, J.L. & Cala, L.A. Evoked potentials, saccadic velocities and computerised tomography in diagnosis of multiple sclerosis. Br. Med. J. 1: 1315–1317 (1977).

McDonald, W.I. Conduction in the optic nerve. Trans. Ophthal. Soc. U.K. 96: 352 (1976).

McDonald, W.I. & Sears, T.A. The effect of experimental demyelination on conduction in the central nervous system. Brain 93: 538–598 (1970).

Moschos, M., Palimeris, G., Panagakis, E. & Pagratis, H. The diagnostic value of the implicit time of VER in the diagnosis of retrobulbar neuritis. Bull. Hell. Ophthal. Soc. (1979).

Authors' address:

Athens University Eye Clinic,

National Ophthalmological Centre of Athens,

170 Messoghion Street,

Cholargos-Athens, Greece

PART THREE

GENETICS AND DEGENERATION

VISUAL EVOKED POTENTIAL (VEP) METHODS OF DETECTING MISROUTED OPTIC PROJECTIONS

D. CREEL, H. SPEKREIJSE & D. REITS

(*Salt Lake City, U.S.A./Amersterdam, The Netherlands*)

ABSTRACT

Misrouting of retinogeniculostriate projections associated with retinal hypopigmentation has been found to be a general phenomenon throughout mammals, including humans. The distinctive finding when testing human albinos is the dramatic change in the VEP between hemispheres when effects of binocular stimulation are compared with monocular stimulation. We have compared the efficacy of luminance and pattern onset/offset, noise modulated light, pattern reversal, and pattern appearance/disappearance stimuli in detecting misrouted optic fibers. Pattern appearance/disappearance were found superior to other stimuli at detecting anomalies of misrouting of retinogeniculostriate projections. As a group, humans with retinal hypopigmentation have poor VEPs to disappearance or pattern reversal stimuli. Acuity and nystagmus seem to be the two variables most indicative of poor pattern reversal responses. Appearance/disappearance (onset/offset) pattern stimuli are more versatile for detection of abnormalities in the visual system than pattern reversal stimuli.

INTRODUCTION

One of the clinical applications of the scalp recorded visual evoked potential (VEP) is to detect pathology of geniculostriate projections. Most clinical abnormalities involving thalamocortical projections are the result of trauma, tumors or vascular accidents. Each patient's disruption of geniculostriate projections is idiosyncratic. Due to the random nature of specific location of the pathology it is difficult to generalize among patients.

A model system for geniculostriate abnormalities is the mammalian albino. The human albino is a model for several concomitant ophthalmological conditions: defects of acuity due to both optics and to foveal hypoplasia, nystagmus, strabismus, and misrouting of retinal ganglion fibers (Coleman, Sydnor, Wolbarsht & Bessler 1979; Creel, O'Donnell & Witkop 1978; Creel, Witkop & King 1974; Taylor 1978). All mammals, including humans, that lack retinal melanin pigmentation have misrouted retinogeniculostriate projections. The misrouted retinal fibers appear to be genetically engineered and consistently expressed throughout albinic mammals.

The original suggestion that anatomical differences may exist between albino and pigmented members of the same species was made by Sheridan (1965). Sheridan observed differences in interhemispheric transfer of visual information among 'split-brain' albino and ocularly pigmented rats. Sheridan hypothesized that, '. . . the paucity of uncrossed fibers that characterized rodents in general is even further reduced in the albino'. This hypothesis was verified anatomically in rats by Lund (1965). Giolli & Guthrie (1969) reported the same phenomenon in albino rabbits. Guillery's (1969) finding that the Siamese cat has an unusual nondecussated optic system prompted Creel (1971a, b) to suggest that since the Siamese cat possesses a mutant albino allele at the C locus, there may be a genetically determined misrouting of optic fibers of albino mammals that is a general trans-species phenomenon which includes humans. The abnormal optic system of albinic mammals has been verified in nine species: cat, ferret, guinea pig, mink, mouse, rabbit, rat, tiger and human (Creel & Giolli 1976; Giolli & Creel 1973; Guillery 1971; Guillery & Kaas 1971, 1973; Guillery, Okoro & Witkop 1975; Guillery, Scott, Cattanach & Deol 1973; Sanderson, Guillery & Shackelford 1974).

Fifteen years of anatomical and electrophysiological investigations have demonstrated that the abnormality is correlated with hypopigmentation of the retina. The misrouted retinal ganglion fibers originate in the first 15–20° of temporal retina. Instead of coursing through the optic chiasm and terminating in the ipsilateral hemisphere, most retinal ganglion fibers from the first 15–20° of temporal retina erroneously decussate and terminate in visual centers of the contralateral hemisphere (Guillery 1974). In the dorsal lateral geniculate nucleus (LGNd) this results in disruption of the normally distinct laminations of decussated and nondecussated retinal ganglion fibers. The misrouted temporal fibers that erroneously decussate at the chiasm terminate in laminae normally occupied only by nondecussating fibers, fragmenting these laminae. The misrouted fibers disrupt the normal point to point register of the retina in the LGNd. The effect of this is to disturb the anatomical substrate for binocular vision, initially in the LGNd and subsequently at the cortex. For a diagrammatic representation of this see Guillery (1974).

It was demonstrated that evoked potentials recorded from the visual cortex of rats, guinea pigs and Siamese cats reflect the misrouting of non-decussated optic fibers (Creel, Dustman & Beck 1970; Creel & Giolli 1972; Creel 1971a, b). The evoked potential technique provides a method for evaluating similar visual anomalies in humans. A significant asymmetry between VEPs recorded from each hemisphere of monocularly stimulated human albinos, as compared to normally pigmented humans, is indicative of misrouted optic projections.

Several studies, with a combined number of 70 oculocutaneous (total) albinos or ocular albinos, have shown that using flash or checkerboard flash stimuli results in evidence of misrouting in 70% of the patients (Coleman, Sydnor, Wolbarsht & Bessler 1979; Creel, O'Donnell & Witkop 1978; Creel,

Witkop & King 1974). The failure to detect misrouting in 30% of patients was interpreted to be due to anatomical and genetic variability or to insensitivity of the scalp recorded VEP (Creel, O'Donnell & Witkop 1978).

Our task in this investigation was to study several methods of visual stimulation to determine the most effective stimulus for detecting misrouted retinogeniculostriate projections in humans with retinal hypopigmentation.

METHODS AND MATERIALS

We tested 8 oculocutaneous albinos and 7 ocular albinos. Fourteen were between ages 16 and 30, and one was 58 years old. Complete clinical examinations included genetic history, hairbulb incubation tests and skin biopsy (Witkop, Quevedo & Fitzpatrick 1978), corrected and uncorrected visual acuities, laser retinometry, TNO random dot stereograms and Ishihara color plates. Five were tested for red/green matching on the Nagel anomaloscope.

During VEP recording all patients were tested with corrected vision. As a group albinos have poor visual acuity that can not be corrected to normal 6/6 (20/20) vision. However, several individuals in this group did have vision which could be corrected to 6/9 in at least one eye. One ocular albino and one oculocutaneous albino were also among those rare albinos without observable binocular nystagmus. Data as a function of the severity of nystagmus will be presented in the Discussion. All 15 albinos failed the TNO stereogram plates. None of the albinos showed defects of color vision except perhaps a minor extended red/green matching range of a few units on the Nagel anomaloscope.

A TV-screen (Sony CVM-1810 E, 50 Hz) subtending $20 \times 15°$ was used to display a white and black checkerboard pattern of 100% contrast with checks ranging from 15' to 110'. During recording of the VEPs to either pattern reversal or pattern appearance/disappearance the subjects were asked to fixate upon a 10' pink square, which was generally positioned in the center of the screen. The size of the fixation square was enlarged for subjects with poor visual acuity.

The VEPs were derived from 5 Ag-AgCl electrodes attached with collodion to the scalp at positions O_1, O_z, O_2 and at positions along the same plane halfway from O_1 to T_5 and O_2 to T_6. We refer to these positions as O_3 and O_4. Reference for all electrodes was linked ears (A_1 and A_2). The common ground electrode was at C_z. The bandwidth of the EEG amplifiers was 0.3 to 35 Hz. The cut-off frequency was set by a fourth-order Butterworth filter. If you wish to estimate the latencies from the figures, the VEP peak latencies should be reduced by 14 msec to adjust for the phase shift introduced by this low-pass filter. An HP-2100 computer was used to average the pattern VEPs. Depending on the stimulus condition 60–300 VEPs were averaged.

The cycle period for both pattern reversal and appearance/disappearance stimuli was 800 msec. For pattern reversal each check was black for 400 msec and white for 400 msec. Two stimulus durations were used for pattern appearance/disappearance: 300 msec of black and white checks, 500 msec

159

of a uniform grey with the same mean illuminance as the checks; and 180 msec black and white checks, 620 msec of grey (150 asb). Stimulus durations are indicated on each Figure. The effect of longer pattern onset in the appearance/disappearance stimulus is only to further separate the 'off' response from the 'onset' response.

A clear indicator of hemispheric laterality of a VEP is to examine the difference between potentials recorded from O_1 versus O_2. For each stimulus condition we subtracted O_2 from O_1 to display the difference potential. These are indicated on each Figure.

RESULTS

Fig. 1 depicts pattern appearance/disappearance VEPs of a normally pigmented subject following binocular and monocular right eye stimulation. In this and all subsequent figures only the data obtained with 50' checks

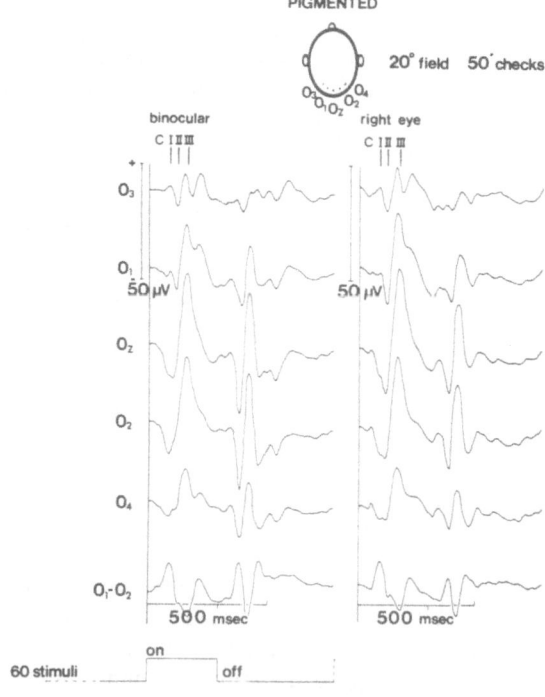

Fig. 1. Pattern onset/offset of a checkboard stimulus. This pigmented subject was atypical in that he has a large asymmetry between hemispheres with binocular stimulation. Note the difference potential between electrodes O_1 and O_2, and that there is no change in the difference potential following monocular stimulation, except for an overall attenuation of the responses.

160

(the check size that proved to be the most effective for generating pattern VEPs in albinos) will be presented. There are several points to note in this Figure. The VEP has a large positive-negative-positive onset response (the so-called CI, CII, CIII components) and a strong 'off' response to disappearance. The CI component has been shown by Jeffreys and Axford (1972) to originate in area 17; the other two components seem to come from prestriate areas. This particular subject has a small CI component which is asymmetrically lateral. Secondly, the O_1-O_2 difference potential indicates considerable hemispheric asymmetry following binocular stimulation, but essentially no change with monocular stimulation. Most individuals show some asymmetry even with binocular stimulation although not usually this much.

Asymmetry is probably a combination of asymmetry of electrode placement and asymmetry of cortical sulci. So asymmetry as such can never be used as a decisive criterion for misrouting. It is the *change* in the asymmetry of the response when comparing binocular versus monocular stimulation that should be considered. This is immediately evident when the effects of monocular versus binocular stimulation in Fig. 1 are compared with those of the albino in Fig. 2. Stimulation of the central $20°$ of the left eye produces a CI component primarily in the right hemisphere, and stimulation of the right eye produces a CI component in the left hemisphere. It is the change in polarity of the CI component (indicated by arrows in Fig. 2) which is indicative of the observation that most retinal fibres originating in the central $20°$ decussate and project to the contralateral hemisphere. Fourteen out of fifteen albinos demonstrated significant hemispheric asymmetry in the CI component using appearance/disappearance stimulation. One ocular albino who had some foveal reflex showed no misrouting with the stimulus techniques used in this study. Secondly, notice that the albino's response is not as complex, and especially notice the poor 'off'' response to disappearance of the pattern.

We were surprised to find that most albinos have both a poor 'off' response, and a poor or nonexistent pattern reversal response. Half of the albinos simply did not have a definitive response to pattern reversal. Fig. 3 depicts an extreme example. This ocular albino was representative of the 'typical' albino in that most albinos have a simple response to checkerboard appearance. Their VEPs mainly have only a strong CI component and very poor CII or CIII. This subject is also typical of albinos in that his VEP has no 'off' response to disappearance, and dramatically in this case, no pattern reversal response. Half the albinos show an absence of both an 'off' response, and an absence of a pattern reversal response. The other half of albinos show some degree of an 'off' response and pattern reversal response. A few, perhaps 20%, have a fully developed (negative-positive-negative complex) pattern reversal response with binocular stimulation, although of a small amplitude compared with their appearance response. Whereas the CI in these appearance responses showed the misrouting, this could not be detected from their reversal responses.

DISCUSSION

The most important result of this study emphasizes the importance of stimulus parameters. In the case of detecting misrouted retinal fibres which

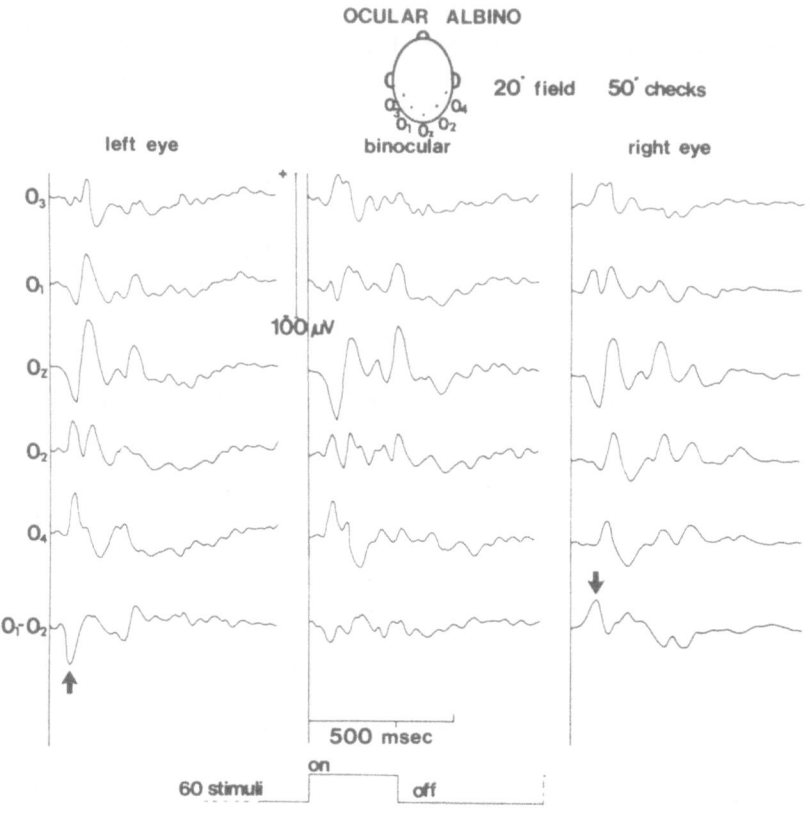

Fig. 2. Pattern onset/offset of a checkerboard stimulus in an albino. This subject demonstrates the more typical symmetry found with binocular stimulation in most people. Note, however, the difference potential between electrodes O_1 and O_2 following monocular stimulation. The first component as indicated by arrows reverses polarity when stimulation is changed from one eye to the other.

correlate with albinism, flash and checkerboard flash stimuli yield a detection rate of approximately 70% among human albinos (Coleman, Sydnor, Wolbarsht & Bessler 1979; Creel, O'Donnell & Witkop 1978; Creel, Witkop & King 1974). However, the present study shows that a detection rate of over 90% can be reached by using appearance/disappearance stimuli. Furthermore, pattern reversal stimulation proved to be even less effective than flash stimulation because it does not clearly indicate misrouting. Therefore, it is not an adequate stimulus for the human albino visual system, even when a larger stimulus field is used. Appearance/disappearance is superior to flash, patterned flash, noise modulated light and pattern reversal in detecting anomalous geniculostriate projections that exist in human albinos.

Pattern reversal stimuli have proven to be very effective for providing an overall measure of integrity of the visual system (Halliday, McDonald & Mushin 1973; Asselman, Chadwick & Marsden 1975; Regan, Milner & Heron

162

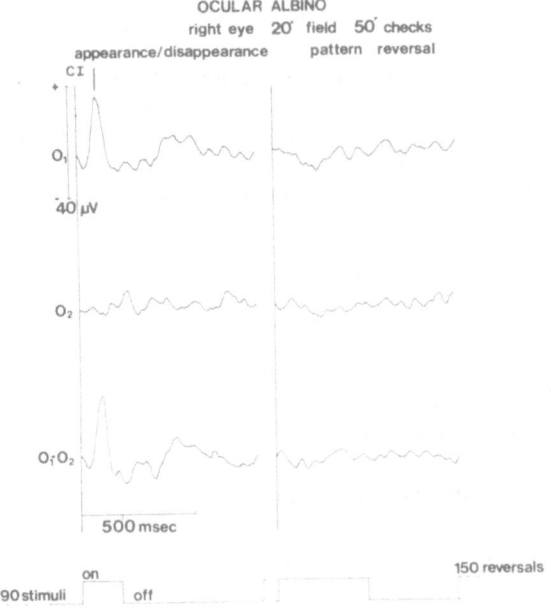

OCULAR ALBINO
right eye 20' field 50' checks
appearance/disappearance   pattern reversal

Fig. 3. Pattern onset/offset and pattern reversal of a checkerboard stimulus. Right eye stimulation produces a simple response in the left hemisphere indicative of misrouted optic fibres in albinos. Note the absence of a pattern reversal response also characteristic of the majority of albinos.

1976; Duwaer & Spekreijse 1978). Its use as a diagnostic indicator of demyelinization, such as in multiple sclerosis, has been the major clinical contribution of scalp recorded VEPs. However, appearance/disappearance seems to be also more effective in testing patients with multiple sclerosis since a definite response can be obtained in more patients with this than with the reversal stimulus (Riemslag, Spekreijse & Van Walbeek, this volume).

There are several effects of visual anomalies associated with albinism in mammals. Albino mammals lack the anatomical substrate for binocular vision which is easily demonstrated by stereogram tests. Albinos also have poor acuity, a high incidence of strabismus, and of nystagmus (Witkop, Quevedo & Fitzpatrick 1978; Taylor 1978). The question is, which of the abnormalities of vision is most closely associated with poor pattern reversal VEPs?

To isolate the critical effect we retested albinos and patients with symptoms similar to albinism: achromatopsia, congenital strabismus and congential nystagmus. All three have poorly developed foveae, poor acuity and often nystagmus. However, they do not demonstrate misrouting of retinogeniculostriate projections, and they also have some stereovision within the limits of their individual acuities. As a group, all patients with poor acuity and nystagmus were found to have at least a clear appearance

163

response. Thus, poor pattern reversal VEPs are probably not most directly related to cortical disorganization.

The best clues for the cause of poor pattern reversal responses were obtained in patients with relatively good acuity (6/9; 20/30). This level of visual acuity is sufficient for normal pattern reversal VEPs to even 20′ checks. One patient was a 10-year-old female with congenital nystagmus. Like most patients with nystagmus, she could reduce her nystagmus by tilting her head to a favourable position. With normal nystagmus she had essentially a non-existent pattern reversal VEP, with reduced nystagmus she had a pattern reversal response. The other patient was a 23-year-old female tyrosinase-positive albino who was exceptional both for her 6/9 visual acuity, and that she had no apparent nystagmus with binocular vision. Covering her left eye produced a fine pendular occlusion nystagmus in her right eye, and covering her right eye produced a coarse pendular occlusion nystagmus in her left eye. Her pattern reversal VEP was normal with binocular stimulation, but barely recognizable when evoked by monocular stimulation with coarse nystagmus. Monocular viewing with fine nystagmus produced an intermediary VEP. We cannot determine, of course, whether the effects of nystagmus are also due to disruption of the response related to nystagmus *per se* or that nystagmus is simply further reducing acuity. The important point is that pattern reversal is an ineffective stimulus for patients with either poor acuity or nystagmus, whereas the appearance stimulus still evokes a clear onset response.

In both research and clinical application pattern reversal and appearance/disappearance stimuli are often used as if they give interchangeable information. They definitely do not. We should reassess the use of pattern reversal stimuli. Appearance/disappearance (onset/offset) pattern stimuli are more versatile, and in all cases studied more efficient at identifying pathology in the visual system.

REFERENCES

Asselman, P., Chadwick, D.W. & Marsden, C.D. Visual evoked responses in the diagnosis and management of patients suspected of multiple sclerosis. Brain 98: 261−282 (1975).

Coleman, J., Sydnor, C.E., Wolbarsht, M.L. & Bessler, M. Abnormal visual pathways in human albinos studied with visually evoked potentials. Exp. Neurol. 65: 667−679 (1979).

Creel, D. Visual system anomaly associated with albinism in the cat. Nature, Lond. 231: 465−466 (1971a).

Creel, D. Differences of ipsilateral and contralateral visually evoked responses in the cat: strains compared. J. comp. physiol. Psychol. 77: 161−165 (1971b).

Creel, D., Dustman, R.E. & Beck, E.C. Differences in visually evoked responses in albino versus hooded rats. Exp. Neurol. 29: 298−309 (1970).

Creel, D. & Giolli, R.A. Retinogeniculostriate projections in guinea pigs: Albino and pigmented strains compared. Exp. Neurol. 36: 411−425 (1972).

Creel, D. & Giolli, R.A. Retinogeniculostriate projections in albino and ocularly pigmented rats. J. Comp. Neurol. 166: 445−456 (1976).

Creel, D., O'Donnell, F.E. & Witkop, C.J., Jr. Visual system anomalies in human ocular albinos. Science 201: 931−933 (1978).

Creel, D., Witkop, C.J., Jr. & King, R.A. Asymmetric visually evoked potentials in human albinos: Evidence for visual system anomalies. Invest. Ophthalmol. Vis. Sci. 13: 430–440 (1974).

Duwaer, A.L. & Spekreijse, H. Latency of luminance and contrast evoked potentials in multiple sclerosis patients. Electroenceph. clin. Neurophysiol. 45: 244–258 (1978).

Giolli, R.A. & Creel, D. The primary optic projections in pigmented and albino guinea pigs: an experimental degeneration study. Brain. Res. 55: 25–39 (1973).

Giolli, R.A. & Guthrie, M.D. The primary optic projections in the rabbit: An experimental degeneration study. J. Comp. Neurol. 136: 99–126 (1969).

Guillery, R.W. An abnormal retinogeniculate projection in Siamese cats. Brain Res. 14: 739–741 (1969).

Guillery, R.W. An abnormal retinogeniculate projection in the albino ferret (Mustela furo). Brain Res. 33: 482–485 (1971).

Guillery, R.W. Visual pathways in albinos. Sci. Am. 230: 44–54 (1974).

Guillery, R.W. & Kaas, J.H. A study of normal and congenitally abnormal retinogeniculate projections in cats. J. Comp. Neurol. 143: 73–100 (1971).

Guillery, R.W. & Kaas, J.H. Genetic abnormality of the visual pathways in a 'white' tiger. Science 180: 1287–1289 (1973).

Guillery, R.W., Okoro, A.N. & Witkop, C.J., Jr. Abnormal visual pathways in the brain of a human albino. Brain Res. 96: 373–377 (1975).

Guillery, R.W., Scott, G.L., Cattanach, B.M. & Deol, M.S. Genetic mechanisms determining the central visual pathways of mice. Science 179: 1014–1015 (1973).

Halliday, A.M., McDonald, W.I. & Mushin, J. Visual evoked response in the diagnosis of multiple sclerosis. Br. Med. J. IV: 661–664 (1973).

Jeffreys, D.A. & Axford, J.G. Source locations of pattern-specific components of human visual evoked potentials. Exp. Brain Res. 16: 1–40 (1972).

Lund, R.D. Uncrossed visual pathways of hooded and albino rat. Science 149: 1506–1507 (1965).

Regan, D., Milner, B.A. & Heron, J.R. Delayed visual perception and delayed visual evoked potentials in the spinal form of multiple sclerosis and retrobulbar neuritis. Brain 99: 43–46 (1976).

Riemslag, F.C.C., Spekreijse, H. & Van Walbeek, H. Contrast evoked potential diagnosis of multiple sclerosis: A comparison of various contrast stimuli. In: 18th ISCEV Symposium. (Ed. H. Spekreijse and P.A. Apkarian) Junk, The Hague. (Doc. Ophthal. Proc. Series Vol. 27) This volume (1981).

Sanderson, K.J., Guillery, R.W. & Shackelford, R.M. Congenitally abnormal visual pathways in mink (Mustela vison) with reduced retinal pigment. J. Comp. Neurol. 154: 225–248 (1974).

Sheridan, C.L. Interocular transfer of brightness and pattern discriminations in normal and corpus-callosum-sectioned rats. J. comp. physiol. Psychol. 59: 292–294 (1965).

Taylor, W.O.G. Visual disabilities of oculocutaneous albinism and their alleviation. Trans. Ophthal. Soc. U.K. 98: 423–445 (1978).

Witkop, C.J., Jr., Quevedo, W.C., Jr. & Fitzpatrick, T.B. Albinism, In: The Metabolic Basis of Inherited Disease, 4th edition. (Ed. J.B. Stanbury, J.B. Wyngaarden & D.S. Fredricksen) McGraw-Hill, New York 282–317 (1978).

Authors' addresses:
D. Creel
V.A. Medical Center,
Salt Lake City,
Utah 84148, U.S.A.

and

H. Spekreijse & D. Reits
The Netherlands Ophthalmic Research Institute,
P. O. Box 6411,
1005 EK Amsterdam, The Netherlands

VISUAL EVOKED POTENTIAL AND PSYCHOPHYSICAL FINDINGS IN DOMINANT HEREDITARY OPTIC ATROPHY

S.J. CREWS & G.F.A. HARDING

(Birmingham, England)

ABSTRACT

Twenty-seven members of families with dominant hereditary optic atrophy were investigated. Visual acuity, Goldmann perimetry, Farnsworth Munsell 100-hue tests, and visual evoked potentials to flash and pattern-reversal were performed. All except the Goldmann perimetry showed a significant association with the presence of optic atrophy. The flash VEP showed a positive-negative-positive response in most of the affected patients.

INTRODUCTION

Dominant hereditary optic atrophy is more common than the Leber's type of optic atrophy with which it is sometimes confused. It has also been confused with congenital tritanopia. The condition has an insidious onset, reduction of vision often being found in the first decade of life. The method of inheritance is autosomal dominant but it shows variable expression, and this, in addition to the difficulty in obtaining accurate family histories, often leads to unnecessary neurological investigation.

Distance vision is often worse than near vision and in some families there is an associated myopia. Studies of the visual fields in these patients frequently show small defects which are difficult to record, the most common of which is a centrocaecal scotoma (Smith, Pokorny & Ernest 1977). The most consistent early diagnostic sign is a blue defect of colour vision which may precede optic nerve pallor. As the condition progresses red-green discrimination may be affected and later complete colour blindness ensues (Krill, Smith & Pokorny, 1971). The optic atrophy is only partial and temporal in distribution, making diagnosis of abnormality difficult if psychophysical tests are equivocal.

In studies of Leber's hereditary optic atrophy abnormalities of the visual evoked potential have been reported (Harding, Crews & Good 1979). These patients frequently show an unusual negative response at a latency of 100 m.secs. It has been suggested by Halliday (1976) that this negative component is related to the presence of a central scotoma.

It appeared sensible therefore to attempt a study of patients with dominant hereditary optic atrophy and to compare the VEP to both flash and pattern-reversal and the psychophysical findings.

METHOD

We have so far studied twenty-seven patients from six families with dominant hereditary optic atrophy, seventeen of whom were affected. Eleven members of one family were studied and in two other families, eight and four members were investigated respectively. In twenty-three of the twenty-seven patients all tests were completed on the same day.

Corrected visual acuity was assessed for both near and distance but for the purpose of this analysis, if the distance vision was worse than 6/12 then the visual acuity was rated as abnormal.

The Goldmann permeter was used to record the visual fields. The scotomata were analysed in terms of the reduction of cortical representation which would ensue as suggested by Drasdo (1977), Fig. 1. Superimposed on

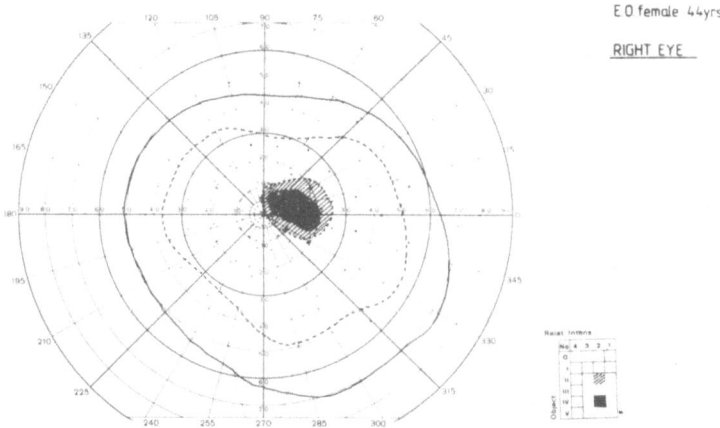

Fig. 1. This figure shows the method of scoring the field defects. Each dot represents a loss of 1% of neural representation. It can be seen that this method of scoring preferentially highlights central scotomata and is clearly the appropriate criteria for quantifying neural loss. The scoring system was developed by Drasdo (1977). The example given is one of the fields of an affected patient of family W.

the fields is a graticule of dots. Each dot represents an area in which a local scotoma would cause a loss of 1% of cortical and neural representation. If the loss was greater than 5% then the fields were rated as abnormal. It will be seen that this method of scoring preferentially rates scotomata which are central since these have a greater cortical representation than those in the periphery. For allowing us to use this method which he has developed we are most grateful to Neville Drasdo.

Colour vision was assessed by the Farnsworth Munsell 100-hue Test. The total error score was compared to the norms for the age and any tritanopic tendency or defect was noted.

The visual evoked potentials were recorded from electrodes placed over the right and left occiputs, referred to the ipsilateral central electrode. Flash stimulation was given monocularly to each eye at an intensity of 1,363 candelas/metre^2. A reversing checkerboard pattern, each check subtending a visual angle of 50' of arc was reversed at a rate of twice per second. The resulting VEPs were compared with normal aged matched controls and the latency, amplitude and symmetry rated as normal or abnormal. The presence of a negative response at 100 m.secs. to either stimulus was particularly noted.

RESULTS AND DISCUSSION

The visual evoked potential was abnormal in every affected patient in the entire series. The most common finding ($p < 0.01$) was a positive-negative-positive (PNP) response at about 100 m.seconds to flash stimulation (Fig. 2). Although similar findings were sometimes seen in the pattern-reversal response, this was not significantly associated with optic atrophy, and a more common finding was a marked reduction in amplitude, particularly in patients with reduced visual acuity. Surprisingly, PNP responses to flash or pattern-reversal were not associated with central field defects. It is difficult to know whether this peculiar triphasic positive-negative-positive or PNP morphology is produced by a negative replacement of the positive P_2 component or a marked delay in the P_1, N_2 and P_2 components of the VEP.

One of the patients (J.Mc) presented initially as a child with slightly reduced vision, constricted visual fields, reduced macular function on the Freidmann Visual Analyser and high Farnsworth error scores.

The family history (Fig. 3) indicated a pattern of dominant hereditary optic atrophy and indeed when these other members were investigated they were shown to be suffering from this condition. Her mother and siblings however did not show diagnostic signs.

On subsequent re-testing, her Goldmann field, macular function and Farnsworth score steadily improved to normal. Her visual evoked potential was consistently normal for the age and did not show a PNP response.

Her two cousins were also investigated. Their ages were only 6 and 11 respectively. The younger child had an abnormal Farnsworth score, but normal visual acuity and Goldmann fields. Her visual evoked potential to flash stimulation was markedly delayed, although the pattern-reversal response was within normal limits (Fig. 4).

The elder child had a slight tritanopic defect, although her total error score on the Farnsworth Munsell Test was within the normal range. Other tests revealed normal results, except the VER which showed marked delay to flash stimulation and a slight delay on pattern-reversal (Fig. 5).

Table 1 shows the summary of the findings on the 27 patients.

170

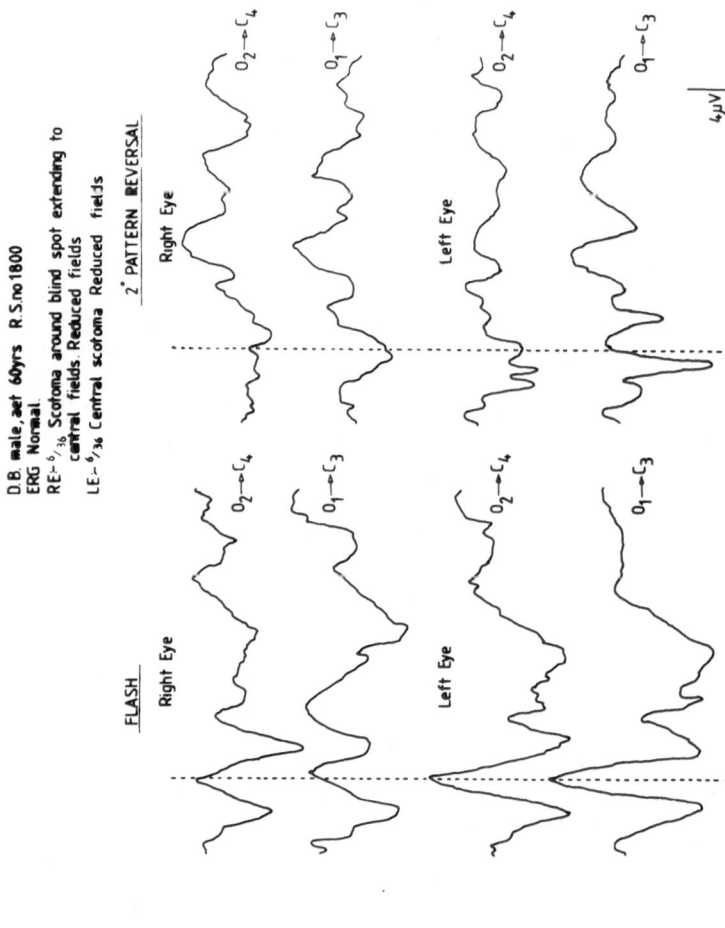

Fig. 2. This figure shows a typical visual evoked potential finding in patients with hereditary optic atrophy of the dominant type. The response to flash stimulation of both the right and left eye is a classical PNP response with the negative component around 100 milliseconds. The responses to pattern reversal are most variable, these from both eyes show a reduction in normal amplitude and only the response from the left occiput on the left eye stimulation shows any evidence of a negativity. These results are from a member of family Be.

FAMILY	SEX	AGE	INITIALS	VA	GOLDMANN	F 100	VEP flash	VEP pattern	OPTIC ATROPHY	COMMENTS
W	M	52	J.W.						+	
	F	44	E.O.						+	
	M	32	P.W.						+	
	F	18	A.O.							
	M	20	S.O.							CATARACTS
	F	10	L.O.						+	
	F	25	D.D.						+	
	F	34	E.B.						+	
	M	6	L.B.						+	LT CONVERGENT SQUINT
	F	4	E.B.							
	F	10	J.D.						+	
Be	M	60	D.B.						+	
	F	40	S.M.						+	
	F	10	J.M.						±	
	M	9	D.M.							
Bo	F	65	C B						+	
	M	35	T B						+	
	F	15	J Mc							FUNCTIONAL
	M	14	Ke.Mc.							LT AMBLYOPIA
	F	12	Ka.Mc.							
	F	43	Jo.Mc.							
	F	11	A. Bo.							
	F	6	J. Bo							
Sp	F	32	K.S.						+	
	F	37	P.B.						+	
F	F	55	F F						+	
Sh.	F	22	C.S.						+	

✕ Both eyes abnormal

╲ One eye abnormal

The families that we have studied are each collated under the family initial. Abnormality on any of the diagnostic tests is shown by a cross. Optic atrophy in the affected members is shown by a plus sign. It can be seen that in all affected patients at least three of the results are abnormal.

The range of defects exhibited by affected members varies between the individuals. It would appear that affected members above 30 years of age show all defects, whereas those up to this age may show a variety of defects

171

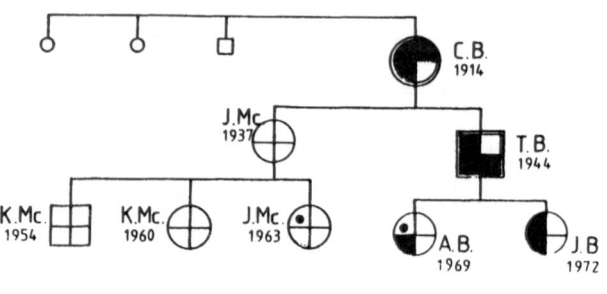

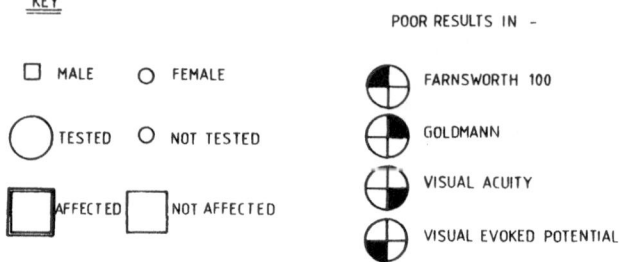

Fig. 3. This figure shows the family Bo. Patient J.Mc. 1963 shows the patient who presented with initially abnormal Farnsworth Munsell F100 Test and since her grandmother showed evideice of hereditary optic atrophy she and her family were thoroughly investigated. Her two cousins (J.Bo and A.Bo) showed some abnormalities on electrophysiological and psychophysical testing.

affecting at most three of the visual acuity, field, F100 or VEP scores. This would support the suggestion of a slowly progressive condition.

In certain of the unaffected patients some of the results are abnormal and in some cases this is due to other ocular conditions.

In young children the visual evoked potential was a most useful objective diagnostic addition to psychophysical testing which requires subjective co-operation. In patient AB the delayed VEP is the only definite abnormal finding in this eleven year old, although the Farnsworth showed early signs and follow-up studies will be necessary to indicate the prognostic value of this finding.

The visual acuity, Farnsworth, flash VEP and pattern reversal VEP results are all significantly related to the presence of optic atrophy ($p < 0.01$). The abnormalities of the Goldmann Field Score were not significantly related.

The visual acuity and Farnsworth scores are also significantly inter-related ($p < 0.01$) an important differentiation with congenital tritanopia in which the visual acuity is not affected.

The flash VEP showed a PNP response in most of the affected patients, but unlike previous suggestions this was not associated with central field loss and cannot therefore be entitled a scotomatous response. The visual evoked potential appears to offer a valuable diagnostic technique for early screening of members of the family with a view to genetic counselling.

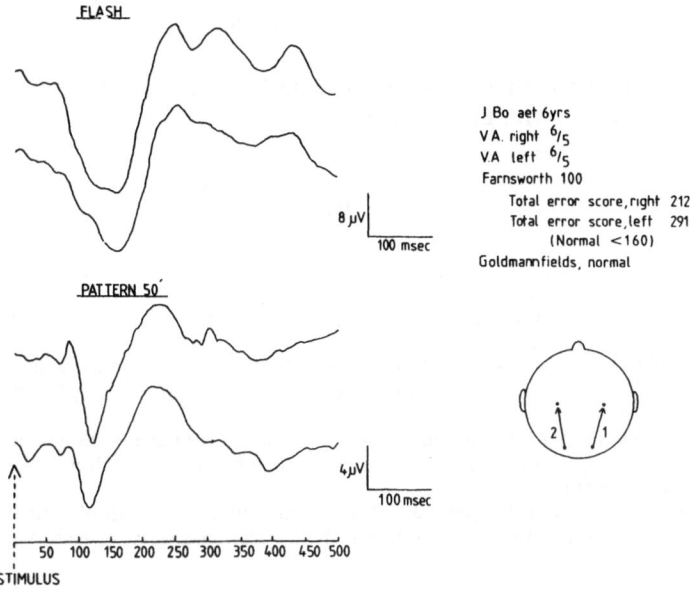

Fig. 4. Patient (J.Bo) aged 6 showed a delayed flash VEP response although pattern-reversal was within normal limits. She also had abnormal F100 score.

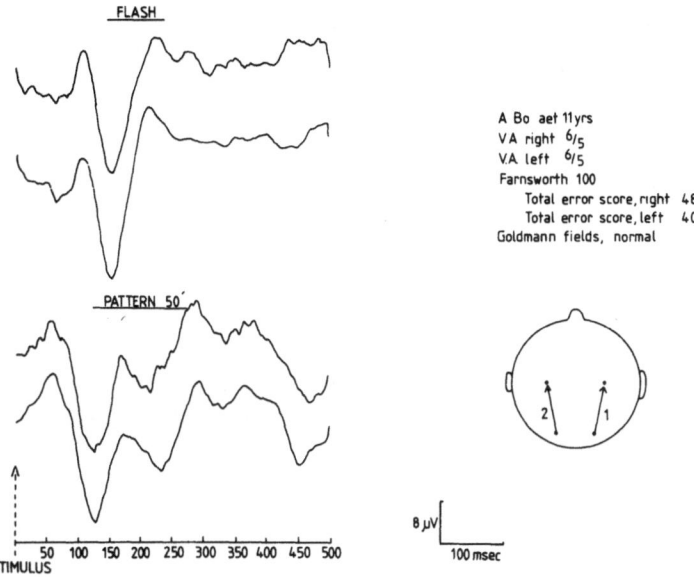

Fig. 5. Patient (A.Bo) aged 11 showed delayed flash and slightly delayed pattern responses. Her Farnsworth Munsell Test revealed a slight tritanopic defect.

ACKNOWLEDGEMENTS

We are grateful to Peter Good for technical assistance and to Miss Jennifer Pullan for her help with the graphics.

REFERENCES

Drasdo, N. The neural representation of visual space. Nature (Lond). 266: 554—556 (1977).

Halliday, A.M. Visually evoked responses in optic nerve disease. Trans. Ophthal. Soc. U.K. 96: 372 (1976).

Harding, G.F.A., Crews, S.J. & Good, P. The VEP as a diagnostic aid in neuro-ophthalmic disease. In: Evoked potentials. (Ed. C. Barber). MTP Press, Lancaster 235—241 (1979).

Krill, A.E., Smith, V.C. & Pokorny, J. Further studies supporting the identity of congenital tritanopia and hereditary dominant atrophy. Invest. Ophthal. Vis. Sci. 10: 457—465 (1971).

Smith, V.C., Pokorny, J. & Ernest, J.T. Primary hereditary optic atrophy. In: Hereditary retinal and choroidal diseases. (Ed. A.E. Krill). Harper and Row, New York. 1109—1134 (1977).

Authors' address:
Clinical Neurophysiology Unit
University of Aston in Birmingham
Birmingham, England

ELECTROPHYSIOLOGICAL STUDIES OF THE VISUAL CAPACITIES AT ADVANCED STAGES OF PHOTORECEPTOR DEGENERATION IN THE RAT

W.K. NOELL, M.C. SALINSKY, R.A. STOCKTON
S.B. SCHNITZER & V. KAN

(Buffalo, N.Y., U.S.A.)

ABSTRACT

Contrary to what one might expect from the histological appearance of the retina, visual abilities persist when all rod cells have disappeared, and surviving cone cells have no outer and inner segments. Visual capacities were measured in the mutant, rdy (RCS-like) rat from the age of 30 to 560 days by behavioral testing of form discrimination, the ERG, single unit optic nerve activity, and cortical potentials from non-patterned and patterned stimuli. The cortical potentials from the surface of the central projection area of the visual cortex provided the most reliable, easily measured indices of the course of the degenerative process. These potentials revealed characteristic changes of latency (prolongation), threshold (increase), and optimal spatial frequency (reduction). Flicker responses of cortex and of recordable ERG components survived remarkably well. Deterioration of visual capacity measured behaviorally at around the age of 10 months, coincided with failing cortical responses and a reduction of the number of optic nerve fibers responsive to light. At the age of 7 months, 95% of the optic nerve axons responded to visual stimulation; receptive fields had antagonistic center-surround organization but on-center units represented a greater fraction of the responsive axons than in the normal rat. The proven photo-responsiveness of severely degenerated retinas should have a major impact on the understanding of vision in patients with retinitis pigmentosa and similar disorders.

INTRODUCTION

A retinal physiologist viewing the histological sections of retinas from the C3H (rd) mouse or the RCS (rdy) rat at an advanced stage of hereditary retinal degeneration is ready to proclaim these animals blind because the outer nuclear layer is reduced to a row of scattered nuclei and the layer of rods and cones is completely absent. This is the typical picture of photo-receptor death and degeneration in a number of animal models of retinitis pigmentosa. Nevertheless, throughout the history of the study of hereditary degeneration in the mouse, there have been claims that behavioral testing reveals the preservation of visual function in these animals (cf. Keeler 1927; Karli, Stoeckel & Porte 1954). More recently these observations have been extended to the rdy rat first studied histologically by Bourne et al. in 1938. LaVail et al. (1974) found that these rats at an advanced stage of degeneration respond to light in a conventional lever pressing test. Kaitz (1976) reported that they are capable of brightness discrimination. Anderson and O'Steen (1972) tested visual function in retinal degeneration produced by exposing young, normal albino rats for 30 days to damaging light. Despite apparently widespread visual cell degeneration, the rats discriminated between black-white patterns and learned new discriminations at 'rates indistinguishable from control animals'.

The histological study of the behaviorally light-responsive rats, $\frac{1}{2}$ to 2 years old revealed a small number of photoreceptor cell bodies located between the inner nuclear layer and the retinal border that is provided by the apical Müller cell processes interdigitating with the apical processes of the pigment epithelium (LaVail, Sidman, Rausin & Sidman 1974). The nuclei of these cells were round to ovoid in shape and had a chromatin distribution 'characteristic of immature rod cells or of cells interpreted as cones in the rat retina.' Most of these cells displayed synaptic ribbons with the typical cluster of synaptic vesicles, either near the cell body or in a presynaptic terminal at some distance from the cell body within the outer plexiform layer. Some terminals were 'simple' making contact with one or two postsynaptic processes. They were described as resembling rod spherules. Other terminals were 'complex' in configuration, with many ribbons and flat post-synaptic contacts resembling cone pedicles. The cell bodies of these units had a residual cilium which in most cells extended beyond the body for no more than 1—2 microns. No outer segment was found. The number of the preserved photoreceptor cell bodies was very low at the rat's age of one year. They were then distributed posteriorly between optic disc and points midway to the ora serrata at either side of the disc. In contrast, conventional and ribbon synapses in the inner synaptic layer were abundant though reduced in number at the age of one year compared to the normal controls.

The histological survival of cone cells lacking outer and inner segments was first observed in studies of the retinal effects of iodoacetate in rabbit, cat and monkey (Noell 1955; 1958). Iodoacetate (IAA) was found to affect preferentially the rod cell population. Following intravenous injection of IAA retinal function immediately disappeared and, depending upon dose schedule, was followed within a few days by the histological disappearance of visual cells throughout the retina. Characteristically, however, a single row of nuclei of the outer nuclear layer, normally 6—12 rows wide, tended to servive in rabbit and cat. There nuclei had a chromatin organization characteristic for the cones of the normal vertebrate retina. Typically, these cone-like cells had lost inner and outer segments.

In rhesus monkeys after iodoacetate poisoning, the cone cells in the central, rod-free region, always survived and had a normal appearance, but just outside this region, where normally rods alternate with cones, outer cone segments were shortened while the inner cone segments were broadened and filled the space vacated by the destroyed rods. At distance 3 to 5 mm. from the fovea, however, inner and outer cone segments had disappeared but the cone cell bodies had servived.

The histological appearance of the retina of rhesus monkeys after iodoacetate was compared with the retina of retinitis pigmentosa patients as described in the literature (Noell 1959; see also Szamier, Berson, Klein & Meyers 1979). The case reports agreed that a single row of visual cell nuclei, representing the remnants of cone cells, survived in patients for some distance from the fovea. This survival, however, did not extend as far into the periphery of the retinas as in the rhesus experiments. Cone cell pathology in advanced human retinitis pigmentosa of long duration seemed more severe than in the animal model. In the iodoacetate affected monkey surviving cone cell bodies also seemed to be reduced in number when the retina was studied 6 months after rod cell death instead of 3 weeks.

Stimulated by the results of the iodoacetate experiments, our laboratory has been involved for many years in studies of the electrophysiology, biochemistry and histology of hereditary photoreceptor degeneration as manifested in the rd mouse and the rdy rat (Noell 1965). More recently, we have undertaken an extensive study of the photoreceptive function of the rdy rat at an age when all rod cells have been destroyed and the surviving elements of the outer nuclear layer are only cone-like cells. This work has not been published in detail. At this time, we present a brief summary of our findings which derive from the recording of the visually evoked cortical potentials, the study of single unit optic tract activities and behavioral form discrimination experiments.

RESULTS AND DISCUSSION

To our initial surprise, flash evoked mass responses of the cerebral cortex, measured by averaging techniques, were found to survive the death of the rod population. The main differences from normal were a prolonged latency by 20 msec or more and a lower amplitude of component potentials (Fig. 1).

Visual cell degeneration in the rdy rat measured by pyknosis and loss of outer nuclei, begins 2 weeks after birth. At the age of 3–4 months the overwhelming majority of the rod cells has disappeared and at the age of 6–8 months all rod cells of the retina have vanished. At this age, the one remaining row of the outer nuclear layer consists of pyknotic nuclei and non-pyknotic nuclei which have the cone cell appearance.

The visually evoked cortical responses were well preserved up to the age of 8 months. Using strong stimuli, they had very similar features as the responses of the normal animal to flashes 2 log units weaker. They follow repetition up to 16/sec while the normal rat followed the same flash at rates of 32/s.

The abnormal retina also was capable of driving synchronous cortical activity in response to patterned stimuli, bar or checker board reversal, but effective spatial frequencies were lower than in the normal rat.

The cortical responses deteriorated after the age of 8 months and were

177

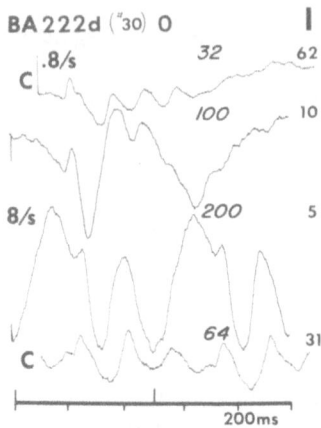

BA 222d ($^\circ$30) 0

.8/s   32   62

C

100   10

8/s   200   5

64   31

C

200ms

Fig. 1. Cortical evoked potentials from a mutant albino rat (BA), 222 days old, in comparison to records (labelled C) from a normal, adult albino rat. The records from the control rat (uppermost and lowest tracings) are transposed on the time scale to the right so that their N_1 potential (first negative, upward deflection) coincides with the (abnormally delayed) N_1 potential of the mutant rat. The 2 upper records are the summed responses (runs) of 32 flashes (for C) and of 100 for BA to wide-field strong xenon-arc flashes delivered by a Grass stimulator at 0.8/s. The calibration mark (upper right corner) indicates the amplitude of the average response denoting $62\,\mu V$ for C and $10\,\mu V$ for BA. The two lower traces are in response to the same flash at 8/s; 200 runs for BA, 64 runs for C; calibration unit is $5\,\mu V$ for BA and $31\,\mu V$ for C. Sweep time is 250 msec.

poorly preserved at 12 months. Measurable responses were obtained up to the age of 18 months.

Hooded rdy rats, 7–9 months old, learned to discriminate between the horizontal and vertical orientation of a white bar. This ability was lost at the age of one year simultaneously with a marked deterioration of the electrical responsiveness of the visual cortex.

Mass responses of the retina (ERG) recorded from the cornea or within the eye were almost undetectable with a single flash after the age of 3 months, but averaging techniques revealed responses up to the age of 12 months. They followed flicker as well as the cortical responses. They were similar in form, amplitude and threshold as the ERG of the normal strongly light adapted rat. The presumed origin of these ERG potentials is the inner synaptic latyer of the retina (Fig. 2).

Unitary activity of optic tract axons in response to white or black stimuli presented on a tangent screen were recorded in the hooded rdy rat at ages ranging from 3 to 18 months (Stockton, Salinsky & Noell 1976). At the age of 7–8 months, the majority of these units had concentric, antagonistic receptive fields indicating that the abnormal retina has one of the basic functions of visual information processing. The most frequently studied units had their receptive field within the central $20°$ (Fig. 3).

The temporal pattern of the discharges of the optic units of the rdy rat

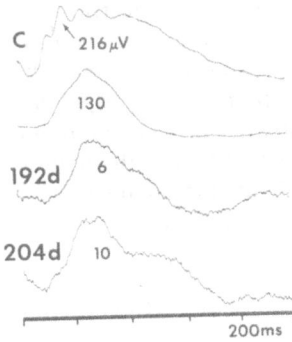

Fig. 2. ERGs of the mutant albino rat at the age of 192 and 204 days (lower traces), in comparison to records from a control rat (upper 2 traces). Stimulus conditions are the same as in Fig. 1, except that stimulus rate is 0.2/s. The 2nd control tracing is obtained in a partially light adapted state which raised ERG threshold by 1.8 log unit. The maximal amplitude of the average response is given in μV.

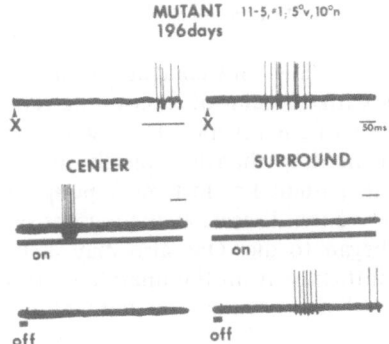

Fig. 3. Single unit responses (axon impulses) from the optic tract of a mutant (pigmented) rat at the age of 196 days. The center of the receptive field of the unit was located 5° ventral and 10° nasal from the projection of the optic disc. The two tracings of the uppermost row are the responses to a diffuse xenon flash (X) recorded at different sweep speed (note horizontal line denoting 50 msec). The two lower rows illustrate the firing in response to the *on* and *off* of a 10° white target applied to either the *center* (left) or the *surround* of the receptive field; the heavy black lines denote the stimulus; *on* coincides with the start of the sweep. The illustrated unit was the first of 8 units encountered during one vertical penetration through the optic tract near the chiasm. Penetration was through the brain.

was similar as observed with the x-cells of the cat when light adapted beyond the scotopic range.

Optic nerve units with on-center responses were at least twice as frequent in the abnormal retinas as in the normal rat. Units which had no on-center excitation rarely showed a brisk response at *off* in contrast to the normal rat. This suggested that retinal feature detection in rdy may differ from normal.

179

Using a combination of direct electrical stimulation of the optic nerve and photic stimulation of the retina, it was found that probably less than 5% of the optic tract axons are unresponsive to retinal light stimulation at the age of 7 months. However, the number of optic axons transmitting visual information decreased rapidly after the age of 8 months.

Histological analysis suggests that the deterioration of the visual functions after the age of 8 months is correlated with a reduction in the number of the remnant cone nuclei and with spotty disorganization of the inner layers.

CONCLUSION

We conclude that the surviving cone-like, but cone-less cells are the photoreceptive elements at an advanced stage of retinal degeneration in the rdy rat. They seem well suited to provide primary visual information to the retinal network through preserved synaptic connections with the second-order neurons. We assume that photopigment synthesis is preserved in these cells, and that the photopigment is incorporated into the plasma membrane of the surviving cell body and enables it to produce an electrical signal in response to light absorption (see also Cicerone 1977; Cicerone, Green & Fisher 1979).

We hope that our findings and conclusions stimulate studies in retinitis pigmentosa patients with the aim of discovering remnant or dormant visual function. On the basis of the rat model one would expect better peripheral vision in retinitis pigmentosa than is typically reported. It may be that the retina of the 'typical' patient has lost most peripheral 'remnant' cone cells during the first years of the disease, as the mutant rat does about 10 months after the rod cells began to die. One also may assume that there is a suppressive, inhibitory influence from the unaffected retinal regions (e.g. fovea) upon severely affected areas where the only photoreceptive elements are surviving (remnant) cone cell bodies. In fact, we have begun to test this hypothesis by psychophysical means on selected retinitis pigmentosa patients (Temme & Noell, unpublished). We will attempt to enhance peripheral vision in these patients by foveal adaptation procedures and by 'training'.

REFERENCES

Anderson, D.V. & O'Steen, W.K. Black-White and pattern discrimination in rats with photoreceptors. Exp. Neurol. 34: 446–454 (1972).
Bourne, M.C., Campbell, D.A. & Tansley, D. Hereditary degeneration of the rat retina. Br. J. Ophthal. 22: 613–623 (1938).
Cicerone, C.M. Cone-driven ganglion cells survive in advanced retinal degeneration. Invest. Ophthalmol. Vis. Sci. 138 (1977).
Cicerone, C.M., Green, D.G. & Fisher, L.J. Cone inputs to ganglion cells in hereditary retinal degeneration. Science 203: 1113–1115 (1979).
Kaitz, M. Effects of light on brightness perception in rats with retinal dystrophy. Vision Res. 16: 141–148 (1976).
Karli, P., Stoeckel, M.E. & Porte, A. Degenerescence des cellules visuelles photoreceptries. Arch. Sci. Physiol. 8: 305–328 (1954).

Keeler, C.E. Iris movement in blind mice. Am. J. Physiol. 81: 107–112 (1927).

LaVail, M.M., Sidman, M., Rausin, R. & Sidman, R.L. Discrimination of light intensity by rats with inherited retinal degeneration: A behavioral and cytological study. Vision Res. 14: 693–702 (1974).

Noell, W.K. Metabolic injuries of the visual cell. Am. J. Ophthalmol., 40: 60–68 (1955).

Noell, W.K. Differentiation, metabolic organization and viability of the visual cell. A.M.A. Arch. Ophthalmol. 60: 702–733 (1958).

Noell, W.K. The visual cell: Electric and metabolic manifestations of its life processes. Am. J. Ophthalmol. 48: 347–370 (1959).

Noell, W.K. Aspects of experimental and hereditary retina degeneration. Biochemistry of the Retina. (Ed. C.N. Graymore) Academic Press, New York 51–72 (1965).

Stockton, R.A., Salinsky, M. & Noell, W.K. Visual functions in advanced hereditary retinal degeneration (rat). Invest. Ophthalmol. Vis. Sci. (Suppl.) 92 (1976).

Szamier, R.B., Berson, E.L., Klein, R. & Meyers, S. Sex-linked retinitis pigmentosa: Ultrastructure of photoreceptors and pigment epithelium. Invest. Ophthalmol. Vis. Sci. 18: 145–160 (1979).

Authors' address:
Dept. of Physiology,
Neurosensory Laboratory,
State University of New York at Buffalo,
2211 Main Street,
Building C,
Buffalo, NY 14214, U.S.A.

OPTIC NERVE CHANGES
IN DOMINANT CONE-ROD DYSTROPHY

J.R. HECKENLIVELY, T. ROSALES & D. MARTIN

(Los Angeles, Calif. U.S.A.)

ABSTRACT

The diagnosis of cone-rod dystrophy is made based on electroretinographic (ERG) evidence; while both are abnormal, the photopic ERG is suppressed more than the scotopic ERG. Because the cone-rod dystrophy group is characterized by progressive visual field loss, and abnormal ERGs, these patients are usually given the diagnosis of retinitis pigmentosa.

The cone-rod dystrophy group has some characteristics that separate it from the rod-cone group; the patients are not nightblind until advanced stages of the disease, and they usually have temporal optic atrophy, and telangiectasia of disc and parapapillary vessels. Usually, there is minimal pigmentary disruption of the retina.

A family with autosomal dominant cone-rod dystrophy is presented which demonstrates these unique features.

INTRODUCTION

Retinitis pigmentosa (RP) is the generic name given to a group of inherited retinal degenerations characterized by progressive visual field loss, abnormal electroretinogram, and other variable clinical and test findings, including retinal pigmentary deposits, vascular attenuation, optic atrophy, and retinal pigment epithelial disturbances or atrophy. Frequently, nightblindness is an early sign, but there are a minority of RP patients whose dark adaptation test is normal or only mildly compromised, and who subjectively do not have nightblindness until their disease is in the advanced stages. One of the groups of RP patients which have exhibited this phenomena of normal or near normal night vision, have been those individuals who can be classified as 'cone-rod dystrophies'.

Cone-rod dysfunction is an electrophysiologic term (Berson 1977) which can be used to sub-classify retinitis pigmentosa on the basis of changes seen on the electroretinogram (ERG). Not all cases of RP have non-recordable ERGs, particularly in the earlier stages of the disease process. If the photopic (light adapted, high intensity flash) ERG which tests the cone system, is more severely affected than the scotopic (dark adapted, low intensity flash) ERG which tests the rod system, and both are abnormal, the classification of cone-rod dystrophy may be considered; other criteria should be met in order to use the term. These would include such items as a positive family history, documentation or history of progression, fundus abnormalities not consistent with any other known enity, and a medical/ocular history not suggestive of another cause for the disorder.

It would be proper to use the phrase cone-rod degeneration just based on the ERG data, but the term dystrophy denotes a disease present from birth; it is inherited, and is progressive in its manifestations (Krill & Deutman 1972). In many cases, it is difficult to establish the classification of cone-rod dystrophy because the ERG becomes non-recordable. If a member of a family can be classified as a cone-rod dystrophy, it is reasonable to assume other members of the same family, who are affected, but who have non-recordable ERGs, have the same genetic defect, and at an earlier stage of the disease would have demonstrated the same ERG pattern.

This paper examines the findings in a dominant pedigree (Fig. 1) of cone-rod dystrophy, looking at six patients in three generations. These patients

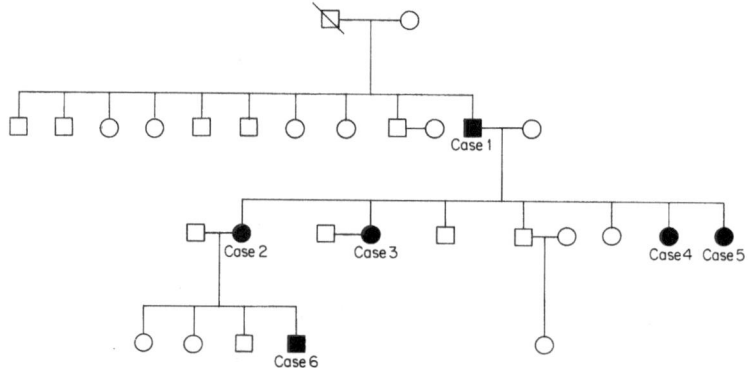

Fig. 1. Pedigree of family with cone-rod dystrophy. All members have been examined. Squares denote males, circles are females, affected members are filled in.

have severe atrophy of the temporal disc, with loss of nerve substance, telangiectasia and preservation of disc and peripapillary vessels, and in several cases, have alterations of the nerve fiber layer, which appears indistinct and swollen at the disc margin, or in the propositus, shows focal opacification throughout the posterior poles.

CASE REPORTS

Case 1 (propositus) is a 55 year old white male who was told of retinal abnormalites on an army physical exam at age 18 when he was diagnosed as having retinitis pigmentosa. The patients states that his visual acuity at that time was 6/12 (20/40). Severe visual problems were noted at age 35, and at age 43 he had bilateral cataracts removed. Slit lamp and external examination were unremarkable with the exception that there was some brown pigment noted in the vitreous. Fundus examination revealed a pale optic nerve with flattening and atrophy of the temporal side of the disc (Fig. 2). There were

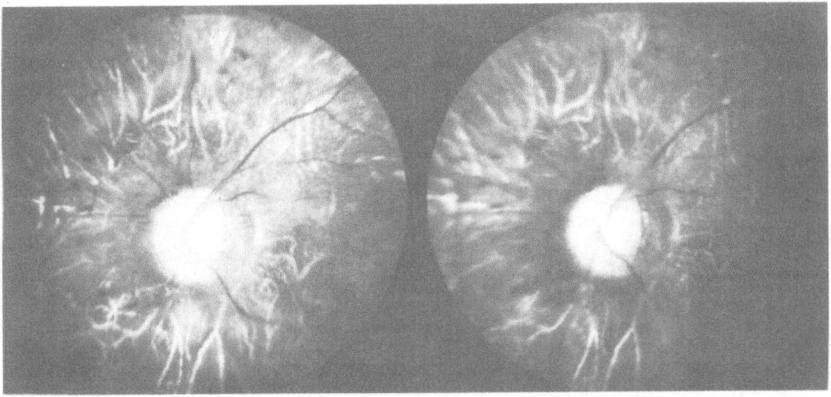

Fig. 2. Case 1, advanced cone-rod dystrophy; stereographic view of left optic nerve demonstrating flattening and atrophy of the temporal side of disc, hypopigmentation and/or diffuse loss of RPE gives tigroid fundus appearance, scattered white elongated lesions of the nerve fiber layer can be seen superior temporal to disc.

Figure can be viewed in stereo with Stereoviewer (Air Photo Supply, Bronx, N.Y.) or by using a set of + 7.00 lens tilted about 15° in toward nose.

large areas of retinal pigment epithelial (RPE) loss and an appearance of choroidal sclerosis in that the choroidal vessels were yellowish and looked under-perfused. The retinal vessels were attenuated. The fluorescein angiogram (Fig. 3) demonstrated peripapillary loss of the RPE and choriocapillaris, with larger choroidal vessels remaining patent. There were multiple telangiectatic surface disc vessels temporally, some of which show persistent fluorescence on late frames.

The most remarkable change was the appearance of the nerve fiber layer; throughout the posterior pole of both eyes, there were small white opacifications which aligned themselves parallel to and within the fibers of the nerve fiber layer (Fig. 2). They resembled 'dry' cotton wool spots, i.e., they did not look edematous. On stereographic examination of the fundus photos, the location of most of the pigment deposits was clearly subretinal at the level of the RPE (Fig. 4). Further clinical data is presented in Tables 1 & 2.

Case 2 is the 33 year old daughter of case 1, who has noticed some mild night-blindness but functionally has not had severe problems. Her past medical history is negative for any significant problems. On slit lamp examination, fine white deposits were seen in the fetal nucleus. Fundus exam was remarkable in that the temporal aspect of the disc was missing with some generalized

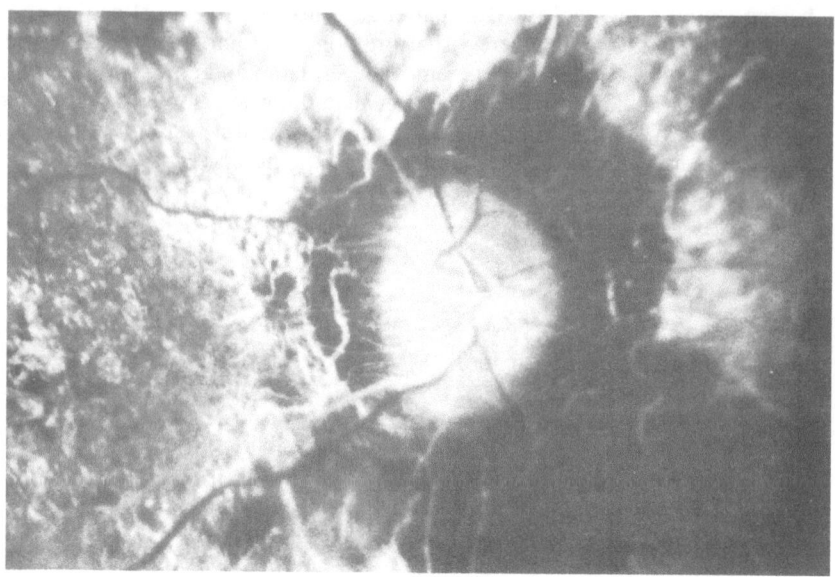

Fig. 3. Case 1, fluorescein angiogram right optic nerve, demonstrating many fine telangiectatic vessels, particularly on the temporal aspect of the nervehead. Peripapillary atrophy of RPE and choriocapillaris is present, but larger choroidal vessels are patent.

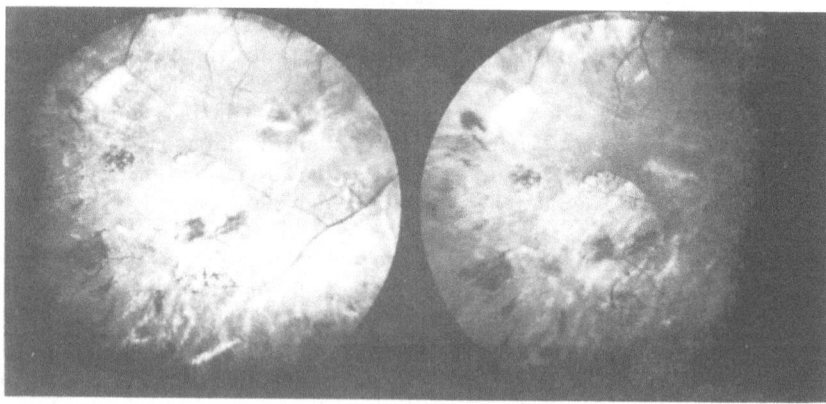

Fig. 4. Case 1 stereographic view of right posterior pole with atrophic macular lesion, loss of retinal pigment epithelium, with pigment deposition mainly at the level of the RPE. Scattered focal lesions of the nerve fiber layer can be seen above and below macula.

186

swelling of the nerve fiber layer overlying the disc (Fig. 5). A golden-yellow deposit could be seen buried in the left disc superior nasally. There was peripapillary atrophy temporally, and on the nasal side of the disc, the retinal pigment epithelium was yellowish tan, giving a partial halo effect to the disc. The retinal vessels were within normal limits. The overall appearance to the fundus was a tigroid pattern from hypopigmentation of the RPE. Electroretinographic testing revealed cone-rod dysfunction; the electrophysiological and clinical details can be seen in Tables 1 & 2.

Table 1. Clinical characteristics dominant cone-rod dystrophy.

Patient	Age	Eye	Visual acuity	Goldmann visual field (I−4)	Color vision Farnsworth* error score/axis	Final rod threshold (log units)
Case 1	55	OD	10/200	barely detects	−	4.30
		OS	10/200	target centrally	−	
Case 2	33	OD	20/30	30°	214 early	0.20
		OS	20/30	15°	208 tritan	
Case 4	16	OD	20/30	15°	67 low dis-	1.30
		OS	20/30	6°	149 crimination	
Case 5	13	OD	20/25	10°	107 early tritan	0.50
		OS	20/30	7°	100 no axis	
Case 6	8	OD	20/50	5°	not done	3.40
		OS	20/60	3°		

* Nagel Anomaloscope was normal in cases 2, 4, 5.

Table 2. Electrophysiological data dominant cone-rod dystrophy family.

Patient	Eye	Electroretinogram Pamp	PBIT	Samp	SBIT	Electrooculogram dark/light ratio
Case 1	OD	non-recordable				not done
	OS	non-recordable				
Case 2	OD	50 uv	36 ms	100 uv	60 ms	156%
	OS	20 uv	36 ms	70 uv	60 ms	148%
Case 4	OD	non-recordable				122%
	OS	non-recordable				135%
Case 5	OD	30 uv	40 ms	50 uv	80 ms	125%
	OS	NR		NR		129%
Case 6	OD	non-recordable				not done
	OS	non-recordable				

Pamp = photopic b wave amplitude; PBIT = photopic b wave implicit time;
Samp = scotopic b wave amplitude; SBIT = scotopic b wave implicit time.

Case 3 is the 27 year old daughter of the propositus, who has complaints of visual difficulties. Extensive documentation of her condition has not been performed, but the examination of fundus photos taken with the portable

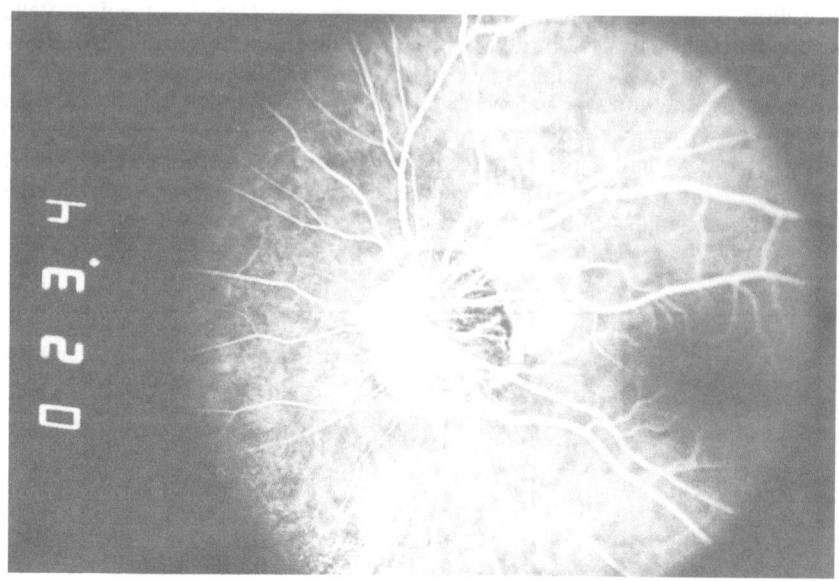

Fig. 5. Case 2, fluorescein angiogram of left eye, 33 year old woman with cone-rod dystrophy and atrophy of temporal disc with telangiectasia of disc vessels.

Kowa camera as part of a linkage analysis study, reveals that she has the same type of optic nerve changes as her sisters.

Case 4 is the 16 year old daughter of the propositis who is asymptomatic, although, on questioning notes some problems with peripheral vision, and possibly some nightblindness. The external and slit lamp examination were unremarkable. Fundus examination revealed a tigroid (blond) fundus, the optic nerve was pink, but the temporal aspect was missing, and there was swelling of the nerve fiber layer overlying the disc margin adjacent to the area of missing disc tissue. Dilatation of surface disc vessels could be seen ophthalmoscopically. The retinal vessel size was within normal limits.

Case 5 is the 13 year old daughter of case 1, and is asymptomatic. Biomicroscopy revealed fine diffuse pigment in the vitreous of both eyes. Fundus exam revealed a tigroid appearance to the retina due to hypopigmentation of the RPE. The disc was pink with a slight tilted appearance. The nerve fiber layer overlying the disc inferiorly looked swollen, and stained on late fluorescein angiogram frames (Fig. 6). Surface vessels on the disc were telangiectatic. The retinal vasculature size was within normal limits. The data was consistent with the diagnosis of cone-rod dystrophy (see Tables 1 & 2).

Case 6 is the 8 year old grandson of the propositus. He is symptomatic from peripheral vision loss, often bumping into objects and has mild reading difficulties. His best corrected vision is OD 6/15 (20/50), OS 6/18 (20/60).

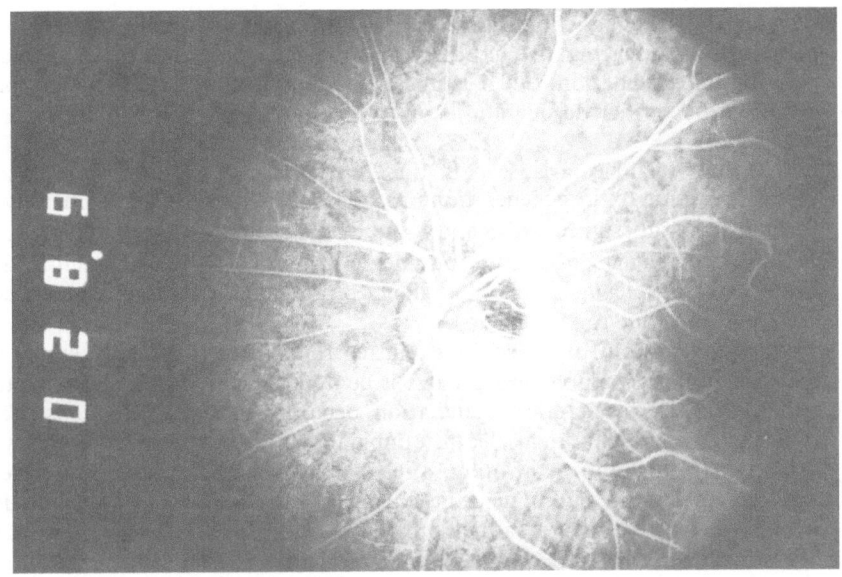

Fig. 6. Case 5, late transit fluorescein angiogram of left eye, 13 year old girl, demonstrating temporal optic atrophy and telangiectasia of surface disc and peripapillary vessels. Inferior disc margin nerve fiber layer is swollen and hyperfluorescent on later frames.

Slit lamp exam revealed fine deposits in the fetal nucleus OU. Ophthalmoscopic examination revealed a tigroid fundus. The optic nerve was pink with some flattening of the temporal side of the disc, and an indistinct appearing nerve fiber layer inferior nasally. There was some attenuation of the retinal vasculature. Dilatation of the disc surface vessels could be seen in both eyes. Further clinical and electrophysiological data is presented in Tables 1 & 2.

DISCUSSION

This dominant cone-rod dystrophy family has a variety of findings which are atypical for retinitis pigmentosa. The photopic ERG is more severely affected than the scotopic ERG, the temporal optic nerves show severe atrophy, the surface disc and peripapillary vessels are telangiectatic, most of the patients demonstrate edema of the disc, and there are minimal pigmentary changes, which are sub-retinal, and present in the advanced stages of the disease process.

This three generation family allows a view of the earlier and late stages of this disease. The temporal optic atrophy was seen early in all affected members. Most of the members had swelling of the nerve fiber layer of the disc, of the type reported to be related to obstruction of axoplasmic flow (McLeod 1976, Minckler, Tso & Zimmerman 1976). As the fluorescein angiograms demonstrate adequate circulation to the nerve head and retina, a

189

vascular or ischemic etiologic process would not seem likely. An intrinsic pathological or degenerative mechanism of the ganglion cell or its axon would be a logical explanation, but it is not clear whether the optic nerve atrophy precedes the retinal degeneration, or vice versa. It may be that they occur concurrently.

The disc telangiectasia seen in these patients may represent a localized vascular reaction to the degeneration process occurring in the nerve fiber layer. Preliminary studies in recessive and X-linked cone-rod dystrophy patients also demonstrate telangiectasia and optic nerve atrophy, of the type seen in this family, so the teleangiectasia most likely represents a common degenerative pattern in the cone-rod group.

One explanation for the various unusual findings in this family would be that the primary pathological process is centered in the bipolar layer of the retina, with trans-synaptic degeneration occuring in both directions. This could explain the abnormal electroretinogram findings, the nerve fiber layer alterations, and the optic atrophy. The fact that the cone system is preferentially affected with subsequent degeneration may account for the relative atrophy in the temporal area of the disc where the heaviest concentration of fibers from the cones are received. Potts et al. (1972) found that these areas, in rhesus monkeys, corresponded to an increased density of fibers, mainly from a higher percentage of small fibers.

However, one of the most unusual aspects in these cases remains the preservation of central vision, which with the loss of the maculopapillary bundle region of the disc, might be expected to be severely compromised.

A panretinal toxic process could conceivably explain the multiple tissue layer involvement in these patients, but other diseases of this type frequently have central and peripheral nervous system effects which have not been observed.

The cone-rod dystrophy group appears to consistently have minimal pigmentary migration and retinal deposition compared to the rod-cone RP dystrophies, and many of the patients would be termed 'retinitis pigmentosa sine pigmento'. Since the rod system is more severely affected electroretinographically in the rod-cone dystrophies, and is less affected sequentially in the cone-rod dystrophies, this may imply that the pigmentary degenerative phenomena seen in many patients may be dependent on some type of rod-RPE degenerative mechanism. Supporting clinical evidence for this concept are the pigmentary changes in the propositus whose rod system undoubtedly was affected after the cone system, in which the majority of the pigmentary deposition is subretinal on stereographic examination of the fundus photos (Fig. 4). This is in contrast to typical RP in which there is migration of pigment to form perivascular cuffs, or bone spicules around retinal vessels (Lucas 1956; Meyer, Heckenlively, Spitznas & Foos 1980 submitted). Further evidence of the persistent functional integrity of the rod system in this family, is their final rod threshold, which is barely affected until advanced stages of the disease.

It might be argued that this family does not truly have retinitis pigmentosa; however they do have a retinal degeneration with progressive loss of visual field, extinguished or abnormal ERG, preservation of central vision, and pigment clumping in the advanced stages of the disease. The acceptance of the diagnostic term 'RP' is dependent on what definition is used. Because of the heterogeneity of these diseases, there has been some difficulty in establishing precise diagnostic criteria.

Since the cone-rod dystrophies appear to have specific findings of telangiectasia and temporal optic atrophy, this may prove useful in making the diagnosis of cone-rod dystrophy, after the ERG is non-recordable. Whether these changes can be used for classification of RP will be dependent on whether other diseases are found that have similar findings, and if they can be differentiated from the cone-rod dystrophy patients.

For instance, telangiectasia of retinal vessels with optic atrophy has been noted as characteristic of Leber's optic atrophy (Smith, Hoyt & Susac 1973) and cases with a slow insidious onset (Nikoskelainen, Sogg, Rosenthal, Friberg & Dorfman 1977) and acute onset (Gittinger, Kelterner, Miller & Burde 1979) have been reported. No report of an electroretinogram being performed in any case of Leber's optic atrophy was found.

Performing an electroretinogram and other electrophysiological/psychophysiological tests should be undertaken in cases of hereditary optic atrophy to insure that none of these patients are confused with the cone-rod dystrophy group.

Four of the six patients in this family showed definite swelling and alterations of the nerve fiber layer, which have been associated with other studies with obstruction of axoplasmic flow. The propositus with advanced disease had focal opacifications of the nerve fiber layer throughout the posterior poles of each eye. Three of the four affected daughters had areas of disc 'edema'. This is a striking similarity to the pseudoedema found in Leber's optic atrophy, so a common degenerative mechanism may be taking place in both types of patients.

The findings of optic nerve atrophy, telangiectasia, and sparse or no pigmentary changes, appear to be a common finding to all inherited types of cone-rod dystrophies (Heckenlively, Martin & Rosales 1981 accepted). This is the first time that specific retinal abnormalities have been found to be consistently present in association with an electroretinographic diagnosis. Looking at the components of the ERG more critically may demonstrate other RP sub-types that may be helpful in localizing the etiologic processes and degenerative mechanisms occuring in retinitis pigmentosa and other hereditary retinal degenerations.

ACKNOWLEDGEMENT

This work was supported in part by the National Retinitis Pigmentosa Foundation, Baltimore, MD, USA.

Robert Fantl, M.D., Fresno, California referred the patients. Mr. Jay Sands and Mr. Dennis Thayer assisted with the fundus photography.

REFERENCES

Berson, E.L. Hereditary retinal diseases: Classification with the full-field electroretinogram. In: 14th ISCERG Symposium (Ed. Th. Lawwill). Junk, The Hague (Doc. Ophthal. Proc. Series Vol. 13) 149–171 (1977).

Gittinger, J.W., Kelterner, J.L., Miller, N.R. & Burde, R.M. Progressive visual loss associated with peculiar disc swelling. Survey Ophthalmol. 24: 117–121 (1979).

Heckenlively, J.R., Martin, D.A., Rosales, T.O. Telangiectasia & optic nerve atrophy in the cone-rod degenerations. Accepted for publication 1981 Arch. Ophthalmol.

Krill, A.E. & Deutman, A.F. Dominant macular degenerations, the cone dystrophies. Am. J. Ophthalmol. 73: 352–369 (1972).

Lucas, D.R. Retinitis pigmentosa, pathological findings. Br. J. Ophthalmol. 40: 14–23 (1956).

McLeod, D. Ophthalmoscopic signs of obstructed axoplasmic transport after ocular vascular occlusions. Br. J. Ophthalmol. 60: 551–56 (1976).

Meyer, K.T., Heckenlively, J.R., Spitznas, M., & Foos, R.Y. A clinicopathological correlation in a dominant retinitis pigmentosa family (submitted for publication).

Minckler, D.S., Tso, M.O.M. & Zimmerman, L.E. A light microscopic, autoradiographic study of axoplasmic transport in the optic nerve head during ocular hypotony, increased intraocular pressure, and papilledema. Am. J. Ophthalmol. 82: 741–757 (1976).

Nikoskelainen, E., Sogg, R.L. Rosenthal, A.R., Friberg, T.R. & Dorfman, L.J. The early phase in Leber hereditary optic atrophy. Arch. Ophthalmol. 95: 969–78 (1977).

Potts, A.M., Hodges, D., Shelman, C.B., Fritz, K.J., Levy, N.S. & Mangnall, Y. Morphology of the primate optic nerve. II. Total fiber size distribution and fiber density distribution. Invest. Ophthalmol. Vis. Sci. 11: 989–1003 (1972).

Smith, J.L., Hoyt, W.F. & Susac, J.O. Ocular fundus in acute Leber optic neuropathy. Arch. Ophthalmol. 90: 349–354 (1973).

Authors' address:
Jules Stein Eye Institute
800 Westwood Plaza
Los Angeles, California 90024
U.S.A.

VISUAL EVOKED POTENTIALS IN PRE-SENILE DEMENTIA

G.F.A. HARDING, C.E. DOGGETT, A. ORWIN & E.J. SMITH

(*Birmingham, England*)

ABSTRACT

Pre-senile dementia is difficult to diagnose due to the variability in behavioural expression. Visser, Stam, Van Tilburg, Op den Velde, Blom & De Rijke (1976) reported the flash visual evoked potential is delayed in patients suffering from pre-senile dementia (Alzheimer type).

Twelve patients with a provisional diagnosis of Alzheimer's disease were studied. In all cases the EEG and flash VEP was obtained and in nine of the cases pattern-reversal stimulation was also used. The EEG showed generalised slowing with reduction of alpha activity in eight cases.

The flash visual evoked potential was delayed in ten cases, the mean latency of the P2 (P100) component was 162.5 m.secs. Surprisingly the pattern-reversal evoked potential was found to be normal in all nine cases studied. The mean latency was 102.7 m.secs.

This finding of a markedly delayed flash VEP co-existing with a normal pattern-reversal VEP has not previously been reported in patients with pre-senile dementia, and is such an unusual finding as to provide a diagnostic criteria for early detection of this condition.

INTRODUCTION

Pre-senile dementia occurs at a relatively early stage of life usually in the 5th and 6th decade. The condition progresses rapidly with cerebral degeneration and mental deterioration in the early stages. Characteristic features are loss of memory, time disorientation and lethargy. Memory loss is usually the most outstanding feature and is often interpreted by family and associates as inattentiveness.

Both Picks and Alzheimer's disease are forms of pre-senile dementia. The former is characterised by lethargy, indifference, and akinesia. Memory retention is better than in Alzheimer's disease where memory loss although severe, is often hidden by the patient's retained intellectual ability. There is often some aphasia and dysarthria and the patients speech becomes slurred, confused and indistinct (Perez, Rivera, Meyer, Gay, Taylor & Matthew 1975).

Although the aetiological factors affecting Alzheimer's disease are unknown, cerebral atrophy with diminished gyri and ventricular dilation are commonly seen. Neurofibrillary tangles are microscopically observed with extracellular senile plaques and the disease differs from senile dementia only in its age of onset.

There have been many studies of EEG findings in this and other pre-senile dementia and senile dementia conditions. In general the EEG in Alzheimer's disease is characterised by diffuse theta activity, with reduction of normal background alpha activity and perseveration of slowing of background activity produced by hyperventilation (Fig. 1). By contrast, patients with Picks disease frequently show a normal EEG (Gordon & Sim 1967).

There have been remarkably few studies of the visual evoked potential in pre-senile and senile dementias. Lee and Blair (1973) described a study on one patient with Jakob-Creutzfeldt disease and Visser et al. (1976) described nineteen patients with either senile or pre-senile dementia of the Alzheimer type. Both authors report delayed components of the visual evoked potential to flash stimulation.

MATERIAL

This study was carried out on twelve patients who were diagnosed as having probable pre-senile dementia of an Alzheimer's or arterio-sclerotic type. There were 3 males and 9 females and the mean age was 62 years, range 53 to 69 years. All patients received a full EEG and in most cases both flash and pattern reversal evoked potential studies were performed. The patients have been studied over a nine year period although all but one patient presented in the last five years.

The flash stimulus was a Grass PS22 stroboscope at intensity 2 producing 1363 candelas per square metre. The pattern-reversal stimulus consisted of a mirror-moved pattern of 56 minute black and white checks in a target of $14°$ radius. Responses to 50 repetitions were averaged using either a PDP8 computer or a Datalab Micro 4. The responses were recorded from right and left occiputs (O_2 and O_1) referred to ipsilateral central electrodes (C_4 and C_3).

RESULTS

The results of the investigation were compared to a group of elderly normal people (age range 65—75 years). Their mean flash evoked response is shown in Fig. 2. The mean latency of the major positive P_2 component is 117.2 milliseconds, standard deviation 10.7 m.secs. The earlier P_1 component is frequently of higher amplitude than the P_2 component in elderly persons, but its mean latency is only 72 m.secs. and it is therefore unlikely to be confused with the P_2 component. The latencies and amplitudes of the components obtained from this control population compare well with those of Dustman and Beck (1969) and Straumanis et al. (1965).

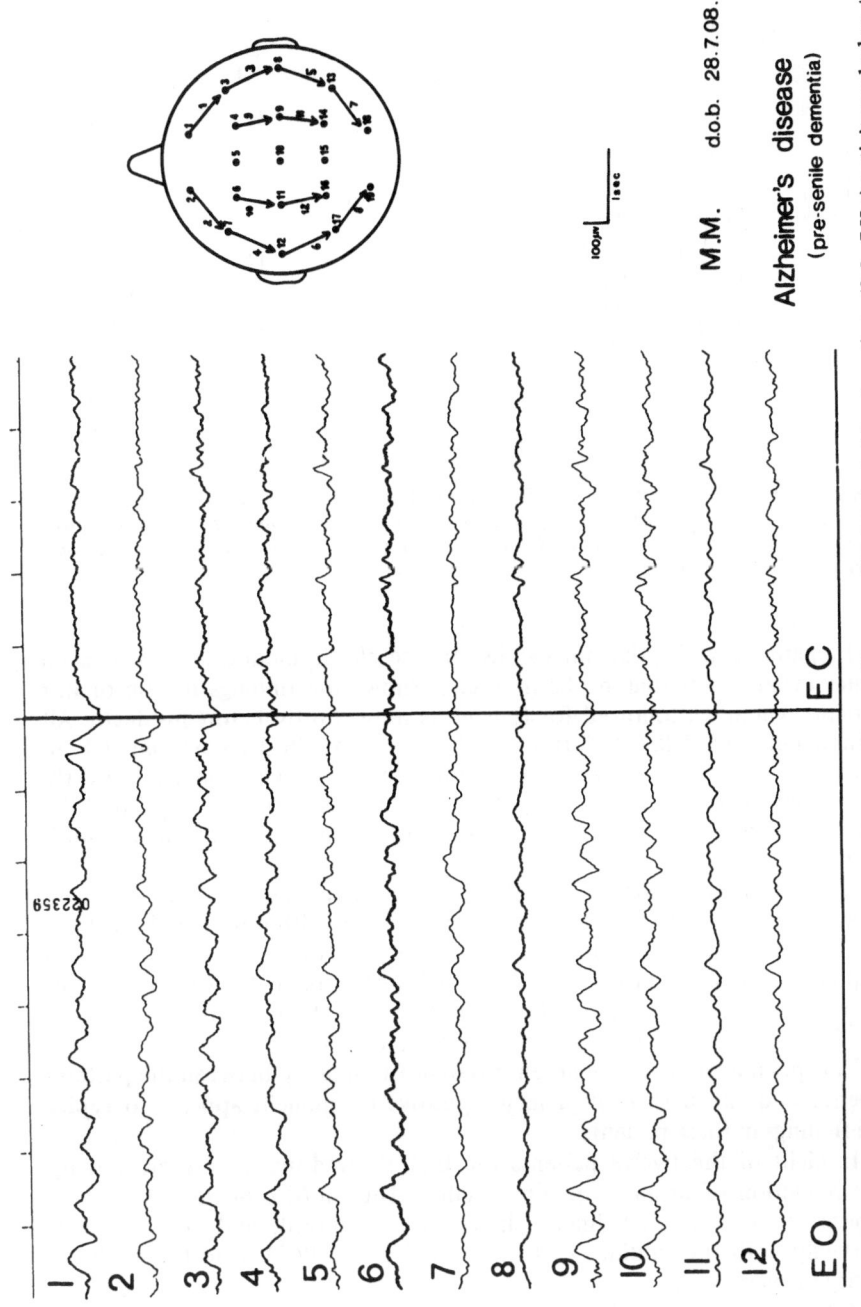

M.M.   d.o.b. 28.7.08.

Alzheimer's disease
(pre-senile dementia)

Fig. 1. This figure shows the classic EEG pattern in Alzheimers disease. The record is dominated by slow theta (3.5–7 Hz.) activity and when the eyes are closed (EC) there is practically no alpha activity observable in the posterior derivations (Channels 5, 6, 7, 8, 11 and 12).

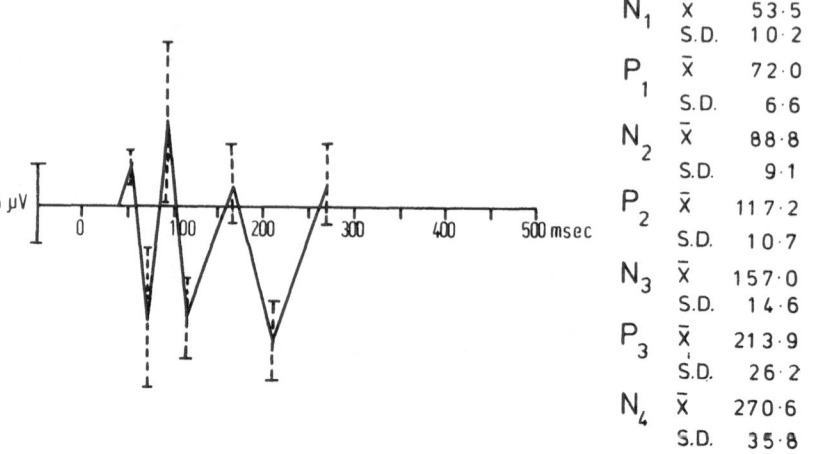

component	latency (m.sec.)	
N_1	$\bar{x}$	53·5
	S.D.	10·2
P_1	$\bar{x}$	72·0
	S.D.	6·6
N_2	$\bar{x}$	88·8
	S.D.	9·1
P_2	$\bar{x}$	117·2
	S.D.	10·7
N_3	$\bar{x}$	157·0
	S.D.	14·6
P_3	$\bar{x}$	213·9
	S.D.	26·2
N_4	$\bar{x}$	270·6
	S.D.	35·8

Fig. 2. Shows the average normal flash evoked potential for an elderly population (65–75 years). The exaggerated P_1 component at 72 milliseconds can be seen, almost equal in amplitude to the later P_2 component (117.2 milliseconds). The standard deviations for amplitude are shown as dotted vertical bars.

In patients with Alzheimer's disease the classic picture is of a delayed visual evoked potential to flash. Fig. 3 shows the findings in one of our patients whom we followed for four years until shortly before his death. All components are delayed, but it can be seen that the P_2 component is in excess of 200 m.secs. latency. The earlier P_1 component remains too early to be identified as a flash evoked P_2 component. It should be noted that the marked delay is present in the earliest recording and persists unchanged until shortly before death.

Surprisingly, although in almost every patient the flash VEP was markedly delayed, the response to pattern-reversal remained within normal limits (Fig. 4). In this example the difference in latency between the pattern-reversal response, and the flash response exhibited by this patient is of the order of 50 milliseconds. The mean difference in latency between pattern reversal and flash responses in these patients was 59.4 m.secs.

This phenomenon of a marked difference in latency between the pattern-reversal and the flash evoked major positive component appears to typify the findings in these patients.

In eight of the twelve patients the EEG showed increased theta activity and reduction of background alpha rythm. Thus in 67% of the patients the typical pattern of Alzheimer's disease was observed, and this contrasts markedly with the findings of Gordon and Sim (1967), who found abnormality in every case.

Table 1 gives the details of the patients, their ages and diagnoses, and the EEG and visual evoked potential findings to flash and pattern reversal

196

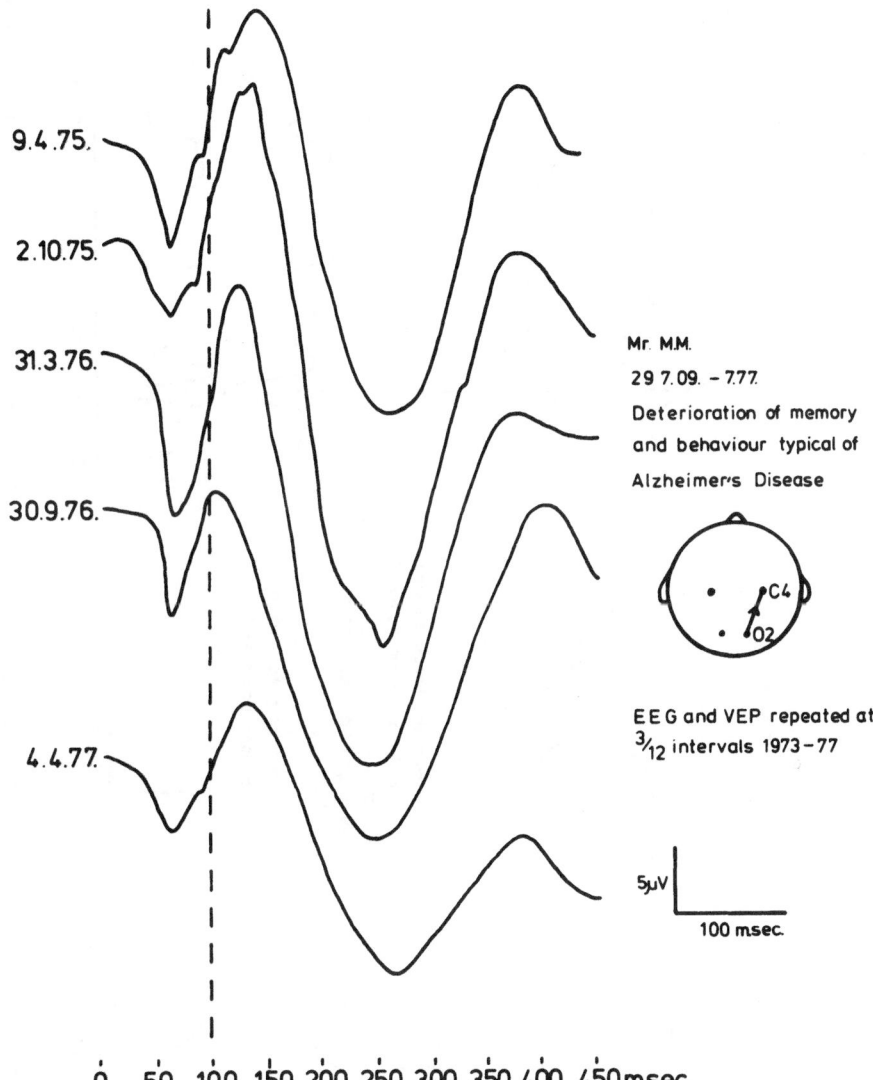

9.4.75.

2.10.75.

31.3.76.

30.9.76.

4.4.77.

Mr. M.M.

29 7.09. – 7.77.

Deterioration of memory
and behaviour typical of
Alzheimer's Disease

EEG and VEP repeated at
³⁄₁₂ intervals 1973–77

5μV

100 msec.

0 50 100 150 200 250 300 350 400 450 msec.

Fig. 3. Alzheimer's disease, serial flash VEP. This patient was studied for 4 years prior to death. He was diagnosed when his dementia was in its early stages, and periodically investigated with EEG and VEPs. As can be seen his flash evoked potential consistently showed a P_1 component around 70 m.secs., N_2 at 140 m.secs. and P_2 at 250 m.secs. This delay remained relatively unaltered during the course of his progressive dementia.

stimuli. It can be seen that although the EEG did not always show abnormality, ten of the twelve patients showed a delayed flash visual evoked potential. In two of the patients (W.C. and M.R.) the latency of the flash evoked potential was just within the upper limits of the normal range for the

197

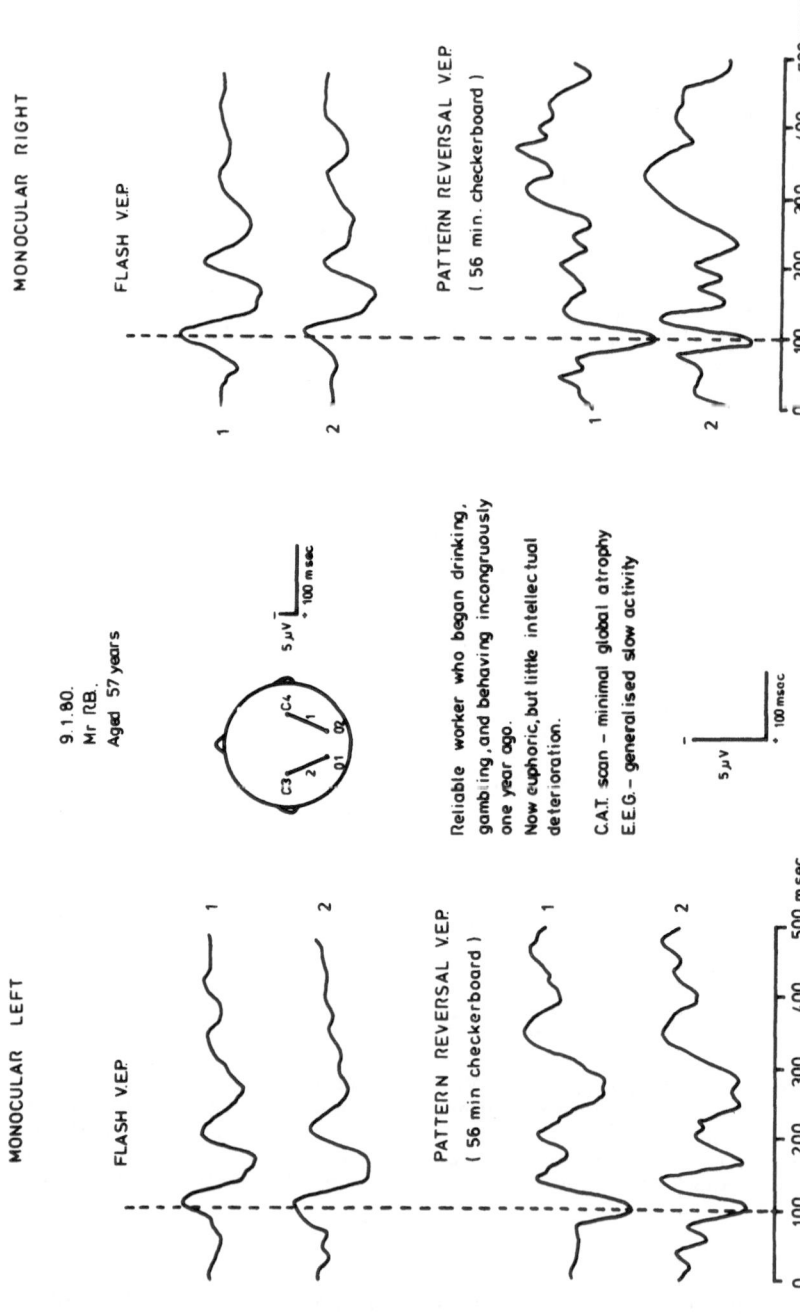

Fig. 4. Pre-senile dementia. The visual evoked potential to flash stimulation of either eye shows a delayed P_2 component at 150 m.secs. Pattern-reversal stimulation reveals a clear major positive at 100 m.secs. exactly at the mean norm.

Table 1. Pre-senile dementia – clinical details of 12 patients investigated between April 1971 and May 1980.

Initial	Age	E.E.G.	Visual Evoked Potential latency of P_2			Diagnosis	Other clinical indications
			Flash	P.R.	Diff		
A.B.	69	Slow	150	–	–	Alzheimer's	Pneumoencephalography – lateral ventricles dilated, illusions, senile paranoia, incontinency
M.M.	66	Slow	250	120	130	Alzheimer's	
E.S.	66	Slow	170	–	–	Alzheimer's	
E.G.	63	EMG artifact	170	(EMG)	–	Alzheimer's	
B.K.	66	Slow low amp	170	100	70	Pre-senile dementia	Pneumoencephalography – diffuse atrophy
K.T.	69	Normal	140	100	40	Arterio sclerotic dementia	1977 – considerable memory deficit
W.C.	61	Normal low amp	130	105	25	Alzheimer's	Progressive deterioration of Alzheimer type. CAT Scan showed cerebral atrophy
M.W.	57	Slow	150	108	42	Alzheimer's	Severely demented
R.B.	57	Slow	150	100	50	Pre-senile dementia	Behaviour changes. CAT-Scan – minimal cerebral atrophy
L.V.	60	Normal	180	105	75	Pre-senile dementia	Forgetfulness
M.R.	53	Slow	130	95	35	Pre-senile dementia	Intellectual impairment forgetfulness
G.W.	60	Slow	160	92	68	Alzheimer's	Severe cognitive impairment – preservation of personality
Means	62.25		162.5	102.7			

age. All the nine patients tested showed a classically normal pattern-reversal response well within the normal range for latency and of normal morphology. The patients who had flash visual evoked potentials just within the normal range, showed a pattern-reversal response 25 or 35 milliseconds earlier.

It is of interest to note that two other patients have been investigated under the heading 'possible Alzheimer's disease', in both cases their findings were atypical and they ultimately were found to be suffering from other conditions.

These patients showed a markedly delayed pattern-reversal response as well as a delayed flash response (Fig. 5).

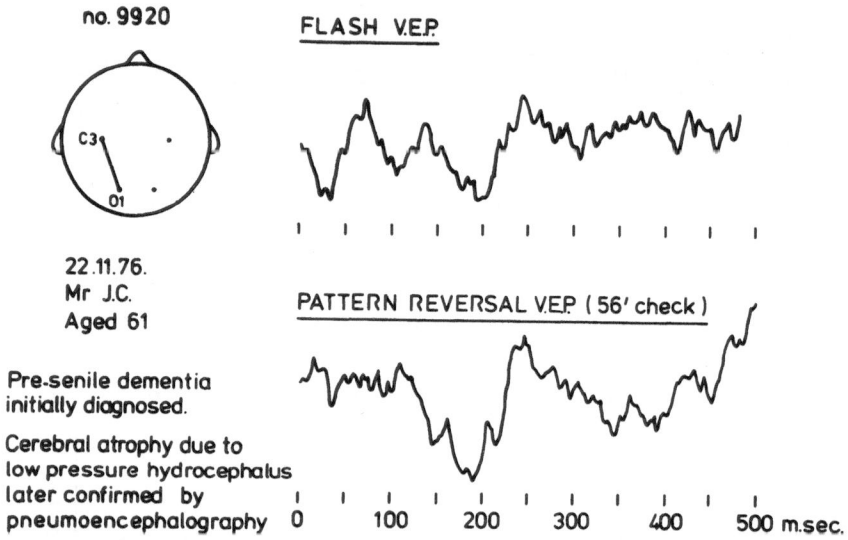

Fig. 5. Low pressure hydrocephalus. The flash and pattern reversal VEP in a patient initially diagnosed as pre-senile dementia. Both the flash and pattern VEP are delayed which is not consistent with the results observed in other patients with pre-senile dementia. Other techniques showed the initial diagnosis to be incorrect, and low pressure hydrocephalus to be the cause of the cerebral atrophy.

DISCUSSION

Fig. 6 summarises the findings of both flash and pattern-reversal and compares the patients to a similarly aged, control population. It can be seen that the latency of the pattern-reversal responses nicely overlaps that of the normal controls, whereas the latency of the flash response shows a clear delay in almost all cases. This latter finding confirms that of Visser et al. (1976), although the presence of this delay coexisting with normal latency pattern-reversal response has not previously been observed. The mechanism for this unusual finding is unknown, but the presence of cerebral atrophy with probable integrity of the visual pathway may be the critical feature.

200

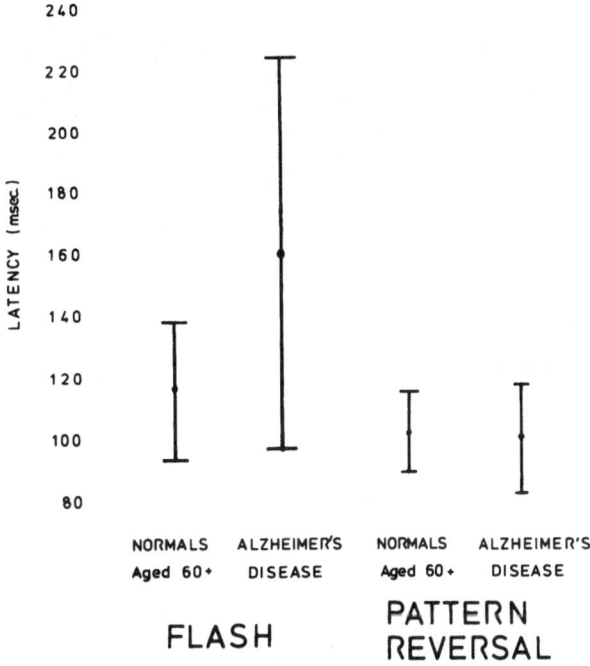

240

220

200

LATENCY (msec.)

180

160

140

120

100

80

| NORMALS | ALZHEIMER'S | NORMALS | ALZHEIMER'S |
| Aged 60+ | DISEASE | Aged 60+ | DISEASE |

FLASH PATTERN REVERSAL

Fig. 6. Latency of P$_2$ component in Alzheimer's disease. Means ± 2 standard deviations of the major positive component of the flash and pattern VEP in a group of 12 patients suffering from pre-senile dementia. Comparison with a group of elderly control subjects shows that the flash VEP is delayed, but the pattern reversal VEP is normal in pre-senile dementia.

This unusual VEP finding may well have diagnostic significance since it appears a better indicator than the EEG of pre-senile dementia of the Alzheimer type. Future studies will include Picks disease and senile dementia and it is hoped that this technique will provide a neurophysiological correlate of the histological and clinical similarities between senile dementia and Alzheimer's pre-senile dementia.

ACKNOWLEDGEMENTS

We are grateful to the various psychiatrists who have referred these patients, and to the patients for their co-operation.

REFERENCES

Dustman, R.E. & Beck, E.C. The effects of maturation and ageing on the wave form of visually evoked potentials. Electroenceph. clin. Neurophysiol. 26: 2–11 (1969).
Gordon, E.B. & Sim, M. The EEG in pre-senile dementia. J. Neurol. Neurosurg. Psychiat. 30: 285–291 (1967).

Lee, R.G. & Blair, D.G. Evolution of EEG and visual evoked response changes in Jakob-Creutzfeldt disease. Electroenceph. clin. Neurophysiol. 35: 133−142 (1973).

Perez, F.I., Rivera, V.M., Meyer, J.S., Gay, J.R.A., Taylor, R.L. & Matthew, N.T. Analysis of intellectual and cognitive performance in patients with multi-infarct dementia, vertibrobasilar insufficiency with dementia and Alzheimers disease. J. Neurol. Neurosurg. Psychiat. 38: 533−540 (1975).

Straumanis, J.J., Shagass, C. & Schwartz, M. Visual evoked cerebral response changes associated with chronic brain syndromes and aging. J. Gerontol. 00: 498−506 (1965).

Visser, S.L., Stam, F.C., Van Tilburg, W., Op den Velde, W., Blom, J.L. & De Rijke, W. Visual evoked response in senile and pre-senile dementia. Electroenceph. clin. Neurophysiol. 40: 385−392 (1976).

Authors address:
Clinical Neurophysiology Unit,
Dept. of Ophthalmic Optics,
University of Aston in Birmingham,
Birmingham, England

POSTOPERATIVE ELECTROPHYSIOLOGICAL FINDINGS IN PATIENTS WITH PITUITARY ADENOMA

W. MÜLLER & E. SCHMÖGER

(Erfurt/D.D.R.)

ABSTRACT

The authors have carried out electrodiagnostic examinations in 12 patients after resection of a pituitary adenoma. In almost every patient changes in the EOG, ERG and VECP could be evinced. The cause of both hormonal effects and mechanical influences on the visual pathway structures is discussed in terms of a disturbance of the equilibrium of centrifugal and centripetal pathways.

INTRODUCTION

We first had the intention to present the problems involved in perimetry by means of visually evoked cortical potentials (VECPs) in patients after resection of the pituitary adenoma. This struck us as being of interest from the aspect of giving proof of incomplete or relative hemianopsia. In addition to the VECP changes, we noticed, incidental to comprehensive investigations, changes in the electro-oculogram (EOG) and in the scotopic electroretinogram (ERG) to a suprisingly high degree. We refer to the results obtained in 12 postoperative patients, but meanwhile we have examined electrodiagnostically other patients falling into this category.

METHODS

Apart from the standard clinical diagnosis in our 12 patients the ERGs were recorded photopically and scotopically as well as the EOGs and VECPs applying a technique described previously (Müller, Haase, Gauß & Jung, 1980). These techniques included automated ERG recording, peak times and amplitudes analogue and digitally computer-recorded; stimulus intensities used were 0.6, 2.0, 6.0, 25 and 50 Joules (J). VECP recording was effected at the hemisphere of the Ilmenau-Erfurt Perimeter I at a stimulus intensity of 0.2 J with a background illumination of 10 lux.

Doc. Ophthal. Proc. Series, Vol. 27, ed. by H. Spekreijse & P.A. Apkarian
© *1981 Dr W. Junk Publishers, The Hague/Boston/London*

The macula and an area of 10° nasally from the macula was stimulated. In order to exclude any artefacts, a great number of examinations were carried out repeatedly.

RESULTS

The clinical results obtained in 12 postoperative patients are represented in Tables 1 and 2. We have established 2 groups:

In group I are those patients who show a combination of normal disc with normal visual fields (5 patients). In group II are those patients affected with visual field defects in both eyes, and in most cases with an optic nerve atrophy of both eyes (7 patients).

Table 1. 12 patients after resection of pituitary adenoma. (9 female, 3 male, mean age 45 — ranging from 27 to 59)

Optic disc		Visual field	
Normal both	7 patients	Normal both	6 patients
Atrophy both	4 patients	Bi-temporal hemianopsia	1 patient
Atrophy of one disc (optic disc of the other eye could not be seen)	1 patient	Incomplete bi-temporal hemianopsia	3 patients
		Amaurosis of one eye, residual visual field of the other eye	2 patients

Table 2. 12 patients after resection of pituitary adenoma. (9 female, 3 male, mean age 45 — ranging from 27 to 59)

Visual acuity	Eyes
0.7 – 1.0	17
0.3 – 0.6	5
blind eye	2

Electrodiagnostic results obtained with group I. Table 3 gives a compilation of results for group I. Table 4 compiles the individual results, that is to say in the 5 patients of this group we found only one whose electrodiagnostic results (EOG, ERG, VECP) could be considered normal.

Electrodiagnostic results obtained with group II. Table 5 indicates the results obtained with group II. Table 6 gives a compilation of the individual results. Of those 7 patients not one showed a normal EOG, ERG and VECP. The scotopic ERG was changed in all of the patients, the EOG in 6 of 7 patients, the peak time of the VECP in 4 of 7 patients was prolonged. The results obtained with 2 patients are demonstrated in Fig. 1 & 2a and b.

Table 3. Group I (normal ophthalmological findings).
5 patients

	Patients
Decreased visual acuity	0
EOG changes	4
ERG changes (scotopic)	4
VECP (prolonged peak time)	4

Table 4. Group I (normal ophthalmological findings).
5 patients

	Changes	Amount	Pat. No.
EOG	Right shifting	2	1 dark trough 12 min. 7 dark trough 13 min.
	Basic value ⩾ light peak	2	5 and 6
	Normal	1	10
ERG scotopic	Subnormal a- and b-wave	2	1 and 7
	Superelevated a- and b-wave	1	5
	Normal a-wave and subnormal b-wave	1	10
	Normal a- and b-wave	1	6
VECP	Prolonged peak time	4	1, 5, 7 and 10
	Normal peak time	1	6

Table 5. Group II (pathological ophthalmological findings).
7 patients

	Patients
Optic disc atrophy	5
Amaurosis of one eye	2
EOG changes	6
ERG changes (scotopic)	7
VECP (prolonged peak time)	4

Irrespective of these 12 patients we should like to show you a patient in whom the pituitary adenoma was clinically diagnosed only; the operation, however, had not yet been done. The patient 38 years of age showed a normal vision, normal discs and a normal visual field. The EOG showed a light peak that hardly exceeded the basic value, and did not show any downward tendency up to the 12th minute (following light onset). The scotopic ERG showed reduced a- and b-waves, and was subnormal. The VECP was

Table 6. Group II (pathological ophthalmological findings).
7 patients

	Changes		Amount	Pat. No.
EOG	Right shifting Dark trough 13. or 14. min.		3	2 (r.e.) left eye: retinal detachment 3 and 4
	Superelevated		2	8 and 9
	Subnormal dark period		1	12
	Normal		1	11
ERG scotopic	Subnormal a- and b-wave		3	3, 4 and 8
	Normal a-wave	subnormal b-wave	1	9
		superelevated b-wave	2	11 12 (l.e.) right eye blind: subnormal b
	No recording of ERG		1	2
VECP	Prolonged peak time		4	2 (left eye blind) 11, 4 and 12 (right eye blind)
	Normal peak time		3	3, 8 and 9

developed satisfactorily, the peak times were normal. Fig. 3 shows the results obtained.

DISCUSSION

In all pituitary adenomas hormonal effects on retinal and visual evoked cortical potentials are theoretically possible. Little is known about such effects as Tota & Cavallacci have already reported in 1970, and Wirth just lately in 1979. According to the animal experiments carried out by Nagata (1959a, b) one may start from the assumption that adenohypophysial hormones are enhancing the retinal potentials, whereas the neurohypophysial hormones are reducing these potentials. Other interesting animal experiments by Olafson & O'Steen (1976), and O'Steen & Kraeer (1977) seem to indicate that hormones of the pituitary gland have a regulatory influence on the severity of light-induced retinal photorecptor damage in rats. Furthermore, mention should be made of the clinical descriptions by Wirth (1968) in 5 cases of 'diencephalic-hypophysis diseases' (incomplete Bardet-Biedl syndrome) in which 'supernormal' electroretinograms were recorded.

Regarding our problem, of importance is the information by Smail (1972) who detected an extinguished ERG in a case of a pituitary adenoma, implicating the intermediate part of the gland. A primary pigmentary degeneration of the retina existed, possibly in relationship to a melanophore-stimulating hormone. In addition to these hormonal influence probabilities, mechanical impairment of the visual pathway should be borne in mind. The functional

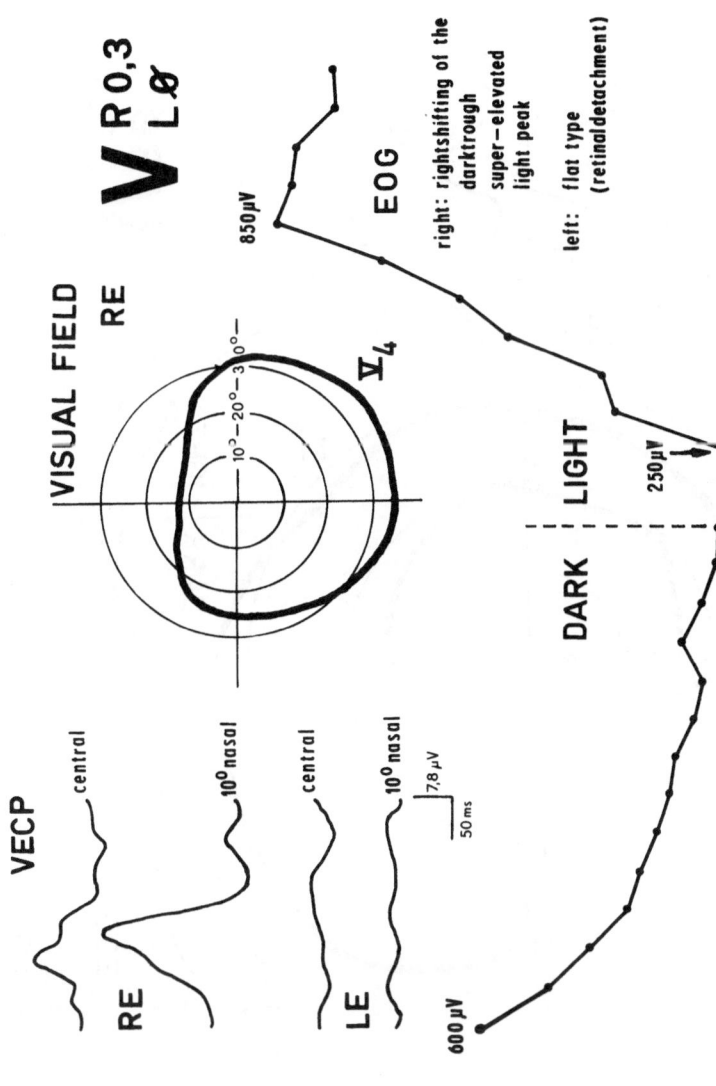

Fig. 1. Data of the patient No. 2 of group II.
Only the right eye must be assessed. The left eye went blind due to a retinal detachment. Remarkable is the shifting to the right in the EOG of the right eye. Dark trough 14th minute. The light peak is very high and must be deemed excessive.

207

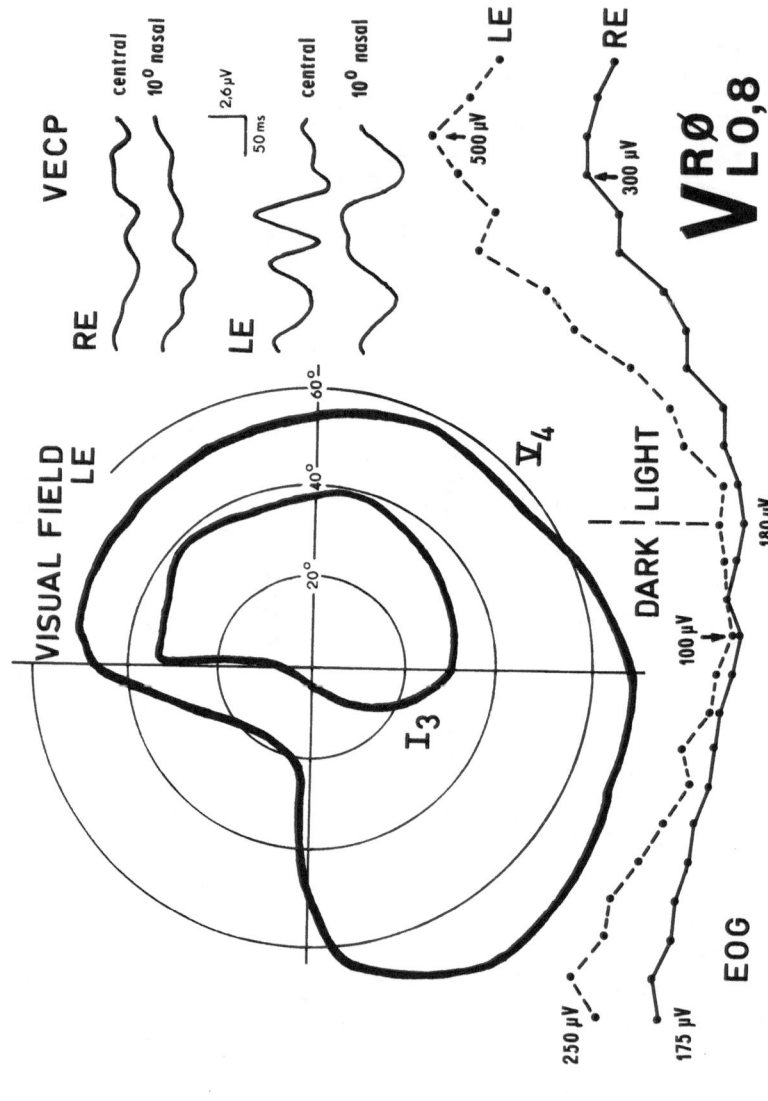

Fig. 2a Data of the patient No. 12 of group II.
The right eye went blind after the operation. The EOG showed a flat dark phase and a distinctly low light peak.
The a-waves in the ERG are bilaterally normal, the b-wave, however, is clearly in the subnormal range.

Fig. 2b. Patient No. 12 (group II)

	ERG		
Stimulus J	right eye (a-wave = normal) b-wave μV	left eye (a-wave = normal) b-wave μV	b (standard) μV
0.4	227	73	440
0.6	340	143	460
2.0	391	173	560
6.0	446	182	600
25.0	430	198	620
50.0	399	208	600

disorders of the visual field caused by this are reflected in the VECP, as shown by Wildberger and co-workers (1976; 1977) in cases of pituitary adenoma.

Also to be considered is an impairment of the hypothetic centrifugal optic fibres which are to have an inhibiting effect on the excitability of the retina (Borg & Knave 1971; Jacobson & Suzuki 1962), especially in progressing dark adaptation. Clinically, adequate observations by Feinsod & Auerbach (1971), as well as by Feinsod, Rowe & Auerbach (1971a, b), support the hypothesis of such centrifugally inhibiting effects on the retina. Among other things, they have reported on 3 patients with pituitary adenoma all of whom showed preoperatively 'subnormal' ERG amplitudes in addition to defective VECPs, and beyond this, at least in two cases they showed optic nerve lesions due to Tuberculum sellae meningioma with preoperatively enhanced retinal responses, the last mentioned of which postoperatively showed great improvement. Although not within the limits of this paper it would be worthwhile to analyse the interesting findings by these authors more accurately.

Due to the fact that our 12 cases could be examined only postoperatively it must be assumed that possible hormonal influences already faded away. This similarly applies to defects of the visual pathway. In the VECP the prolonged peak times, available in $\frac{2}{3}$ of all instances, are relevant. They may help to explain disinhibited retinal potentials on the assumption that there is damage to the hypothetic centrifugal optic fibres together with optic disc atrophy. We were able to discern increased ERG amplitudes only three times whereas decreased ERG amplitudes were discerned seven times; these results really cannot be explained by optic disc atrophy. The changes in the EOG, concerning almost every case involved, are also hard to explain unless all the reduced retinal potentials are traced back to hormonal influences by the intermediate pituitary part of the gland or neurohypophysis and on the assumption that these were not reversible by means of an operation.

In this connection the pre-operative results obtained in the previously discussed patient are certainly of interest. These results provide evidence of a subnormal scotopic ERG and clear EOG changes at normal VECP peak times.

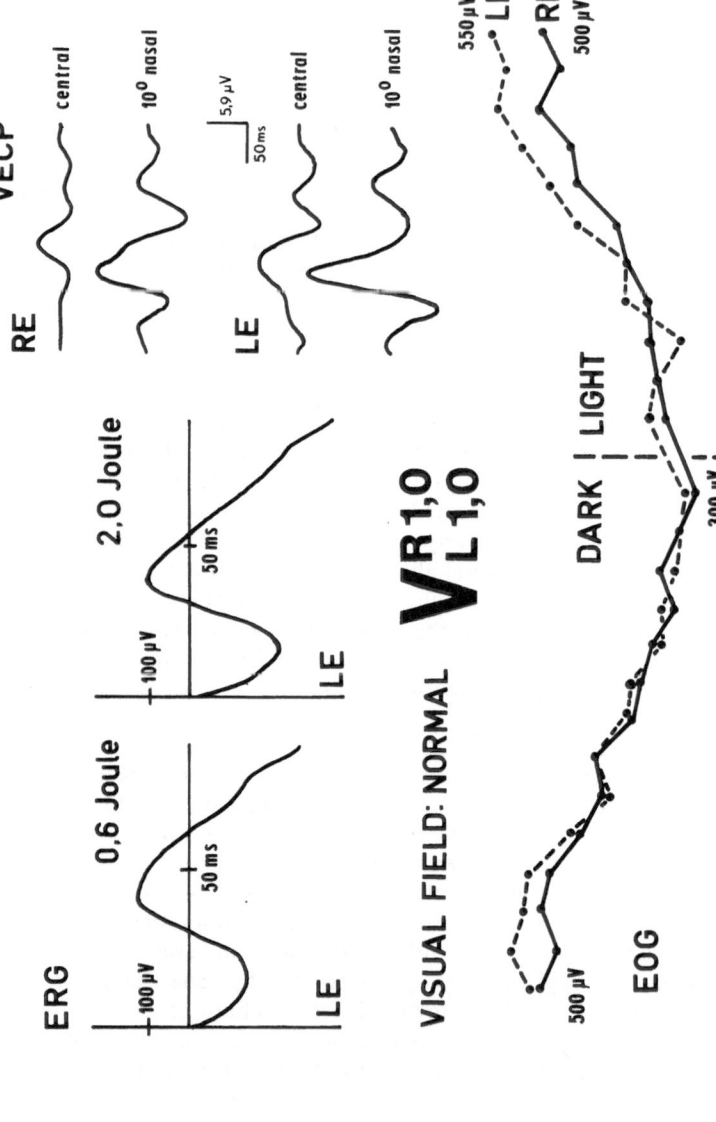

Fig. 3. Data of patient No. 13. Pituitary adenoma clinically secured. Operation has not yet been carried out. EOG: Basic value approximately at the same level as the light peak. ERG (scotopic): a- and b-wave subnormal. VECP: normal.

The problematic nature of the interesting and important issues concerning pituitary adenoma suggest further comprehensive investigations in this area.

REFERENCES

Borg, E. & Knave, B. Long-term changes in the ERG following transection of the optic nerve in the rabbit. Acta Physiol. Scand. 82: 277–281 (1971).

Feinsod, M. & Auerbach, E. ERG and visuell ausgelöste Rindenantwort bei 2 Patienten mit Meningiom des Tuberkulum sellae vor und nach Druckentlastung des N. opticus. Ophthalmologica 193: 360–368 (1971).

Feinsod, M., Rowe, H. & Auerbach, E. Changes in the electroretinogram in patients with optic nerve lesions. Docum. Ophthal. 29: 169–200 (1971a).

Feinsod, M., Rowe, H. & Auerbach, E. Enhanced retinal responses without signs of optic nerve involvement. Docum. Ophthal. 29: 201–211 (1971b).

Jacobson, J.H. & Suzuki, T.A. Effects of optic nerve section on the ERG. AMA Arch. Ophth. 67: 791–801 (1962).

Müller, W., Haase, E., Gauß, J. & Jung, N. Investigation by means of VECP in patients with chronic nephropathy. Docum. Ophthal. Proc. Ser. 23: 171–175 (1980).

Nagata, M. Experimental studies on the influence of pituitary hormones an thiamine on the retina action current. III. The influence of the loading of the pituitary hormones combined with vit. B 1 upon the ERG of rabbits. Acta Soc. Ophthal. Jap. 63: 613–623 (1959a).

Nagata, M. Experimental studies on the influence of pituitary hormones an thiamine on the retina action current. IV. The influence of posterior pituitary hormone of simple use or combined load with vitamin B 1 on ERG in rabbit. Acta Soc. Ophthal. Jap. 63: 1030–1041 (1959).

Olafson, R.P. & O'Steen, W.K. Hormonal influences on photoreceptor damage: the pituitary gland and ovaries. Invest. Ophthalmol. Vis. Sci. 15: 869–872 (1976).

O'Steen, W.K. & Kraer, S.L. Effects of hypophysectomy, pituitary gland homogenates and transplant, and prolactin on photoreceptor destruction. Invest. Ophthalmol. Vis. Sci. 16: 940–946 (1977).

Smail, J.M. Primary pigmentary degeneration of the retina and acromegaly in a case of pituitary adenoma. Br. J. Ophthal. 56: 25–31 (1972).

Tota, G. & Cavallacci, G. Fisiopatologia dell'elettroretinogramma nelle mattie endocrine. Ann. Ottal. 96: 553–577 (1970).

Wildberger, H.G., Van Lith, G.H.M., Wijngaarde, R. & Mak, G.T.M. Visual evoked cortical potentials in the evaluation of homonymous and bitemporal visual field defects. Br. J. Ophthal. 60: 273–278 (1976).

Wildberger, H.G., Van Lith, G.H.M., Wijngaarde, R. & Mak, G.T.M. Differential diagnostic aspects between optic neuritis and chiasm tumors. Ophthalmologica 174: 106–110 (1977).

Wirth, A. ERG and endocrine disorders. In: ISCERG Symposium 1966; The clinical value of electroretinography. (Ed. J. François) Karger, Basel. 260–266 (1968).

Wirth, A. Electroretinogram in general medicine. Ophthalmologica 178: 273–288 (1979).

Author's address:
Eye Clinic
Medical Academy
Nordhäuser Str. 74
DDR -- 506 Erfurt

PART FOUR

PATTERN EVOKED POTENTIAL LATENCY

PATTERN REVERSAL AND APPEARANCE-DISAPPEARANCE RESPONSES IN MS PATIENTS

F.C.C. RIEMSLAG, H. SPEKREIJSE & H. VAN WALBEEK

(Amsterdam, The Netherlands)

ABSTRACT

The contrast reversal response seems to be related to the contrast decrease response (Estévez & Spekreijse 1974). Therefore, the response to the appearance and disappearance of a pattern, which consists of 4 identifiable components probably of different cortical origin, should be a better diagnostic tool for discriminiating patients with possible demyelinating diseases than the response evoked by pattern reversal. We have thus far examined 65 MS patients with both stimulus conditions. On the basis of a 3 SD criterion we tested the latency of the major positive peak of the reversal responses, and the latencies of CI, CII, CIII and the major positive peak of the disappearance component in the appearance-disappearance responses. The detection of an increased latency, particularly for the group diagnosed as definite MS (N = 41), was highest for the appearance-disappearance condition. In addition all patients having an increased latency for the reversal condition also showed an increased latency for the appearance-disappearance condition. The results suggest that the appearance-disappearance stimulus, being more effective in evoking a significant contrast response, should be preferred for clinical diagnosis.

INTRODUCTION

Two stimulus conditions are frequently used for the generation of contrast evoked potentials. The one, in which the two sets of spatial elements in the pattern (e.g. black and white checks) are interchanged abruptly every time, is called pattern reversal; the other, in which the pattern is abruptly replaced by a homogeneous field of preferably the same mean luminance as the pattern, is called appearance-disappearance or pattern onset-offset. Typical responses to both stimulus conditions as measured with an electrode 2.5 cm above the inion and referenced to linked ears, are plotted in Fig. 1. With a spatially symmetric pattern the responses to pattern reversal consist of identical waveforms to the two reversals generally depicted in a record.

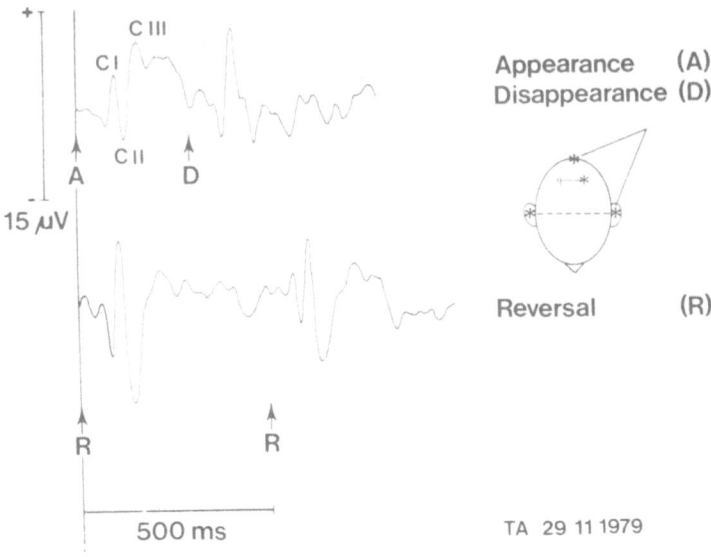

+ ‾

C III

C I

A

C II   D

15 μV

R   R

500 ms   TA 29 11 1979

Appearance   (A)
Disappearance (D)

Reversal   (R)

Fig. 1. Typical responses to appearance-disappearance (top record) of a pattern and to pattern reversal (bottom record) as measured from a midline electrode 2.5 cm above inion and referenced to linked ears. The presentation time in the appearance-disappearance condition was 300 ms every 800 ms; pattern onset and offset are marked by arrows. The reversal rate was 2 reversals per second at instants indicated by arrows. Positivity is upwards in this and subsequent figures.

These waveforms (NPN complex) consistently contain 'a major positive peak' at about 100 ms (Halliday, McDonald & Mushin 1972). In the appearance-disappearance situation two different responses are found; one that is characteristic of the appearance of the pattern, and the other characteristic of the disappearance. The appearance response to a checkerboard pattern very often consists of three distinguishable components (PNP complex). The first, rather weak, positive peak with a latency of about 80 ms is generally indicated as CI, the second, strong, negative peak as CII and the third, positive peak, which is favoured by binocular presentation as CIII (Jeffreys & Axford 1972). The waveform of the disappearance response is generally less complicated and does not vary as much with the spatial parameters of the pattern as the appearance response. It consists mainly of a major positive peak, which, according to Estévez & Spekreijse (1974) is related to the reversal response.

The reversal stimulus was successfully introduced by Halliday in 1972 in the clinic for the differential diagnosis of multiple sclerosis (MS) (Halliday, McDonald & Mushin 1972). These researchers measured the latency of the major positive peak in the reversal response and proved it to be increased in a high percentage of MS patients, even in those without any visual complaints. The success of the work by Halliday's group has prompted commercial fabrication of the pattern reversal stimulus, which is now routinely used in many clinics (see e.g. Spekreijse, Duwaer & Posthumus-Meyjes 1979).

216

Since with the present low-cost micro-processors pattern appearance-disappearance stimuli can be generated as easily as pattern reversal stimuli, an appraisal of both methods for the diagnosis of MS seems indicated.

METHODS

A TV screen (Sony CVM-1810 E, 50 Hz) subtending 6° x 4°, was used to display, at a luminance of 200 asb, a black and white checkerboard pattern with either 20' or 55' checks of nearly 100% contrast. In order to record transient reversal responses, the reversals were presented at a rate of two reversals per second. In the appearance-disappearance condition the pattern was presented for 300 ms every 800 ms. This long presentation time of 300 ms was chosen to be certain that the appearance responses would not be contaminated by the disappearance responses. The recording was typically performed with Ag-AgCl electrodes positioned on the midline 2.5 cm above the inion and referenced to linked ears. The bandwidth of the EEG amplifiers was set at 0.5 to 75 Hz. The EEG was also fed through a low-pass fourth-order Butterworth filter (Barr & Strout EF: cut off frequency 70 Hz), which introduced a total increase of peak latency of 9 ms in the records. If one wishes to estimate peak latency from the responses depicted in this paper, this correction should be made. A combined HP 21MX-HP 2100 computer system was used for averaging the EEG signals. Sixty-five patients classified according to the McAlpine criteria (McAlpine, Lumsden & Acheson 1972) were tested with both reversal and appearance-disappearance stimuli. As a control 24 healthy subjects, 14 to 68 years of age also were tested with both stimulus conditions.

RESULTS AND DISCUSSION

At first the range of normal values was established in order to determine the usual criterion of 3 standard deviations (SD) above the mean. Table 1 presents these normative data and gives the mean peak latencies and the Standard Deviations of the several identifiable components in the contrast responses upon stimulation of the right eye of all subjects studied. The interocular latency differences (latency of the left eye minus that of the right eye) also are given as measured by fitting the monocular responses for best correlation by visual inspection. These data show that the choice by Halliday of the reversal response for clinical practice is a good one, because the standard deviation of the peak latency of the major positivity in the reversal response is smaller than that of any of the components in the appearance response. The smaller the standard deviation, the sharper of course, the discrimination between normal and abnormal response profiles.

It should be emphasized that these latency values may not be considered as normative for other stimulus situations, because peak latencies are influenced by several stimulus parameters including mean luminance, contrast of

217

Table 1. Normal values.

	Mean (ms)	S.D. (ms)	N
Checksize 20'			
Reversals	98	8	23
CI	76	10	21
CII	116	16	24
CIII	175	25	22
Disappearance	116	14	23
Interoc. diff. rever.	0	4	22
Interoc. diff. app. dis.	1	4	21
Checksize 55'			
Reversals	100	8	24
CI	84	11	18
CII	116	11	22
CIII	159	19	20
Disappearance	112	9	21
Interoc. diff. rever.	0	4	23
Interoc. diff. app. dis.	1	4	22

the pattern, field size and check size (Spekreijse, Duwaer & Posthumus-Meyjes 1979; Cant, Hume & Shaw 1978). Furthermore, it should be realized that all these parameters can be modified by (pathological) circumstances including cataract, opacities in the eye media, astigmatism, etc. The influence of refractive error for example, is illustrated in Fig. 2, which shows the

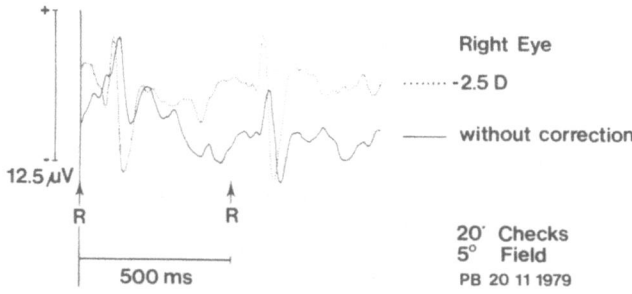

Fig. 2. Reversal responses of a normal eye of a healthy 58 year-old subject, with and without optical correction of − 2.5 diopters. If this refractive error latency difference is incorrectly interpreted as an interocular difference the response classification would be pathological (see Table 1).

reversal responses from a healthy 58 year-old subject who required only − 2.5 diopters of correction to reach a Snellen acuity of 5/5. The responses are shown with and without correction. If for instance the latency difference in these two conditions would have been interpreted as an interocular difference (see Table 1), then the uncorrected response would certainly have been classified as pathological. The results suggest that all patients should have a

Table 2. Detection of increased latencies.

Criterion 3 S.D.	Pattern reversal	Pattern on/offset	Both outside normal range	Both within normal range
Definite (41)	20	26	19	10
Probable (15)	9	10	9	4
Possible (9)	4	4	4	5

a full ophthalmological examination before being tested with pattern stimulation.

Table 2 summarizes the incidence of latency increases in the three groups of MS patients as estimated on the basis of a 3 SD criterion. It can be seen that in the definite MS group the appearance-disappearance condition gives a much higher detection rate than the reversal condition (63% versus 49%). It is to be noted that all patients, except one, with an increased latency for the reversal response also have an increased appearance-disappearance latency. The reason for the lower detection rate of the reversal response is exemplified in Fig. 3, in which the reversal and appearance-disappearance responses of a

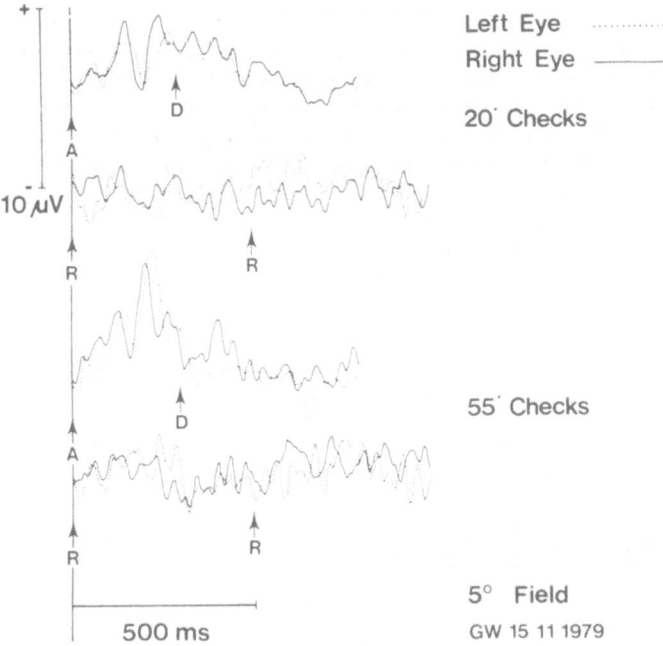

Fig. 3. Appearance-disappearance (first and third traces) and reversal (second and fourth traces) responses from the left and right eye of a definite MS Patient. For all responses the same number (80-100 averages) is used. Note that in the reversal condition the responses can not be discriminated from the background activity with either small or large checks. For the appearance-disappearance condition, however, clearly distinguishable responses are obtained.

definite MS patient are plotted. It is obvious that in the reversal condition no significant responses at all are found for either the 20' check size or the 55' check size. The appearance-disappearance condition, however, evoked clear responses with both check sizes. The same number of averages were used for the reversal and the appearance-disappearance, which can be seen from the comparable background activity in all 8 response traces. Since the appearance responses of either eye in this example are increased in latency by 50 to 70 ms above normal mean, this test confirmed the MS diagnosis.

There were only two patients with no significant contrast evoked potentials for either of the eyes. At the time of the test these two patients had visual acuity of finger counting level. The lowest acuity for which we succeeded in recording *normal* appearance EPs was 1/6. Two patients in our sample showed no significant responses for either the appearance or the reversal stimulus upon stimulation of one eye, but showed normal responses upon stimulation of the other. In literature on VEP diagnosis of MS no attention is drawn to the absence of significant reversal responses. It may be argued that the differences between our reversal stimulus conditions and those of other investigators, e.g. Halliday, account for the higher percentage of non-significant reversal responses. For instance, we use a field of 5° instead of the 32° field used by Halliday. Our data show, however, that stimulation with this small field yields a detection rate comparable to the rates reported in the literature (Spekreijse, Duwaer & Posthumus-Meyjes 1979). Furthermore, Matthews et al. in their 1977 study of a large sample (156) of MS patients, also reported patients showing no significant reversal responses, although they used the same techniques as Halliday. Finally, the absence of a significant response as a positive criterion for MS (e.g. Matthews, Small, Small & Pounney 1977) should be avoided. This is exemplified by the two patients in our sample showing no significant responses to one eye and *normal* responses to the other eye. The absence of an evoked response, per se, should not be used in the differential diagnosis of MS.

CONCLUSION

Our comparative study shows that the appearance-disappearance stimulus generates a significant response in a larger percentage of subjects than the reversal stimulus. Being more effective in generating a contrast evoked potential, the appearance-disappearance stimulus should be favoured above the reversal stimulus in clinical diagnosis.

REFERENCES

Cant, B.R., Hume, A.L. & Shaw, N.A. Effects of luminance on the pattern visual evoked potentials in multiple sclerosis. Electroenceph. clin. Neurophysiol. 45: 496−504 (1978).
Estévez, O. & Spekreijse, H. Relationship between pattern appearance-disappearance and pattern reversal responses. Exp. Brain Res. 19: 233−238 (1974).

Halliday, M., McDonald, W.I. & Mushin, J. Delayed visual evoked responses in optic neuritis. Lancet. 1: 982–985 (1972).
Jeffreys, D.A. & Axford, J.G. Source location of pattern specific components of human visual evoked potentials. I. & II. Exp. Brain Res. 16: 1–40 (1972).
Matthews, W.B., Small, D.G., Small, M. & Pounney, E. Pattern reversal evoked potential in the diagnosis of multiple sclerosis. J. Neuro. Neurosurg. Psychiat. 40: 1009 (1977).
McAlpine, D., Lumsden, C.E. & Acheson, E.D. Multiple sclerosis: a reappraisal. Churchill-Livingstone, Edinborough (1972).
Spekreijse, H., Duwaer, A.L. & Posthumus-Meyjes, F.E. Contrast evoked potentials and psychophysics in Multiple Sclerosis. In: Human evoked potentials, applications and problems (Ed. D. Lehman & E. Callaway). Plenum Press, New York. 363–381 (1979).

Authors' address:
F.C.C. Riemslag and H. Spekreijse
The Netherlands Ophthalmic Research Institute,
Dept. of Visual System Analysis
P.O. Box 6411,
1005 EK Amsterdam.

and

H. van Walbeek
The Alexander van der Leeuw Clinic,
Overtoom 363,
1054 JN Amsterdam,
The Netherlands

ON- AND OFF-CONTRIBUTION TO THE COMBINED OCCIPITAL ON-OFF RESPONSE TO A PATTERNED STIMULUS

G.H.M. VAN LITH, L. CREVITS & S. VIJFVINKEL-BRUINENGA

(Rotterdam, The Netherlands)

ABSTRACT

The hypothesis, derived from previous studies, that the off-response forms the main part of the second positive wave (P_2) in the occipital response to patterned presentations was tested by using stimuli of various durations.

It was found that the off-response confluences with P_2 of the on-response in the combined on-off response. The question, whether the on-response or the off-response contributes more to the combined on-off response could not be answered, though the on-responses were usually higher than the off-responses. By applying hemifield stimulation, the experiments furthermore confirm the conception of a double dipole in the hemisphere contralateral to the stimulated side.

INTRODUCTION

Pattern stimuli can be given as a pattern reversal stimulus or as a pattern presentation stimulus. If pattern presentations are of a long duration, the pattern appearance and disappearance responses, also labelled 'on- and off-' responses, can be separately recorded. With short presentations they melt together. Whether the responses to these various stimuli represent the same systems or structures, is certainly not only of theoretical interest, but also important from a clinical point of view.

To attack this problem, in principle, several methods are at our disposal. Variation of luminance, colour and frequency, so effective in the study of the electroretinogram, provides results when applied to pattern stimulation, that seem too complicated for our problem.

A rather simple measure is to look at waveform or latency. Even then problems may arise, for latencies depend highly on the methods used. Comparing Halliday's papers on this subject with those of Jeffreys, it appears that the main positive peaks of Halliday's reversal response and of Jeffreys' pattern flash response have approximately the same latencies (Halliday & Michael 1970; Michael & Halliday 1971; Jeffreys & Axford 1972a, b). In our set-up, however, they are quite different, viz. for a pattern reversal response 90–110 msec and for a pattern on-off response 160–180 msec.

Another method to investigate the relation between various responses is to follow carefully waveform and latencies going gradually from one stimulus form into another one. This method was applied by Estévez & Spekreijse (1974) to investigate the relation between a pattern reversal response and the response to a pattern appearance-disappearance stimulus. Their conclusion was that, 'the data of Michael and Halliday (1971), obtained with a pattern reversal stimulus seem to be mainly related to the decrease in contrast, whereas the data of Jeffreys and Axford are related to the contrast-increase' response. The first part of this conclusion was recently confirmed by Kris & Halliday (1980).

To identify various peaks, Jeffreys and Halliday applied the method of dipole localization, by stimulating parts of the visual field. From this method it appeared that the dipole of Halliday's reversal response had a different direction and location as compared to that of Jeffreys' pattern flash response. Applying hemifield stimulation, Halliday's main positive peak was highest at the ipsilateral occipital electrode, whereas Jeffreys' positive peak C_I was highest contralaterally. Last year we could provide an addition to these findings (van Lith, Henkes & Vijfvinkel-Bruinenga 1980); applying a TV-system, a pattern on-off response showed two distinct positive peaks of which the first, smaller one, behaves like Jeffreys' C_I and the second, more prominent one, like Halliday's main positive peak.

Combining the conclusion of Estévez and Spekreijse that Halliday's response is more related to the off-response, with ours, we wondered whether the off-response contributes mainly also to our second positive component. This supposition was checked with the three methods aforementioned, viz. latency measurement, transition from one stimulus form into the other one and determination of the dipole direction.

METHOD

A TV-system was used; the visual field subtended 12° by 17.5°. The check size was 40′, the contrast between light and dark checks 40% and the mean luminance 40 cd/m², which remained constant during and between the pattern presentations. Duration of the pattern presentations was nominally varied between 20 and 500 msec. It has to be realized that a stimulus duration of 20 msec, obtained by TV-techniques, presents only one frame with all problems inherent, such as a coarser line pattern and a very short actual presentation to the foveal region (Van Lith, Van Marle & Van Dok-Mak 1978; Van Lith, Van Marle & Vijfvinkel-Bruinenga 1979). The presentation frequency was maintained at 1 presentation per second. Ten normal subjects were examined. Leads according to Halliday, as well as to Jeffreys were applied.

RESULTS

The combined on-off response as well as the isolated on-response always consisted of a complex with two positive peaks (Fig. 1A), the mean latency

224

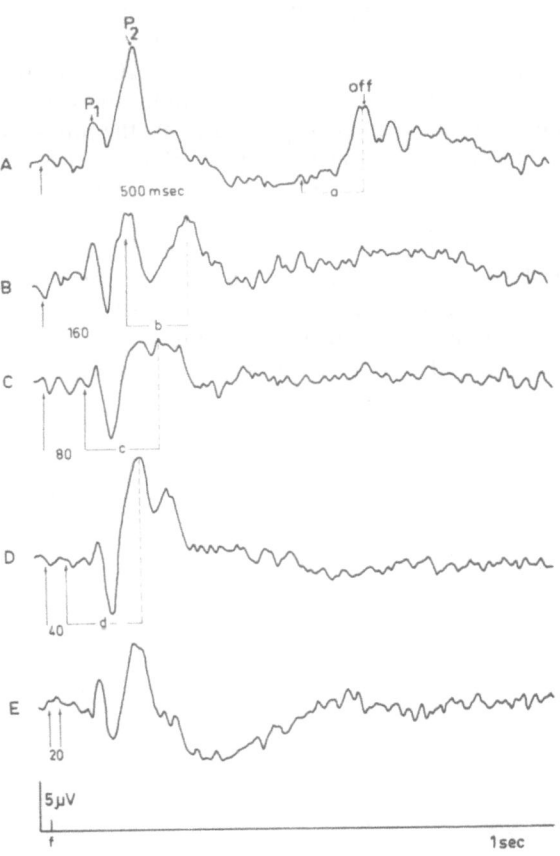

Fig. 1. Occipital potentials to a pattern appearance-disappearance stimulus of various durations: A: 500 msec, B: 160 msec, C: 80 msec, D: 40 msec, E: 20 msec. The first arrow below each recording points to a pattern on-set, the second to the pattern off-set. Latency times of the off-responses: a: 118 msec, b: 117 msec, c: 140 msec, d: 141 msec.

of the first positive peak (P1) being approximately 120 msec and that of the second positive peak (P2) 180 msec. The isolated off-response often was very small, usually only one positive peak being recognizable and measurable. Its mean latency was approximately 120 msec. From this result one might conclude that the off-response would contribute to P1 rather than to P2 of the combined on-off response. Comparing the amplitudes of the responses, however, it was P2 of the combined on-off response instead of P1, that was always substantially higher than that of the isolated on-response. This supports the idea of a contribution of the off-response at short presentations to P2.

What actually happens, can be followed going from a long pattern presentation time to a short one (Fig. 1). At 500 msec and 160 msec (A and B), the on- and off-responses are clearly separated; at 80 msec (C) they melt together resulting in a broad P2, whereas at 40 msec P2 becomes narrower again and much higher. Apparently, there is a summation of the off-response with P2 of the on-response. This summation was consistently present in all subjects, though it could occur at 80, 40 or 20 msec stimulus duration. It is possible that at shorter stimulus durations the off-response could shift further onwards and summate with P1 of the on-response. As already mentioned, however, this did not occur; P1 did not increase in height at a shorter stimulus duration, though sometimes P2 became smaller again as seen in Fig. 1 at 20 msec.

Applying hemifield stimulation, the results of last year were comfirmed. The reversal response, as well as P2 of the combined on-off response was highest at the ipsilateral occipital electrode, P1 at the contralateral side. Though less conspicuous, the same results were obtained for the isolated on-response (Fig. 2). As to the isolated off-response, it is obvious that it

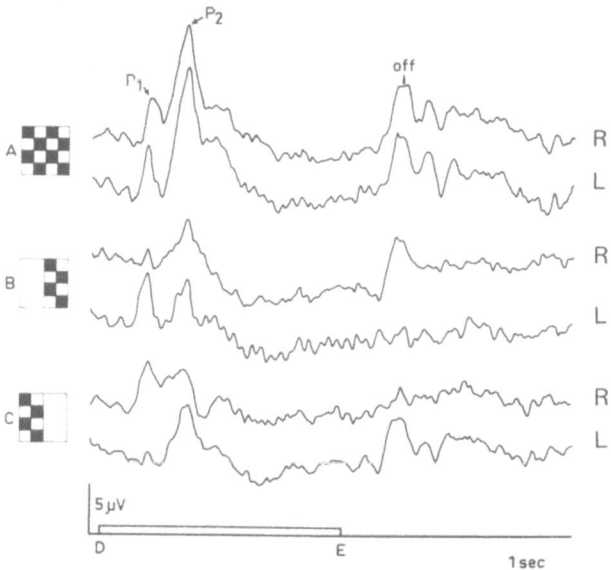

Fig. 2. Occipital potentials to a pattern appearance-disappearance stimulus of 500 msec. R/L stand for right and left electrode. A: full field stimulation, B: right hemifield stimulation, C: left hemifield stimulation, D: pattern on-set, E: pattern off-set.

is also better developed at the ipsilateral electrode, the reverse never being met in the 10 subjects. The conclusion of van Lith et al. (1980) therefore, can be extended (Fig. 3). The reversal response, P2 of the pattern on-response and of the pattern on-off response as well as the off-response, are highest at the ipsilateral electrode whereas P1 in the on-response and in the on-off response is highest at the contralateral electrode.

DISCUSSION

The amplitude measurements, as well as the dipole determinations, point to a contribution of the off-response to P2 of the combined on-off response,

226

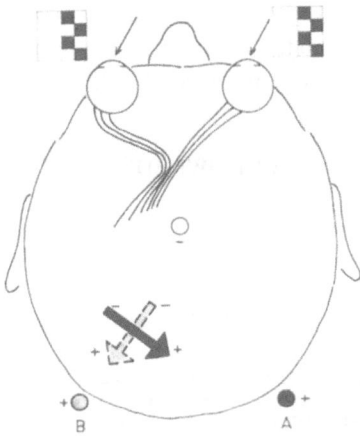

Fig. 3. Direction of the dipoles, evoked by right hemifield stimulation. A: Reversal response, P2 of a pattern on-response and of a pattern on-off response, pattern on-off response. B: P1 of a pattern on-response and of a pattern on-off response.

which is in accordance with our supposition. There remains a question, however, as to the latency measurements, because the off-response with a latency of 120 msec appears to contribute to a peak in the on-off response at 180 msec. Further study is needed regarding the off-latency time as a function of stimulus duration.

A question, which cannot be answered yet, is whether the on-response or the off-response contribute most to the combined on-off response. In Table 1, results of amplitude measurements are shown. In 6 of the 10 subjects

Table 1. Upper part: comparison of the amplitudes of P2 in the on-responses with those of the off-responses.
Lower part: comparison of the amplitudes of P2 in the combined on-off response with the sum of the amplitudes of P2 in the on-response and of the off-response.

on P2	>	off	6
	=		3
	<		1
on-off P2	>	on + off	6
	=		2
	<		2

the on-response was higher than the off-response, from which one could think that the on-contribution to the combined on-off response usually would be the highest. However, when the amplitudes of the combined on-off response are compared to the sums of the amplitudes of the isolated on- and off-responses, the former are higher than the latter in 6 cases as well. It was peculiar, however, that even when no clear off-response could be recognized, P2 could become clearly higher at short stimulus durations. Therefore, the

227

real contribution of the off-response could not be exactly established. This latter problem can be related with Jeffreys' observation that shorter presentations generally evoke larger responses (1972).

ACKNOWLEDGEMENT

We thank Prof. L.H. van der Tweel for revising the manuscript.

REFERENCES

Estévez, O. & Spekreijse, H. Relationship between pattern appearance-disappearance and pattern reversal responses. Exp. Brain Res. 19: 233–238 (1974).

Halliday, A.M. & Michael, W.F. Changes in pattern evoked responses in man associated with the vertical and horizontal meridians of the visual field. J. Physiol. 208: 499–513 (1970).

Jeffreys, D.A. Component analysis of transient pattern VEP's. In: Spatial Contrast (Ed. H. Spekreijse & L.H. Van der Tweel) North-Holland Pub. Co., Amsterdam 80–84 (1974).

Jeffreys, D.A. & Axford, J.G. Source locations of pattern-specific components of human visual evoked potentials. Exp. Brain Res. 16: 1–21 (1972a).

Jeffreys, D.A. & Axford, J.G. Source locations of pattern-specific components of human visual evoked potentials. Exp. Brain Res. 16: 22–40 (1972b).

Kriss, A. & Halliday, A.M. A comparison of occipital potentials evoked by pattern onset, offset and reversal by movement. In: Evoked potentials (Ed. C. Barber) MTP Press, Lancaster. 205–212 (1980).

Van Lith, G.H.M., Van Marle, G.W. & Van Dok-Mak, G.T.M. Variation in latency times of visually evoked cortical potentials. Br. J. Ophthal. 62: 220–222 (1978).

Van Lith, G.H.M., Van Marle, G.W. & Vijfvinkel-Bruinenga, S.M. Interference of 50 Hz electrical cortical potentials evoked by TV-systems. Br. J. Ophthal. 63: 779–781 (1979).

Van Lith, G.H.M., Henkes, H.E. & Vijfvinkel-Bruinenga, S. Asymmetric pattern evoked responses and stimulus parameters. In: Visual electrodiagnosis in systematic diseases. 17th ISCEV Symposium. (Ed. E. Schmöger & J.H. Kelsey). Junk, The Hague (Doc. Ophthal. Proc. Series Vol. 23) 249–253 (1980).

Michael, W.F. & Halliday, A.M. Differences between the occipital distribution of upper and lower field pattern-evoked responses in man. Brain Res. 32: 311–324 (1971).

Authors' address:
G.H.M. van Lith and S. Vÿfvinkel-Bruinenga
Eye Department, Erasmus University
Eye Hospital
Schiedamsevest 180
3011 BH Rotterdam, The Netherlands

L. Crevits
University Hospital,
Ghent, Belgium

PATTERN EVOKED POTENTIALS AS INDICATORS OF FUNCTIONAL VISUAL FIELD ASYMMETRIES

C. BARBER & N.R. GALLOWAY

(Nottingham, England)

ABSTRACT

It has long been known that the pattern VEP elicited by stimulation of the upper half of the visual field differs in form from that elicited by stimulation of the lower half. It has been suggested that this is due to polarity inversion of components (Michael & Halliday 1971; Jeffreys & Axford 1972; Jeffreys & Smith 1979). An alternative view is that it is due to changes in component latency (Eason, White & Oden 1967; Lehmann, Meles & Mir 1977; Lehmann & Skrandies 1979). The latter authors have also suggested that their results indicate different properties of human lower and upper hemi-retina systems.

Transient VEPs have been recorded to the appearance of stimuli comprising small checkerboard patterns, presented in different parts of the visual field. Results indicate that the observed waveform differences between upper and lower field responses are due to different component latencies associated with stimulation of different areas of the visual field and they indicate a step, rather than graded boundary. They do not, however, support the idea of a fundamental distinction between upper and lower field properties but may rather be interpreted as indicating that a basic distinction between central and peripheral responses can, due to functional asymmetry, give rise to an apparent upper/lower field difference.

INTRODUCTION

The retina is markedly heterogeneous in structure and this is reflected in the properties of the visual field. The changing population density of the rods and cones and the increasing receptive field size with increasing eccentricity were pictured by Schultz (1866) in his 'sunflower head' model of the retina; although such a simple model of contrast processing is no longer current its fundamental circular symmetry is generally assumed, either explicity or implicitly, in the measurement of visual field properties. For example, it is quite common for results from measurements made along, say, the horizontal meridan to be taken as representative of a general eccentricity relationship.

In more recent years some measurements of the visual evoked potential

(VEP) have indicated that there may be a fundamental difference in behaviour between the upper and lower halves of the visual field (strictly, between the lower and upper halves of the retina). Certainly, VEPs to stimulation of the two halves are very different in form and upper field responses are invariably of lower amplitude. This was described by Eason et al. (1967) who noted that the VEP to flash stimulation in the lower half of the visual field was of shorter latency than that for stimulation in the upper half. Later they carried out similar work using a patterned stimulus (Eason, White & Bartlett 1971) and again attributed the waveform differences to a latency shift, although in this case the lower field responses appeared to be of longer latency than those from the upper field. Similar waveform differences were observed in studies carried out by Michael & Halliday (1971) and by Jeffreys & Axford (1972). In these cases though, they were ascribed to amplitude inversion of components which were assumed to have constant latencies. This view, which was recently confirmed by Jeffreys & Smith (1979), needs no assumption of functional differences in the two halves of the retina; the waveform changes are explicable in terms of the topography of their cortical projections. However, the alternative view has been taken by Lehmann et al (1977) who argued, on the basis of spatio-temporal maps of surface electrical activity, that the waveform changes were due to latency changes and the VEPs to stimuli presented in the lower half of the visual field occurred earlier than those to stimuli presented in the upper half. Subsequently Lehmann & Skrandies (1979) also observed a difference between the two halves of the field in their behaviour as a function of stimulus frequency and suggested that this indicated a functional difference between the two.

METHOD

The approach adopted was a simple one: VEPs were measured to small stimulus test fields presented at various locations along, or near, the horizontal and vertical meridians of the visual field. The test fields used in these measurements subtended either $4°$ or $2°$ at the subject and comprised high contrast checkerboard patterns of various check sizes ranging from $10'$ to $120'$ of arc. The luminance of the bright checks was $10\,cdm^{-2}$. The pattern was presented every $1.3\,s$ and remained on the screen for $500\,ms$; thus the VEPs were of the pattern-onset type. The stimulus system, which has been described previously (Barber & Galloway 1978) utilised a projection television. The stimulus test field was located at the desired position within the visual field of the subject by means of a suitable-located fixation spot and this, rather than the test pattern, was moved during the course of the experiment thus avoiding the possibility of any change in pattern luminance or contrast being caused by non-uniformity of the screen. Binocular stimulation was used throughout.

The measurements were carried out on four normal subjects. Standard silver/silver chloride EEG electrodes were used; the active electrode was placed 2.5 cm anterior to the inion, on the mid-line, a mid-frontal position was used as reference, and the ear lobes were connected to the equivalent of ground. The bandwidth of the (Medelec Van Gogh) amplifier was 0.1–35 Hz and the signals were averaged on a Nicolet MED-80 computer, using a simple amplitude criterion for artefact rejection. For test field stimulation 128 responses were averaged.

The experimental procedure was designed to minimise the effects of gradual changes in adaptation and attention during the course of the measurements. The subject was comfortably seated in a high-backed chair and allowed to become adapted to a low level of room illumination (illuminance at the subject equal to the stimulus illuminance) for a period of 10 minutes immediately prior to the test. First, the VEP to a standard stimulus, consisting of a $20°$ field of $30'$ checks, was recorded. Then VEPs were recorded to the test field in its required location, for each of the different check sizes being used and finally the VEP to the standard stimulus was measured again. This completed the first half of a measurement session: after a short rest the second half replicated the first except that the order of presentation of the test fields was reversed. The responses from the two test halves were summed and the amplitudes and latencies of the peaks CI, CII and CIII (Fig. 1) were recorded direct from data memory. Amplitudes were measured from a baseline which comprised the mean value of the response in the first 35 ms post-stimulus. In order to facilitate inter-session comparison they were expressed as a percentage of the mean amplitude of CIII in the standard responses. Latencies were measured in ms from the appearance of the test field.

RESULTS

Some typical VEPs are shown (Fig. 1) for the $2°$ stimulus field as it was moved horizontally and vertically from the centre of the visual field. Examination of the responses to a $15'$ check at vertical eccentricities of $+1°$ and $-1°$ shows the characteristic differences in form between upper and lower field responses respectively. It was noted that those peaks which could be interpreted as the inverted CI and inverted CII in the upper field responses, whilst appearing from visual inspection to coincide in latency ($60'$) with CI and CII in the lower field responses, never actually did so. This was clear when accurate latency values were obtained direct from the computer. It was also clear, particularly in the case of stimulation by the larger checks, that the responses were more similar to one another for stimuli of greater eccentricity, regardless of whether they were upper or lower field. The relationship with eccentricity was shown quantitatively by plotting CIII amplitude for $4°$ and $2°$ stimulus fields at various check sizes (Fig. 2). In general, the amplitude decreased with eccentricity and the rate of decrease was sharper for smaller checks. In a horizontal direction, maximum CIII amplitude occurred for a central stimulus. However, this was not so in a vertical direction; in this case CIII was maximised for a stimulus centred $1°$ below the horizontal meridian. Similar results were obtained when CI amplitude was plotted against eccentricity (Fig. 3) although the dependence

232

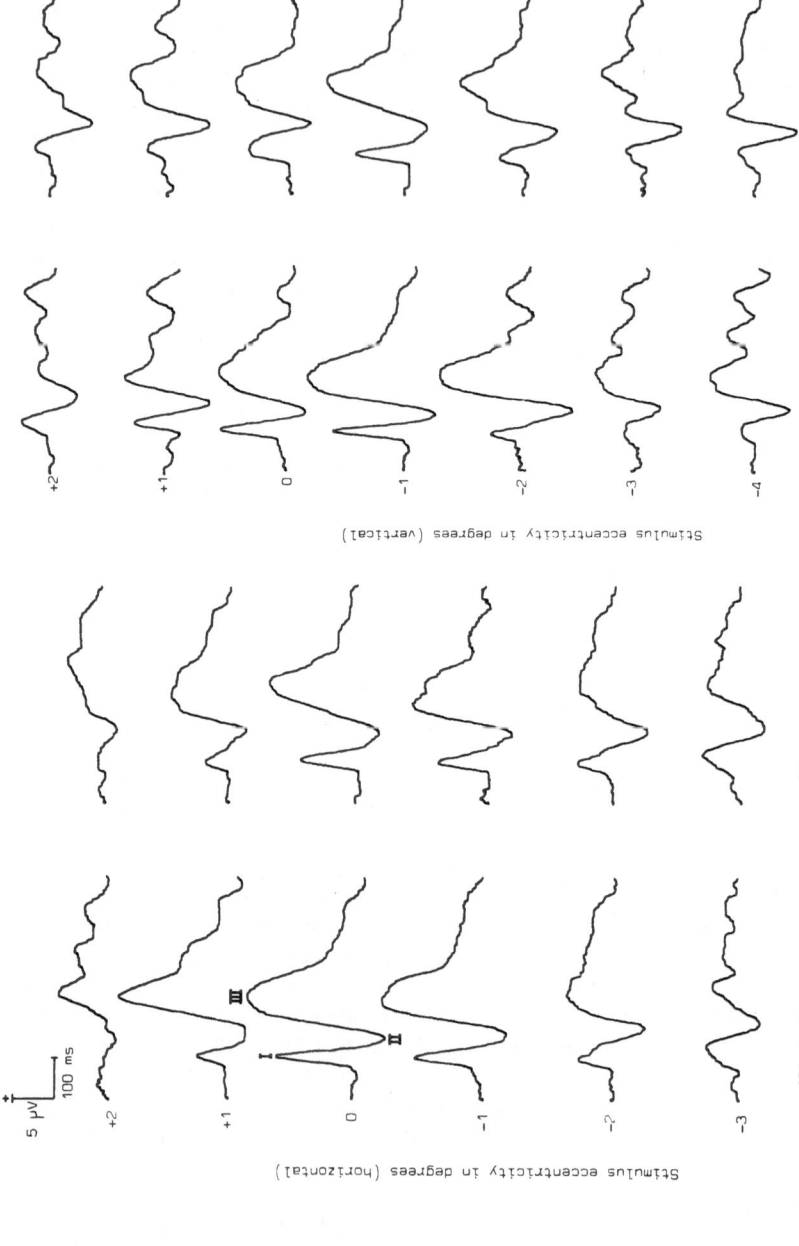

Stimulus eccentricity in degrees (vertical)

Stimulus eccentricity in degrees (horizontal)

60' checks

15' checks

60' checks

15' checks

Fig. 1. Some typical VEPs to stimulation with a checkerboard pattern of 2° total size at various locations along the vertical meridian of the visual field (right half of figure) and along a line parallel to the horizontal meridian but 1° below it (left half of figure).

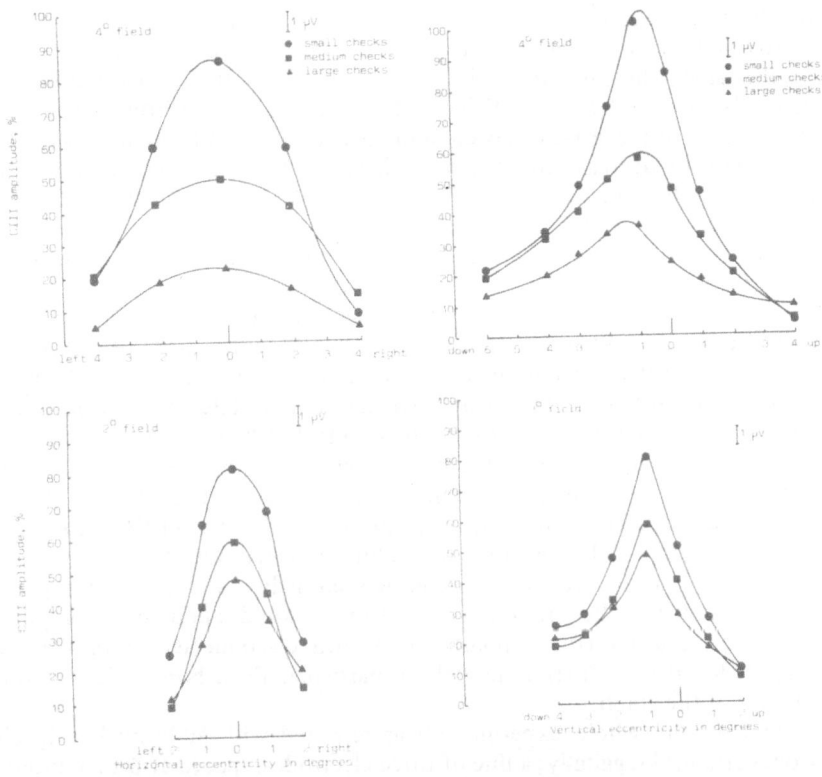

Fig. 2. CIII amplitude as a function of eccentricity in horizontal and vertical directions for 4° and 2° stimulus field. Checks of 15′, 20′, 30′, 40′, 60′ and 120′ of arc were used; the mean value from adjacent pairs of check sizes are shown in this and subsequent figures.

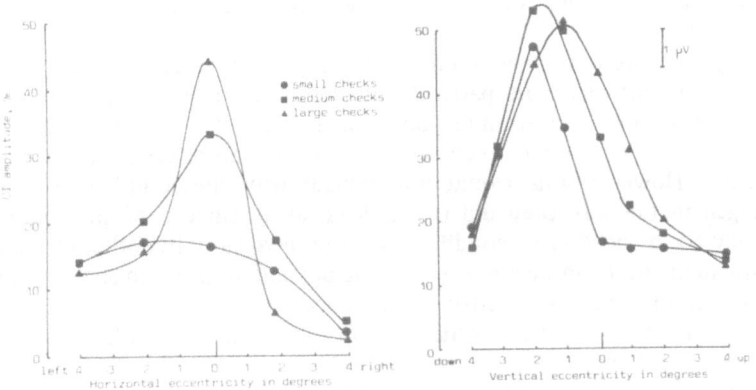

Fig. 3. CI amplitude as a function of eccentricity in horizontal and vertical directions for different check sizes.

on check size was different. We have previously reported (Barber & Galloway 1976) that, with a central stimulus, CIII is maximised for small checks and CI for large. The present results showed that for CIII the relationship held generally across the visual field, but that for CI it was true only for the special case of a centrally-viewed stimulus. It appeared to be due to a differential rate of decrease for different check sizes as the stimulus was moved away from the centre of maximal EP production. Hence, the most efficacious stimulus centre for EP production appeared to be on the vertical meridian, but $1°$ below the horizontal meridian; for brevity we have termed this the 'epicentre'.

An indication of the size of the epicentral area was obtained through consideration of CI latency. If a straightforward identification of components was used (involving an implicit assumption of constant polarity) an area could be identified, within which CI had a short latency (approx. 90 ms) and outside which it had a long latency (100–120 ms). There appeared to be a step, rather than graded, change in latency as the stimulus was moved outside this area, though this could easily be masked if too large a stimulus field were used. Thus, the sharp transition was apparent in the responses to the $2°$ stimulus field but this was 'blurred' when the $4°$ field was used, presumably due to overlap. This can be seen in Fig. 4 in which points were also plotted for the latency values which would apply had component inversion occurred (these points are shown disconnected from the main graph); for the small stimulus field in particular these bore little relation to the rest of the graph.

Finally, the whole experiment was repeated with additional scalp electrodes arranged saggitally; a line of three electrodes, spaced at 2.5 cm intervals and running anterior from the inion, was used, with the same result.

DISCUSSION

These results suggest that the centre of the visual field, so far as elicitation of VEP is concerned, was displaced relative to the physical centre of the visual field.

Any interpretation based on VEP component amplitudes is open to a number of criticisms. In particular it could be argued that, if component inversion occurred, a stimulus positioned just below the meridian would give a larger VEP than a central one, due to partial cancellation of components. However, this would not explain why the components latencies changed in the way they did (or, indeed, at all since constant component latency is a necessary condition of the inversion hypothesis). Also, if component inversion occurs it should be possible to position a small stimulus such that the opposing contributions cancel out; no such position could be found. The fact that CIII, which is generally acknowledged not to undergo inversion, exhibited this asymmetry even more strongly than CI is good evidence that component inversion does not provide an explanation.

It could also be argued that the results are nothing more than an artefact of electrode placement; that the electrode simply was optimally placed to

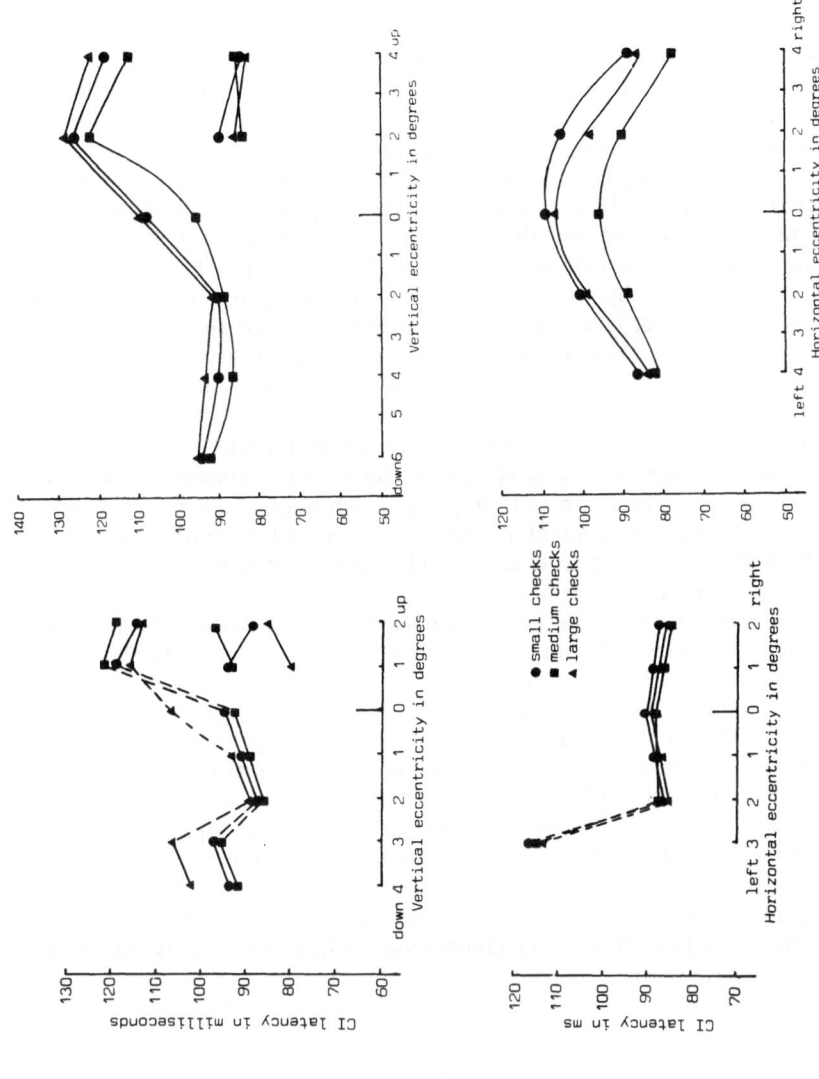

Fig. 4. CI latency as a function of horizontal and vertical eccentricity for a 2° stimulus field (left half of figure) and a 4° stimulus field (right half of figure). In the upper graphs points are shown for two different identifications of CI in the case of upper field stimulation: assuming no component inversion (upper pairs of points) or assuming component inversion (lower pairs of points).

record from the cortical projection of this part of the visual field. Given the broad spread of current in passing from cortex to scalp (Nunez 1977), this seems an unlikely explanation and the fact that identical results were obtained from a saggital row of 3 electrodes shows that this was not so. It is more difficult to directly refute the suggestion that although the results are valid for VEPs, they merely reflect cortical topography; the location which we have termed the epicentre being projected onto the visual cortex such that current spread to nearby electrodes is maximal. The intersubject consistency of this asymmetry, compared with much more variable lateral asymmetries found suggests that this can not be a complete explanation. Finally, a similar vertical asymmetry has been shown in other work using psychophysical methods (Barber, in preparation).

In summary, then, these results indicate the existance of a functional asymmetry of vision. It is envisaged that the epicentre represents, not a 'peak' in visual function, but the centre of a 'plateau' which extends rather more into the lower part of the visual field than the upper. It may also have a somewhat steeper edge in the upper part of the field. It is known that the development of visual function in the brain depends upon the visual environment (Blakemore & Cooper 1970); it may be that this asymmetry reflects the relative contrast richness of the visual environment in the formative stage.

It is difficult to directly compare the present VEP findings with those of other workers since appropriately sized and located stimulus fields have rarely been used. There are some reports of findings which may be interpreted in line with the present results (e.g. Regan 1972; Bartl, Van Lith & Van Marle 1978) but in general the stimulus fields which have been used are too large to permit comparison of results.

The use of large stimulus fields may also be a contributing factor in the conflicting results regarding upper and lower field properties. In further work (Barber, in preparation) the existance of a non-linear interaction between epicentral and peripheral responses has been shown; it appears that stimulation of the epicentral area inhibits production of a peripheral VEP. Thus the asymmetry described above means that a lower field stimulus will elicit mainly an epicentral type of response, whilst an upper field stimulus will elicit a peripheral one. The differences observed between upper and lower field VEPs may, therefore, be due to an underlying epicentral/peripheral distinction; an expression in VEP terms of the basic differentiation between foveal and peripheral retina. Some results on spatio-temporal interactions across the visual field (Barber, in preparation) indicate that this is indeed the case.

ACKNOWLEDGEMENTS

This study was supported in part by a grant from the Trent Regional Health Authority. We acknowledge with thanks the technical assistance of Mrs. C.B. Sills.

REFERENCES

Barber, C. & Galloway, N.R. A pattern stimulus for optimal response from the retina. In: Doc. Ophthal. Proc. Series Vol. 10. (Ed. R. Alfieri & P. Solé). Junk, The Hague. 77–86 (1976).

Barber, C. & Galloway, N.R. A versatile stimulus system for the investigation of visual evoked potentials. J. Physiol. 276: 22P (1978).

Bartl, B., Van Lith, G.H.M. & Van Marle, G.W. Cortical potentials evoked by TV pattern reversal stimulus with varying check sizes and visual field. Br. J. Ophthal. 6: 216–219 (1978).

Blakemore, C. & Cooper, G. Development of the brain depends on the visual environment. Nature, 226: 477–478 (1970).

Eason, R.G., White, C.T. & Bartlett, N. Effects of checkerboard pattern stimulation on evoked cortical responses in relation to check size and visual field. Psychon. Sci. 2: 113–115 (1971).

Eason, R.G., White, C.T. & Oden, D. Averaged occipital responses to stimulation of sites in the upper and lower halves of the retina. Percept. Psychophys. 2: 423–425 (1967).

Jeffreys, D.A. & Axford, J.G. Source locations of pattern-specific components of human visual evoked potentials. Exp. Brain Res. 16: 1–40 (1972).

Jeffreys, D.A. & Smith, A.T. The polarity inversion of scalp potentials evoked by upper and lower half-field stimulus patterns: latency or surface distribution differences? Electroenceph. clin. Neurophysiol. 46: 409–415 (1979).

Lehmann, D., Meles, H.P. & Mir, Z. Average multichannel EEG potential fields evoked from upper and lower hemi-retina: latency differences. Electroenceph. clin. Neurophysiol. 43: 725–731 (1977).

Lehmann, D. & Skrandies, W. Multichannel evoked potential fields show different properties of human upper and lower hemiretina systems. Exp. Brain Res. 35: 151–159 (1979).

Michael, W.F. & Halliday, A.M. Differences between the occipital distribution of upper and lower field pattern-evoked responses in man. Brain Res. 32: 311–324 (1971).

Nunez, P. The dipole layer as a model for scalp potentials. T.-I.-T. J. Life Sci. 7: 65–72 (1977).

Regan, D. Evoked potentials in psychology, senory physiology and clinical medicine. Chapman and Hall London 311 (1972).

Schultz, M. Zur anatomie und physiologie der retina. Arch. Mikrosk. Anat. 2: 175–186 (1866).

Authors' address:
Departments of Medical Physics and Ophthalmology
Queen's Medical Centre,
Nottingham,
U.K.

VECTOR ANALYSIS OF PATTERN VEP

Y. OGUCHI & M. TOYODA

(Tokyo, Japan)

ABSTRACT

A special new method of vector analysis of visually evoked potentials by pattern reversal stimulation was devised. The initial major vector component acquired by half-field stimulation was an *ipsilateral* and anterior-posteriorly tilted vector. The initial major component acquired by full-field stimulation showed a large vertical vector stretching from anterior to posterior. The vector VEP obtained from a patient with left homonymous hemianopsia showed a tilted vector from left anterior to right posterior after full-field stimulation.

INTRODUCTION

Visually evoked potentials (VEPs) are a very useful method of examining the visual pathway. There have been lots of papers about VEPs. Among them (Biersdorf 1974; Blumhardt, Barrett & Halliday 1977; Chiba, Chiba, Kuroda & Adachi 1979; Jeffreys 1977; Müller, Haase, Höhne, Schmöger & Heeing 1974; Schreinemachers & Henkes 1969; Wildberger, Van Lith, Wijngaarde & Mak 1976) the relation between the VEPs and the visual field has proven a very interesting subject. In a previous study (Oguchi & Toyoda 1979), the authors reported a special vector analysis of VEPs on three hypothetical planes. This vector component was called a vector VEP. In the present study one hypothetical plane at the head is applied for a special vector analysis of the pattern VEP. The relation between the results of the vector analysis after half-field stimulation and the anatomical visual pathway is studied in normal subjects. The vector analysis of the VEPs of a homonymous hemianopic patient is also demonstrated.

METHOD

Nine healthy subjects (4 males and 5 females from 23 to 43 years of age) and an 8 year-old boy with left homonymous hemianopsia participated in this study.

Doc. Ophthal. Proc. Series, Vol. 27, ed. by H. Spekreijse & P.A. Apkarian
© 1981 Dr W. Junk Publishers, The Hague/Boston/London

Chloride silver cup electrodes were fixed to the scalp with electrode cream. As seen in Fig. 1, one pair of electrodes, which was placed on the middle of T_4 and T_6 and on the middle of T_3 and T_5 created an X-axis. Another pair of electrodes on C_Z and the inion formed a Y-axis. These two axes (X, Y) formed a hypothetical plane at the head. The electrodes on the middle of T_4 and T_6 and C_Z were fed to the positive lead of the pre-amplifier and electrodes on the middle of T_3 and T_5 and the inion were fed to the negative lead. An electrode was placed on the earlobe as ground.

In the experiment for normal observers, the subject was asked to look at the fixation point. There were three fixation points on the TV-screen, one in the center, the second and the third on the left and right middle edges of the screen. Consequently full-field, right and left half-field stimulation on the screen were carried out. The pattern generator used was the Medelec visual stimulator. The TV-monitor was a Sony Monitor screen, Model 20 vs. The stimulus used was a black and white reversal checkerboard pattern made up of 92 minute squares. For full-field stimulation the field, subtended 28 degrees horizontally and 15 degrees vertically when viewed from a distance of 75 cm. For half-field stimulation the screen subtended the visual angle of 28 degrees either on the temporal field or on the nasal field. The mean luminance was $51.0\,cd/m^2$. The contrast was 80%. The refractive error of the subject was corrected with glasses. No cycloplegics were used. Responses on both X and Y axes were amplified by a biophysical amplifier (Nihonkohden RB-5) with a band pass of 0.5 to 100 Hz and simultaneously recorded with a data recorder (Sony DFR 3513) with a trigger pulse from the visual stimulator. Both responses on the X and Y axes were averaged by a data processor (Nihonkhoden ATAC-450). In each recording one-hundred unilateral stimuli were applied every second. Subsequently, the VEPs were analyzed by the same data processor. The height of amplitude on X and Y axes were continuously plotted on an X-Y plane. This formed a vector loop. The VEPs on X and Y axes and the vector loop were printed out on an X-Y plotter (Fig. 1).

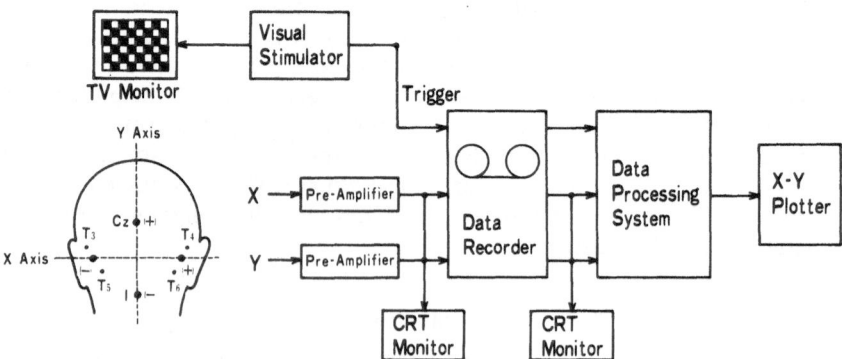

Fig. 1. Block diagram of apparatus. Schematic arrangement for the recording and processing of vector VEPs.

240

RESULTS AND DISCUSSION

VEP after half-field pattern stimulation in normal subjects

Fig. 2 and 3 demonstrate VEPs and vector VEPs after half-field pattern stimulation of the right and the left eye. The above two waves demonstrate scalar VEP waves simultaneously recorded on the X and Y axes. On the bottom vector VEPs analyzed between the vertical bars on the scalar waves are demonstrated. The small square in the vector VEP indicates the starting point of analysis time. In this experiment, we did not chose the analysis time from the onsets of the pattern reversal stimulation as our attention was directed to the components from around 50 to 120 msec. If an analysis time of 256 msec is chosen, the vector loops are more complicated. The solid line indicates nasal half-field stimulation, the dotted line temporal half-field stimulation. As shown in Fig. 2, the two scalar waves on the X-axis show reversed polarity on the base line. But on the Y-axis neither of the VEP waves from the nasal and temporal half-field stimulation are reversed. Vector VEPs from nasal and temporal half-field stimulation demonstrate almost reversed loops on a vertical line. In the initial major component of the vector VEP from right eye stimulation, the vector loop from 79.9 to 106.8 msec. tilts left posteriorly after nasal half-field stimulation. After temporal half-field stimulation, the vector from 71.7 to 101.9 msec. is toward right posteriorly. In the initial major component of the vector VEPs for left eye stimulation, the vector loop from 58.9 to 101.1 msec. tilts right posteriorly after nasal half-field stimulation. After temporal half-field stimulation the vector loop from 66.9 to 99.6 msec. is toward the left posteriorly.

VEP after full-field pattern stimulation in normal subjects

Fig. 4 and 5 show the VEPs and vector VEPs after full-field stimulation of the screen for the right and left eyes. The scalar VEP waves are shown in the upper traces and the vector VEP is demonstrated in the lower. The evoked potentials on the Y-axis are high in amplitude compared with those on the X-axis. The initial major vector component is towards a vertical posterior direction. For the right eye, the analysis time of the vector component is from 71.7 to 120.7 msec. and for the left eye from 70.1 to 114.2 msec.

VEP after full-field pattern stimulation in a patient with homonymous hemianopsia

Figure 6 demonstrates the VEPs and vector VEP of a patient with homonymous hemianopsia. The patient is an 8-year old boy who was suffering from cerebral complication with hemolytic uremic syndrome. The perimetry study showed left homonymous hemianopsia as shown in Fig. 6. When the left eye was stimulated, the evoked potentials more than $10 \mu V$ in amplitude are recognized in the X-axis. However in the Y-axis the initial major component of VEP is not as high in amplitude. In the vector VEP, the initial major vector component tilts right posteriorly in spite of full-field

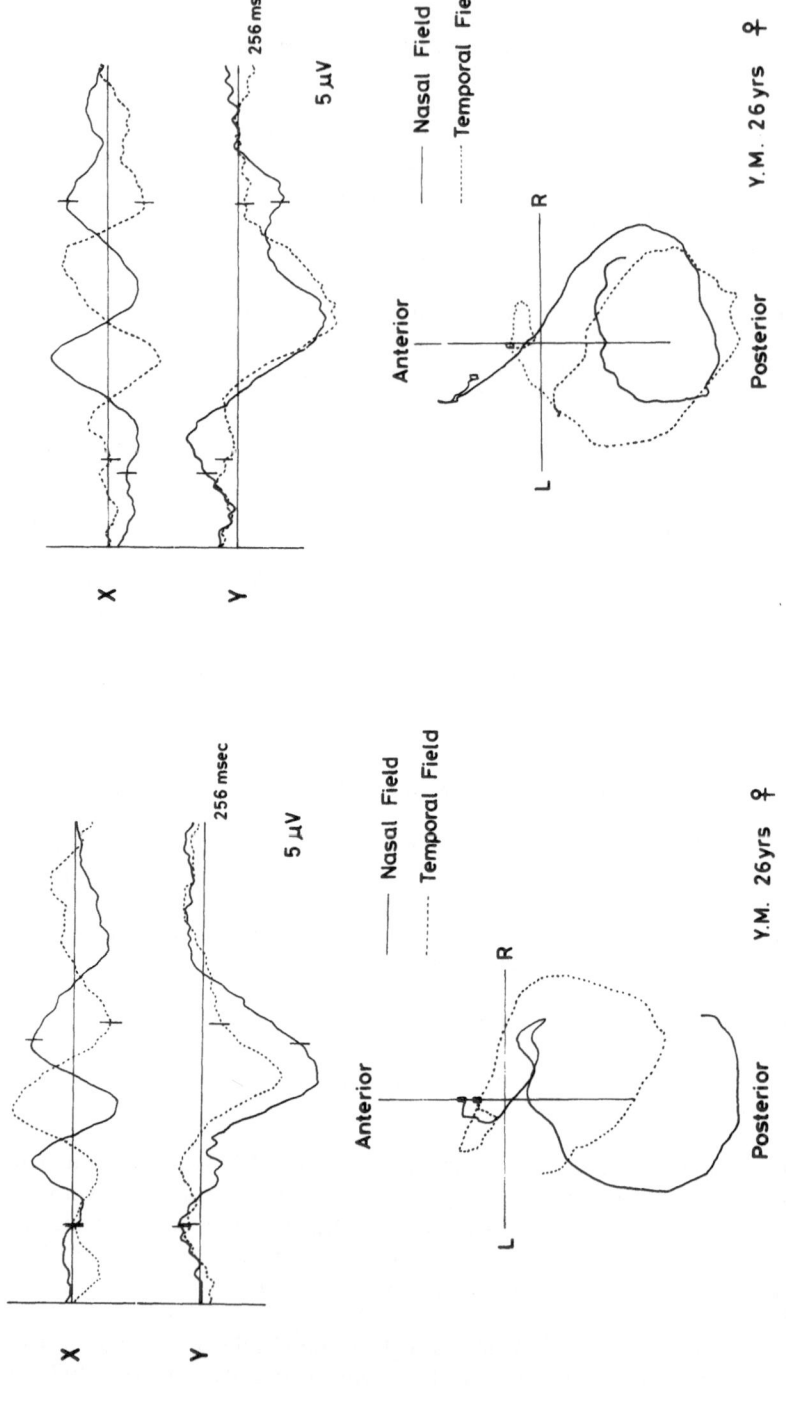

Fig. 2. The upper two recordings show the scalar VEP waves on the X and Y axes. The vector VEPs are shown below. The right eye was stimulated (half field of the screen in the R-eye).

Fig. 3. The upper two recordings show the scalar VEP waves on the X and Y axes. The vector VEPs are shown below. The left eye was stimulated (half field of the screen in the L-eye).

242

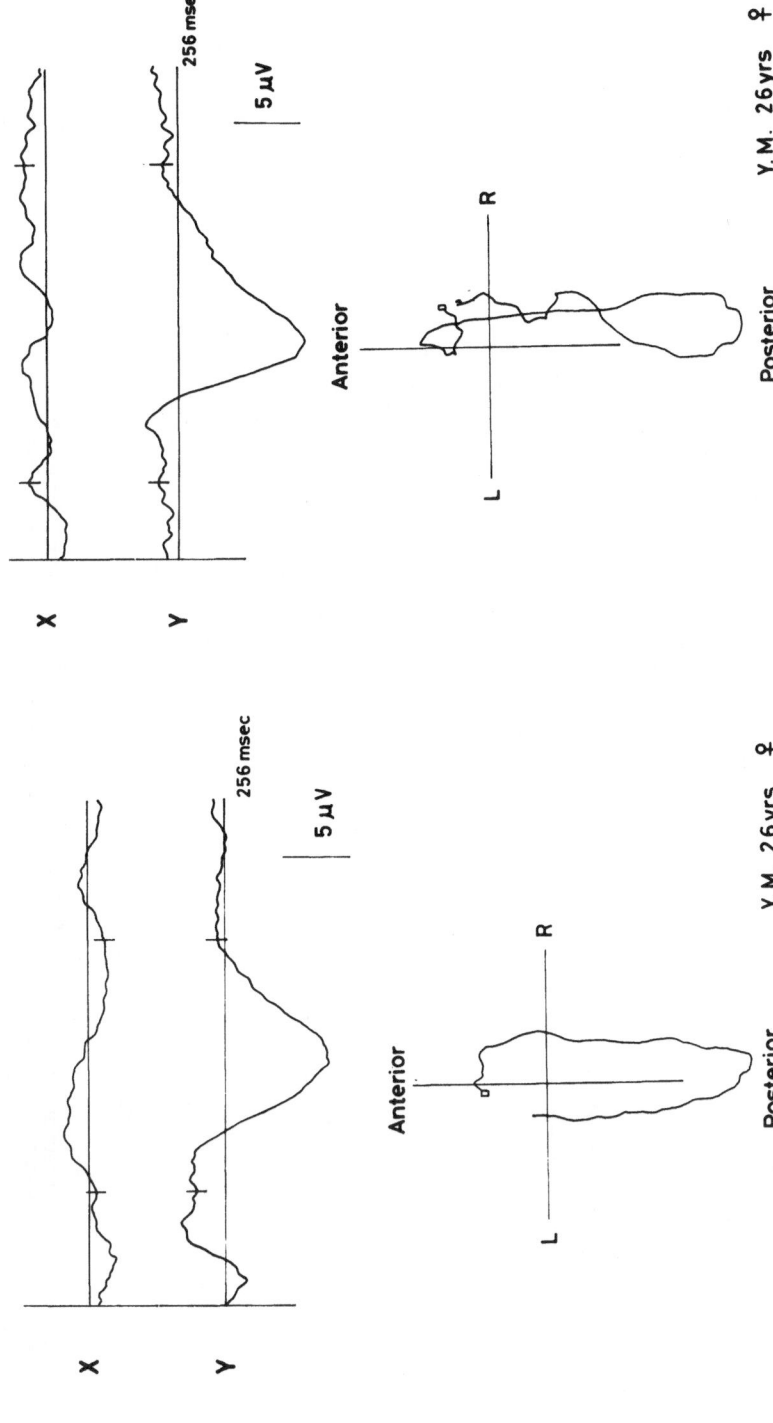

Fig. 5. The upper two recordings show the scalar VEP waves on X and Y axes. The vector VEP is shown below. The left eye was stimulated (full screen in the L-eye).

Fig. 4. The upper two recordings show the scalar VEP waves on X and Y axes. The vector VEP is shown below. The right eye was stimulated (full screen in the R-eye).

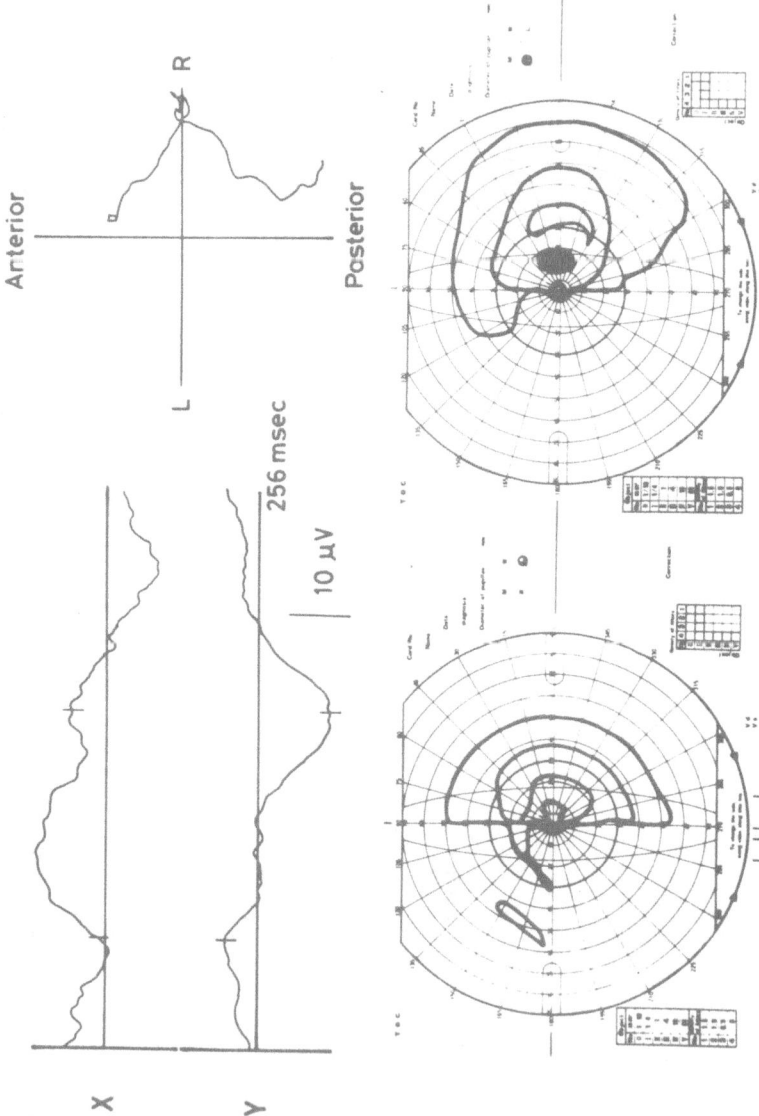

Fig. 6. The left two recordings show the scalar VEP waves of a patient with homonymous hemianopsia (L-eye--. The vector VEP of this patient is shown at the right. The left eye was stimulated. The perimetry results of this patient are shown below.

stimulation. The initial major vector component has no vertical direction of from anterior to posterior. An explanation of the rightward tilt is that the visual field defect of left hemianopsia gives almost no evoked potentials after full-field stimulation, while the right visual field gives good evoked potentials. Therefore the vector VEP tilts right posteriorly. With the right eye stimulated, the initial major vector component also tilts right posteriorly after full-field stimulation.

From this study the vector VEP shows an almost vertical vector component from anterior to posterior after full-field stimulation for nine normal subjects. On the other hand the half-field stimulation gives a large oblique vector component. Moreover large oblique vector components after nasal and temporal half-field stimulation are almost symmetrical. Therefore it is reasonable to obtain a large vertical vector component from anterior to posterior after full-field stimulation. As for the half-field stimulation, the initial major component of the vector VEP tilts to the posterior ipsilateral direction. After left half-field stimulation, the initial major vector component always has a posterior left oblique direction. After the right half-field stimulation, it always has the posterior right oblique direction. Therefore it may be suggested that there is some relation between the electromotive force of the generator and the component of the vector VEP. The result of the vector VEP obtained from the patient of homonymous hemianopsia further suggests that this method of vector VEP analysis might be clinically useful for detecting visual field defects.

REFERENCES

Biersdorf, W.R. Cortical evoked responses from stimulation of various regions of the visual field. In: 11th ISCERG Symposium. (Ed. E. Dodt & J.T. Pearlman). Junk, The Hague (Doc. Ophthal. Proc. Series Vol. 4) 249–259 (1974).

Blumhardt, L.O., Barrett, G. & Halliday, A.M. The asymmetrical visual evoked potential to pattern reversal in one half field and its significance for the analysis of visual field defects. Br. J. Ophthal. 61: 454–461 (1977).

Chiba, Y., Chiba, J., Kuroda, N. & Adachi, E. VECPs to checkerboard pattern reversal stimuli in human-Hemisphric asymmetry, Electrodes positions and half field stimulation-Folia. Ophthalmol. Jpn. 30: 669–673 (1979).

Jeffreys, D. The physiological significance of pattern evoked potentials. In: Visual evoked potentials in man: new developments (Ed. J.E. Desmedt) Clarendon Press, Oxford 134–167 (1977).

Müller, W., Hasse, E., Höhne, W., Schmöger, E. & Heeing, G. Contribution to objective perimetry by means of the VER. In: 11 ISCERG Symposium. (Ed. E. Dodt & J.T. Pearlman). Junk, The Hague (Doc. Ophthal. Proc. Series Vol. 4) 323–327 (1974).

Oguchi, Y & Toyoda, M. Vector VECP – Preliminary report – Folia. Ophthal. Jpn. 30: 655–656 (1979).

Schreinemachers, H.P. & Henkes, H.E. Relation between localized retinal stimuli and visual evoked responses in man. Ophthalmologica. 155: 17–27 (1969).

Wildberger, H.G.H., Van Lith, G.H.M., Wijnaarde, R. & Mak, G.T.M. Visually evoked cortical potentials in evaluation of homonymous and bitemporal visual field defects. Br. J. Ophthal. 66: 273–278 (1976).

Authors' address:
Dept. of Ophthalmology
School of Medicine
Keio University
Shininomachi, Shinjuku-ku
Tokyo 160, Japan.

245

THE VISUAL EVOKED RESPONSE LATENCY IN OPTIC NEURITIS

T.A. COX, H.S. THOMPSON, H.E. KOLDER & J. SNYDER

(Iowa City, U.S.A.)

ABSTRACT

One can estimate the degree of optic nerve dysfunction in optic neuritis, using the pupil as an indicator, by holding neutral filters of increasing density over the unaffected eye until the relative afferent pupillary defect can no longer be seen. We compared the pupillary defect, measured in this way, to the visual evoked response in 13 patients with recovered unilateral optic neuritis. We found that the afferent defect correlated with the difference in visual evoked response (VER) latency between the affected and unaffected eyes, but not with the change in VER amplitude. In nine of the 13 patients the difference in VER latencies between the two eyes was significantly greater than the latency delay induced in normal eyes by a filter equal to the afferent defect. We conclude that (1) balancing the pupil defect with filters in patients with optic neuritis does not balance the VER latency, and (2) in recovered optic neuritis the VER latency predicts the amount of nerve fiber loss more accurately than does the VER amplitude.

INTRODUCTION

The relative afferent pupillary defect is one of the most useful clinical signs in ophthalmology. A bright light is shined on one eye and the pupillary reaction is observed; the light is then quickly moved to the opposite eye and a similar observation is made. The light is alternated from one eye to the other several times, allowing it to remain on each eye for three or four seconds. If one pupil consistently dilates more than the other while the light is held on it, that eye is said to have a relative afferent pupillary defect. Until recently this test was quantified subjectively, usually using a 1 + to 4 + scale. A 4 + afferent pupillary defect is large and easily seen; a 1 + afferent defect is minimal.

Recently we have been quantifying the relative afferent defect by placing neutral density filters over the normal eye (Fineberg & Thompson 1979). We increase the filter density until the afferent defect is neutralized. We can thus provide a measure of the pupil defect in patients with optic nerve disease.

Introducing neutral density filters in front of an eye also delays the pattern-shift visual evoked response (VER) (Halliday, McDonald, & Mushin 1973). The filter over the unaffected eye that balances the pupil defect in optic neuritis will also induce a VER delay in that eye. We wanted to know if that delay would be comparable to the VER delay caused by the optic neuritis in the affected eye. We were also interested in the correlation between VER latency and amplitude and the afferent pupillary defect.

METHODS

We measured the afferent defect and the pattern-shift visual evoked response in patients with unilateral optic neuritis. We studied only those patients who had had VER and pupil studies more than 60 days after an attack of optic neuritis (see Table 1). No patient had evidence of optic neuropathy involving the other eye. Two patients with unrecordable VERs in the affected eye were excluded. Thirteen patients remained; their ages ranged from 23 to 39 years. The visual acuity in the affected eye was 6/7.5 or better in 12 patients and 6/9 in one patient at the time of these studies.

Table 1. Time of VER and pupil studies.

Months after attack	No. of patients
2 – 4	6
4 – 12	3
12 – 24	3
> 24	1

We measured the relative afferent pupillary defect by increasing the filter density over the normal eye in 0.3 log unit steps until the afferent defect was neutralized. Occasionally these steps were too large, so intermediate values were estimated. We bleached both retinas between successive filter changes, and we judged the pupil reactions during the first four swings of the light. We confirmed the measurement by increasing the filter density still further, reversing the afferent defect, and working down.

The visual evoked response was produced using 48 min checks generated on a television screen subtending $11°$ of visual angle horizontally and $8°15'$ vertically. The intensity of the light checks was 34 foot-Lamberts; the contrast ratio was 100%. Pattern reversal rate was 1 Hz; 128 reversals were averaged. Latency was measured to the peak of the major positive wave. The recording electrode was placed 5 cm above the inion and referred to the vertex. The ground was placed on the right earlobe. The subject sat 125 cm from the screen. The pupils were not dilated.

We quantified the VER delay induced by neutral density filters in 17 normal subjects using filters of various densities, ranging from 0.3 to 2.4 log unit decrease in transmittance. The normal eyes of three patients with optic neuritis were also tested with filters. In addition, we tested the normal eye of one other patient with 12 min checks and with a dilated pupil. The neutral density filters were introduced in front of the eye immediately before pattern reversal started and removed at the end of the averaging sequence.

RESULTS

All of the patients had a measurable pupillary defect in the eye that had recovered from optic neuritis. Two patients had normal VERs; five had delayed VERs with normal amplitude; six had delayed VERs with abnormally decreased amplitudes.

The result of plotting the afferent defect against the latency delay is shown in Fig. 1. The pupil defect was weakly correlated with the VER delay

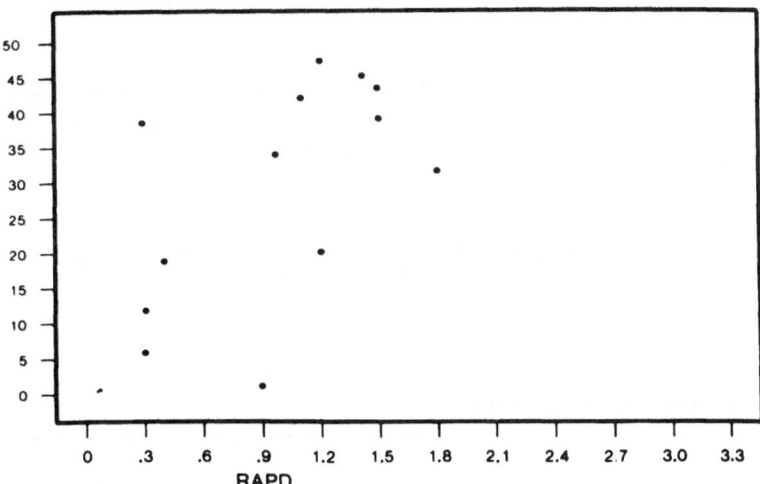

Fig. 1. Comparison of VER latency delay with measured relative afferent pupillary defect (RAPD) in 13 patients with unilateral optic neuritis.

$(0.02 < p < 0.05)$. No significant correlation was found between the pupil defect and the change in amplitude of the VER $(0.3 < p < 0.4$, Fig. 2).

Neutral density filters in our normal subjects caused a linear increase in VER latency with decrease in intensity (Fig. 3). The slope of the regression line for our data (18.6 msec/log unit) agrees closely with the slope (16.4 msec/log unit) calculated from Halliday's data (Halliday, McDonald, & Mushin 1973). The delay induced by filters over the normal eye of three patients was similar to that induced in the controls. Similar delays were induced also when the pupil was dilated and when smaller checks were used.

In nine of 13 patients, significantly more neutral density filter would be required to balance latencies than was required to balance the afferent defect (Fig. 4). For example, one patient had an afferent defect balanced with a 0.3 log filter, but a latency delay of 38 msec in the affected eye. A filter of approximately 2.4 log unit density would be necessary to induce a 38 msec delay in the unaffected eye, thus balancing the VER latencies.

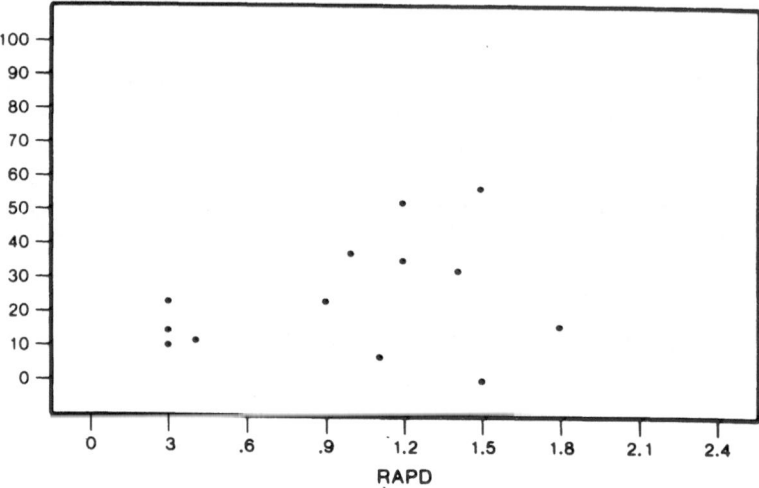

Fig. 2. Comparison of relative afferent pupillary defect with change in amplitude of the VER. Amplitude is plotted as percent reduction in the affected eye.

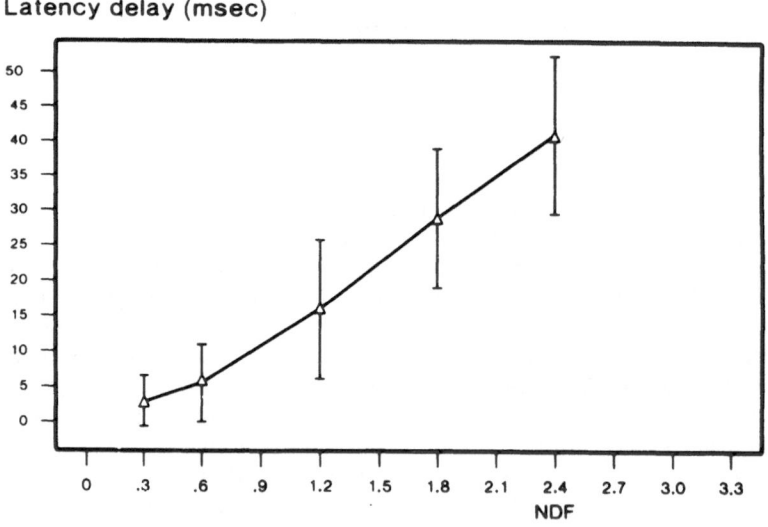

Fig. 3. VER delay induced in 17 normal subjects by filters of increasing density. The range plotted represents two standard deviations above and below the mean.

Latency delay (msec)

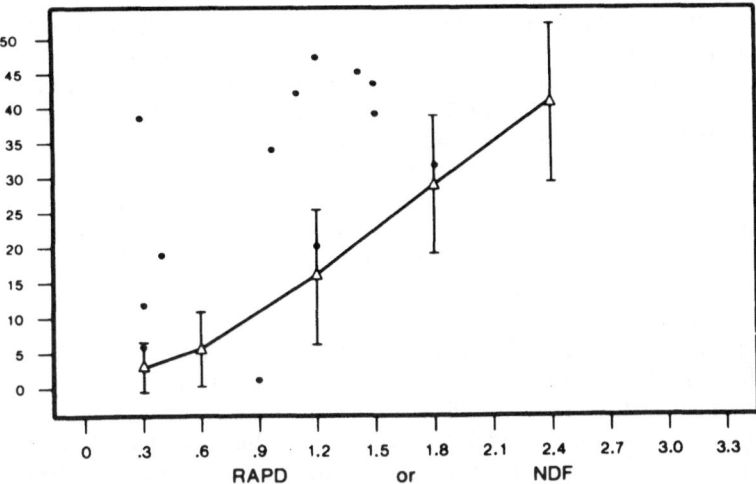

Fig. 4. Data from Fig. 1 and 3 combined. In nine patients significantly more neutral filter would be required to balance the VER latency than was required to balance the afferent pupillary defect.

DISCUSSION

Our VER results using neutral density filters show that the VER latency delay in optic neuritis cannot be simulated in most patients by placing a filter equal to the afferent pupillary defect over the unaffected eye. Other disease processes may show a closer relationship between the two types of VER delay.

Ellis (1979) recently compared the afferent pupillary defect to the VER in 22 patients with optic neuritis. He found a significant correlation between the afferent defect and the VER *amplitude* and no correlation between the afferent defect and the VER latency. The VER was measured with a technique similar to ours, but the afferent defect was measured by comparing the amplitude of the light response in the two eyes using pupillography. Ellis studied all his patients in the acute phase and during recovery, usually making repeated observations on the same patient at different stages of the disease.

We found in our group of patients with recovered optic neuritis that there was no correlation between the afferent defect and VER amplitude, and a fair correlation between the afferent defect and VER latency. The reason for our different conclusions seems to be a matter of statistical method. Ellis studied patients at various times during the course of the disease, and used all of the data from all of the patients to arrive at his conclusions. Halliday, McDonald & Mushin (1974) have shown that the VER amplitude recovers in the recovery phase of optic neuritis. We have noted in our patients that the relative afferent pupillary defect improved during recovery as well. Thus, by using data collected at different times in the same patient one can show a correlation between afferent defect and VER amplitude; they both improve. Using data from several such patients one will again show a correlation between the two measurements. However, the only valid conclusion from such an analysis is that recovery of VER amplitude is correlated with recovery of the pupil defect. Such a conclusion does not mean that the afferent defect and the VER amplitude will be correlated in a group of patients studied only after recovery occurred.

Halliday, McDonald & Mushin (1974) have also shown that the VER latency does not recover after optic neuritis. Since the afferent defect tends to improve somewhat with recovery, data collected at various times from one patient will show no correlation between latency and the afferent defect. Again, the two measurements may still be correlated in patients studied only after recovery occurs.

Thompson, Watzke & Weinstein (1981) compared the relative afferent defect to the visual field in patients with another optic nerve disease, ischemic optic neuropathy. They found that the size of the afferent defect varied with the amount of visual field loss. We presume that the changes in the visual field in ischemic optic neuropathy are due to nerve fiber loss. Thompson, Watzke & Weinstein's study is evidence for the assertion that the measured afferent defect is a quantitative assessment of nerve fiber loss in any unilateral optic neuropathy.

The correlation between the VER latency and the afferent pupillary defect in optic neuritis suggests that the latency is correlated with nerve fiber loss in this disease. One possibility is that nerve fiber loss and conduction block increase with increasing conduction delay in individual axons. That is, larger lesions that presumably have larger and longer segments of demyelinated nerve may have both slower axonal conduction and a greater number of fibers that do not conduct impulses at all. Another possible explanation is based on the assumption that nerve fiber loss alone will delay the VER with no conduction delay in individual axons. If this is true, then increased fiber loss would presumably cause the increased VER latency. Axonal conduction delay might then be constant, regardless of the size of the lesion.

ACKNOWLEDGEMENT

Dr. Cox is supported by a grant from the Heed Ophthalmic Foundation.

REFERENCES

Ellis, C.J.K. The afferent pupillary defect in optic neuritis. J. Neurol. Neurosurg. Psychiatry 42: 1008–1017 (1979).

Fineberg, E., & Thompson, H.S. Quantitation of the afferent pupillary defect. In: Neuro-opthalmology Focus 1980 (Ed. J.L. Smith) Masson Publishing co., New York 25–29 (1979).

Gartner, S. Optic neuropathy in multiple sclerosis. Arch. Ophthal., 50: 718–726 (1953).

Halliday, A.M., McDonald, W.I., & Mushin, J. Delayed pattern-evoked responses in optic neuritis in relation to visual acuity. Trans. Ophthal. Soc. U.K. 93: 315–324 (1973).

Halliday, A.M., McDonald, W.I., & Mushin, J. The dissociation of amplitude and latency changes in the pattern-evoked response following optic neuritis. Electroencephal. clin. Neurophysiol., 36: 218 (1974).

Thompson, H.S., Watzke, R.C., & Weinstein, J.M. Pupillary dysfunction in macular disease. Trans. Am. Ophthal. Soc. in press (1981).

Authors' address:
Department of Ophthalmology,
University of Iowa,
Iowa City, Iowa 52242, U.S.A.

INFLUENCE OF PUPILLARY SIZE ON $\overline{P100}$ LATENCY TIME OF PATTERN-REVERSAL VEP

A. PENNE & S. FONDA

(Modena, Italy)

ABSTRACT

The relation existing between exit pupil of the eye and latency time of pattern-reversal VEP's major positive component was evaluated. VEP recordings were performed on 5 healthy subjects. The exit pupil of the eye was varied either pharmacologically or by placing stops in front of the eye. We ascertained that with small exit pupils $\overline{P100}$ latency time increases.

Therefore, in order to minimize diagnostic errors, we suggest that pupil size should always be considered when analysing latency time.

INTRODUCTION

Measurement of latency time of the major positive component ($\overline{P100}$) of visually evoked potentials produced by pattern-reversal stimulation (checkerboard) at low frequency offers a clinically useful method for the study of optic neuritis and of multiple sclerosis (MS) (Halliday, McDonald & Mushin 1972; 1973a, b). A prolonged latency time appears to be closely connected with demyelination and is generally found in cases of optic neuritis, multiple sclerosis, and in some other conditions like progressive spastic paraparesis, hereditary spinocerebellar ataxias, and compressions of the optic pathways (Halliday, McDonald & Mushin 1974; Asselman, Chadwick & Marsden 1975; Halliday, Halliday, Kriss, McDonald & Mushin 1976). Delayed latency has also been described in glaucoma, ischemic optic neuropathy, tropical amblyopia, and congenital nystagmus (Cappin & Nissim 1975; Asselman, Chadwick & Marsden 1975; Halliday, McDonald & Mushin 1977; Hennerici, Wenzel & Freud 1977). Furthermore, latency time evaluation is important for the study of newborns' visual system maturation (Porciatti, Vizzoni & Von Berger 1979; Sokol & Jones 1979). Therefore, considering the importance of latency time evaluation, especially in connection with the diagnosis of MS where VEPs are able to indicate silent lesions (Halliday, McDonald & Mushin 1973b, 1977), and in the study of newborns' vision, it appears to be very important to establish parameters that might influence the latency. A possible cause of delay is ascribable to the use of TV systems instead of projector systems. According to Van Lith et al. (1978) the standard error is twice as high with the TV system they use compared with that of the projector system. Refractive errors are a second cause of latency time increase (Duwaer & Spekreijse 1978; Collins, Carroll, Black & Walsh 1979). Furthermore, the conduction time augments as spatial frequency increases (Jones & Keck 1978; Parker & Salzen 1977). At contrast levels close to subjective threshold latency varies with contrast (Spekreijse & Van der Tweel 1974). A decrease of the stimulus' average luminance causes a latency increase as well. On the strength of this last consideration we decided to carry out research into the variation of $\overline{P100}$ latency time as a result of varying the exit pupil of the eye, bearing in mind that the light flux incident on the retina depends not only on the luminance of the stimulus but also on the area of the pupil. The relative difference of retinal illumination between a pupil of 2 mm and one of 8 mm amounts to more than 1 logarithmic unit and consequently there is good reason to presume that there might be a different latency time according to pupillary size (Van Lith, Van Marle & Van Dok-Mak 1978). As a matter of fact, it is known that in cases of anisocoria the Pulfrich phenomenon is present (Sokol 1976). This is due to the fact that light intensity of the stimulus reaching the retina of the eye with the miotic pupil is lower and so there is a delay in transmission of the visual impulses to the cortex. The brain interprets this disparity in time as a disparity in space causing the well-known stereo-illusion.

Even though on this theoretical basis a latency variation related to pupil size is to be expected and in spite of its possible practical consequence we were not able to find any previous work in literature covering this topic.

MATERIALS AND METHODS

We examined 5 volunteers, ranging from 26 to 45 years of age, healthy both from an ophthalmological and a general point of view. They were emmetropic or slightly myopic (maximum ametropia: -2 sph); refractive errors were corrected with adequate lenses. As a stimulus we used a black and white checkerboard pattern generated on a circular screen of a TV monitor (HP 1321A X–Y), subtending a visual angle of $18°$ at the viewing distance of 1 m, with a check size of $75'$. A fixation point was provided at the screen center, which the subject had to fixate monocularly. Checkerboard reversal took place every 313 msec (rate of reversal: 3.2 Hz). Luminance levels were 21 cd/m^2 for the white and 1.5 cd/m^2 for the black squares, with a contrast (Lmax $-$ Lmin/Lmax $+$ Lmin) of 0.87. Experiments were made in a dark room. Bipolar recording was employed; conventional silver-silver chloride electrodes were placed 3 cm above the inion and 12 cm above the nasion on the mid-line. The rear electrode was connected to the negative input of the differential amplifier. The right earlobe was grounded. The impedence was kept below 5 kΩ. After differential amplification (filter bandwidth: 2–70 Hz, 40 dB/decade) the signals were transmitted to an Ortec Averager giving an average of 128 responses that were shown on an oscilloscope and recorded on paper by an X–Y plotter.

The experiments were carried out in the following manner: A preliminary VEP recording under natural conditions of the subjects was made in order to determine the eye giving the most ample response and the better definable $\overline{P100}$ latency. That eye was chosen for the experiments. We then proceeded to the dilation of the pupil with drops of 0.5% tropicamide and 10% phenylephrine. When the maximum mydriasis was obtained, we checked the visual acuity again at the distance of 1 m and, whenever necessary, we used corrective lenses. Then aperture stops of decreasing diameters (14–7–4–2–1 mm) were placed in front of the eye of the subject, at a distance of 12 mm from the cornea. We made sure that they were well centered with the visual axis and asked the subject to keep his lids well open during the stimulation. With each diaphragm one averaged VEP recording was carried out. Finally a few drops of 2% pilocarpine were instilled in order to obtain a gradual miosis. During this period VEPs at various pupillary diameters (8–6–4–2.5–1.5 mm) were performed. The pupillary diameter was always measured by the same person by comparison with a series of black disks of different sizes (Fig. 1). Before each recording we checked the visual acuity at the distance of 1 m and it was returned to the initial values, correcting the myopia induced by pilocarpine with negative lenses of adequate power. The peak latency time (culmination time) of the major positive component ($\overline{P100}$) was evaluated.

RESULTS

The mean latencies and S.D. of the major positive component ($\overline{P100}$) for each aperture stop tested are given in Table 1. The graph (Fig. 2) summarizes these

Table 1. Mean latency and S.D. (msec) of the major positive component ($\overline{P100}$) with different diaphragms.

Aperture stop (mm)	$\overline{P100}$ latency (msec)
14	108.8 ± 2.6
7	111.4 ± 3.0
4	117.6 ± 7.9
2	130.4 ± 5.2
1	147.5 ± 8.7

results. It shows the $\overline{P100}$ latency as a function of the stop size. It can be noted that there is a clearly visible increase of latency as the stop size decreases. Passing from the diaphragm of 14 mm to that of 1 mm this delay difference reaches a mean value of 38.7 msec. Let us now consider the results obtained by pharmacological contraction of the pupil. The mean latencies and S.D. of the $\overline{P100}$ for different pupil sizes are listed in Table 2 and plotted in Fig. 3. As the graph shows in this case too, there is a clear increase of latency times as pupillary diameter decreases. When the pupil size passes from

Fig. 1. Pupillary diameter is measured by comparison with a series of black disks.

a diameter of 8 to 1.5 mm, the mean latency increase amounts to 17.8 msec. This delay is evident mainly when the pupil contracts to 2.5 and 1.5 mm, whereas it is very light when it passes from 8 to 4 mm (3.6 msec).

Fig. 4 shows the VEPs of one of the subjects with different aperture stops and pupillary sizes. The increased latency of the major positive component, as a result of reducing the exit pupil of the eye, is clearly visible.

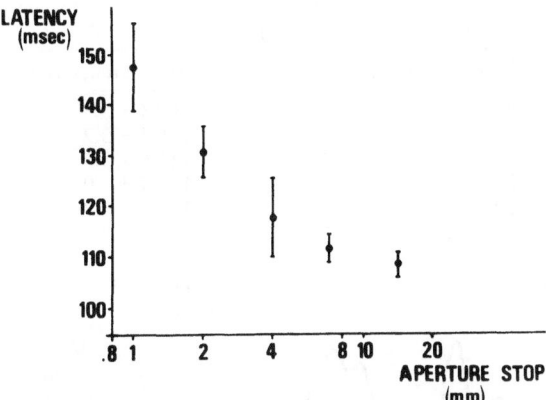

Fig. 2. Latency on $\overline{P100}$ as a function of aperture stop. Mean value and S.D. are indicated. Semi-logarithmic scale.

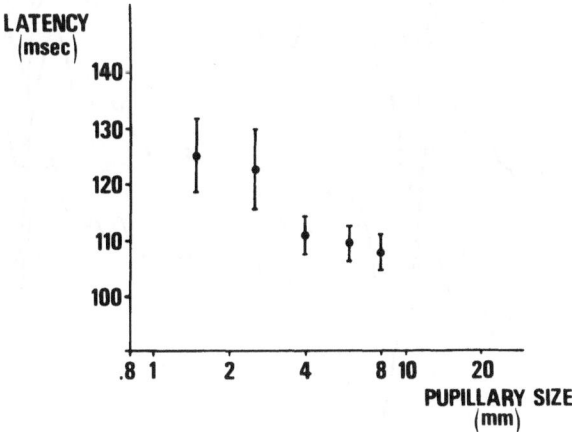

Fig. 3. Latency of $\overline{P100}$ as a function of pupil size. Mean value and S.D. are indicated. Semi-logarithmic scale.

DISCUSSION

The data presented here lead us to conclude that $\overline{P100}$ latency time is influenced by the exit pupil, as we expected from the theoretical premises.

The results obtained with diaphragms placed in front of the eye and those produced with pharmacological miosis are in agreement. The use of miotic agents is at a disadvantage compared to diaphragms, because the myopia induced by the spasm of accomodation has to be corrected frequently and the visual acuity must be checked immediately before each recording. If this

Table 2. Mean latency and S.D. (msec) of the major positive component ($\overline{P100}$) at different pupil sizes.

Pupil size (mm)	$\overline{P100}$ latency (msec)
8	107.4 ± 3.3
6	109.5 ± 3.2
4	111.0 ± 3.5
2.5	122.7 ± 7.0
1.5	125.2 ± 6.7

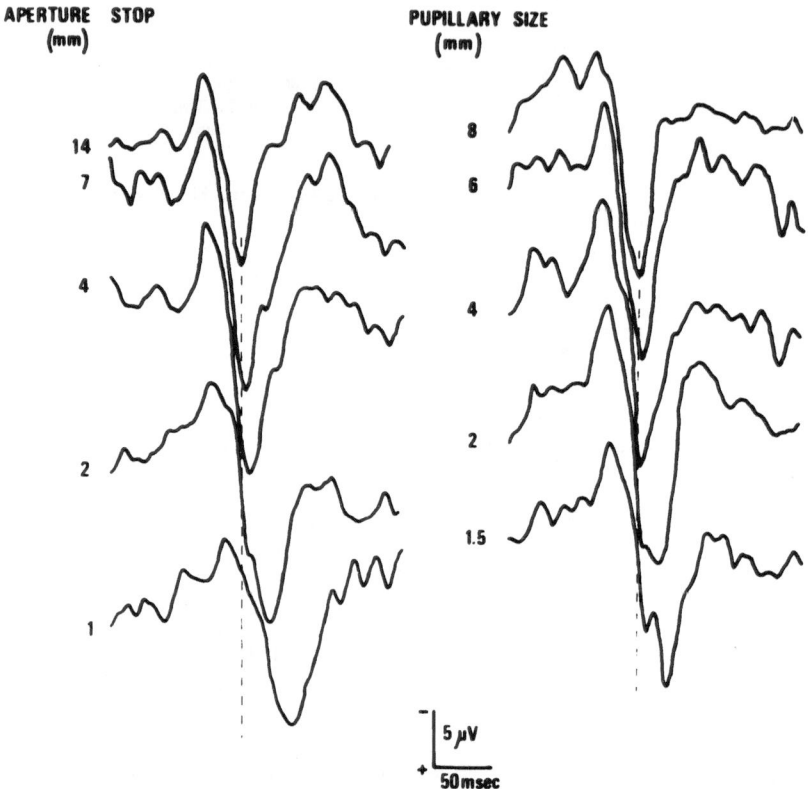

APERTURE STOP (mm)

PUPILLARY SIZE (mm)

Fig. 4. The effect of reducing the exit pupil of the eye by means of aperture stops or pharmacological miosis. The $\overline{P100}$ latency is progressively prolonged.

is carefully performed, the method does not cause other inconveniencies and seems to be adequate.

The effect of pupil size on the $\overline{P100}$ latency is relevant to any investigation of conduction time. If the pupillary diameter is disregarded we run the risk of misinterpreting the VEP results. For instance, a bilateral miosis, whatever its nature may be, producing bilateral delayed responses can cause a diagnositc error.

Perhaps the physiological miosis is one of the possible reasons why

260

newborns' and old people's VEPs show a longer latency (Sokol & Jones 1979; Asselman, Chadwick & Marsden 1975; Halliday, McDonald & Mushin 1973b). Anisocoria could also lead to diagnostic errors, causing a difference of latency between the two eyes. It is known in fact that this difference is minimal in a normal person (Asselman, Chadwick & Marsden 1975).

Probably the influence of the pupil size on the $\overline{P100}$ latency would be less pronounced if the mean luminance of the stimulus was great enough to give a saturation effect. Projector systems, which are usually brighter than TV systems, are probably better in this respect, being possibly less sensitive to variations of pupil size.

CONCLUSIONS

On the basis of our data we conclude that $\overline{P100}$ latency time is dependent on pupil size. Therefore, in order to minimize diagnostic errors, we suggest that pupil size should always be considered when analysing latency time.

ACKNOWLEDGEMENT

This work has been supported by CNR, Progetto Finalizzato Tecnologie Biomediche (Sens 2).

REFERENCES

Asselman, P., Chadwick, D.W. & Marsden, C.D. Visual evoked responses in the diagnosis and management of patients suspected of multiple sclerosis. Brain 98: 261–282 (1975).

Cappin, J. & Nissim, S. Pattern visual evoked responses in the detection of field defects in glaucoma. Arch. Ophthal. 93: 9–18 (1975).

Collins, D.W.K., Carroll, W.M., Black, J.L. & Walsh, M. Effect of refractive error on the visual evoked response. Br. Med. J. 1: 231–233 (1979).

Duwaer, A.L. & Spekreijse, H. Latency of luminance and contrast evoked potentials in multiple sclerosis patients. Electroencephal. clin. Neurophysiol. 45: 244–258 (1978).

Halliday, A.M., McDonald, W.I. & Mushin, J. Delayed visual evoked response in optic neuritis. Lancet 1: 982–985 (1972).

Halliday, A.M., McDonald, W.I. & Mushin, J. Delayed pattern-evoked responses in optic neuritis in relation to visual acuity. Trans. Ophth. Soc. U.K. 93: 315–324 (1973a).

Halliday, A.M., McDonald, W.I. & Mushin, J. Visual evoked response in diagnosis of multiple sclerosis. Br. Med. J. 4: 661–664 (1973b).

Halliday, A.M., McDonald, W.I. & Mushin, J. Delayed pattern-evoked responses in progressive spastic paraplegia. Neurology 24: 360–361 (1974).

Halliday, A.M., Halliday, E., Kriss, A., McDonald, W.I. & Mushin, J. The pattern-evoked potential in compression of the anterior visual pathway. Brain. 99: 357–374 (1976).

Halliday, A.M., McDonald, W.I. & Mushin, J. Visual evoked potentials in patients with demyelinating disease. In: Visual evoked potentials in man: new developments. (Ed. J.E. Desmedt) Clarendon Press, Oxford 438–449 (1977).

Hennerici, M., Wenzel, D. & Freud, H.J. The comparison of small-size rectangle and checkerboard stimulation for the evaluation of delayed visual evoked responses in patients suspected of multiple sclerosis. Brain 100: 119–136 (1977).

Jones, R. & Keck, M.J. Visual evoked response as a function of grating spatial frequency. Invest. Ophthalmol. Vis. Sci. 17: 652–659 (1978).

Lith, G.H.M. van, Marle, G.W. van & Dok-Mak, G.T.M. van. Variation in latency times of visually evoked cortical potentials. Br. J. Ophthal. 62: 220–222 (1978).

Parker, D.M. & Salzen, E.A. Latency changes in the human visual evoked response to sinusoidal gratings. Vis. Res. 17: 1201–1204 (1977).

Porciatti, V., Vizzoni, L. & Von Berger, E.P. The neurological age determination by evoked potentials. 2nd Meeting of the International Society of Paediatric Ophthalmology — Vibo Valentia (Italy), in press (1979).

Sokol, S. The Pulfrich stereo-illusion as an index of optic nerve dysfunction. Surv. Ophthal. 20: 432–434 (1976).

Sokol, S. & Jones, K. Implicit time of pattern-evoked potentials in infants: an index of maturation of spatial vision. Vis. Res. 19: 747–755 (1979).

Spekreijse, H. & Tweel, L.H. van der. Stimulus and visually evoked potential. In: 11 ISCERG Symposium. (Ed. E. Dodt & J.T. Pearlman). Junk, The Hague (Doc. Ophthal. Proc. Series Vol. 4) 269–284 (1974).

Authors' address:
Eye Clinic
University of Modena
Via Vivaldi 30
I-41100 Modena
Italy

VER AND PUPILLARY REFLEX

J. CHARLIER & J.C. HACHE

(*Lille, France*)

ABSTRACT

Visual evoked responses and pupillary reflex have been recorded simultaneously with the automatic perimeter PERIMATIC. Results are reported from normal patients and several cases of visual pathway disturbances. These results are compared to the subjective responses obtained with the same instrument.

INTRODUCTION

There are presently several techniques available to the clinician for the evaluation of light perception. The visual field subjective examination and the visual evoked responses (VER) are now currently used in the neuro-ophthalmic clinic. The pupillary responses have not been so successful but there is some evidence that they can give very interesting information. Each of these methods has its specific interests and limitations. The visual field subjective evaluation gives precise information on the localisation of perception thresholds but it is very dependent on the cooperation, understanding and fatigue of the patient.

The VER are extremely valuable as objective measurements which are little affected by the patients's behavior. There is much evidence that these measurements are relevant to the 'quantity of visual information' received. Several attempts in using VER for the objective evaluation of the peripheral visual field have not really been successful and many reports indicate that stimuli received by the peripheral retina do not elicit occipital VER (Hache 1974; Henkes 1974; Van Lith 1976; Adachi 1977).

Pupillary responses can also be qualified as objective measurements. They involve different visual mechanisms and pathways and have been shown to be very sensitive at the fovea as well as at peripheral retinal locations. (Harms, Aulhorn & Ksinsik 1949; Lowenstein, Kawabata & Lowenfeld 1964).

These three methods provide correlative and complementary informations and their confrontation should be extremely valuable for the establishment of a diagnosis. Such confrontations have already been carried out (Hellner, Hamann, Jensen, Muller-Jensen & Zschoke 1979). However, the use of different instruments and examination conditions is not well adapted to such comparative studies.

METHOD

We have developed a new automatic instrument specifically designed for the clinical investigation of subjective visual field and objective electric and pupillary responses. This instrument is composed of a hemispherical screen, 1 m in diameter, of a stimulation projector providing an adjustable background illumination level and a light spot of controlled size, position, luminance, displacements and presentation time. This projector can generate the different stimuli used in subjective kinetic and static perimetry. It can also generate stimuli adapted to objective examinations. Stimulus sizes up to 10 degrees are obtained, structured patterns (images) can be projected and presentation times can be reduced down to 10 ms with stimulation frequencies up to 50 Hz.

The eye is monitored during the examination with an infrared camera located behind the screen through the blind spot of the eye. The video signal is analysed by a microprocessor which determines the pupil surface area and the fixation point from the position of the corneal reflection relative to the pupil.

VER are recorded with standard amplifiers (A6/B from E.C.E.M.) and averaged with a specific microprocessor. The examination protocol is entirely controlled by a supervising processor. In such conditions, the operator involvement is kept to a minimum and reproduceable standard examination procedures can easily be followed. Examination time is also considerably reduced and patient's fatigue minimized. The fixation point of the eye is controlled throughout the examination and the procedure automatically interrupted when deviation of fixation occurs.

Stimulation parameters and examination protocol are chosen according to two important considerations:

1. to obtain the maximum information within the minimum examination time.

2. to use similar conditions for subjective and objective examinations, which will inprove the comparative evaluation of their results.

The same photopic background level of 10 Asb is used for both subjective and objective examinations. The stimulation parameters are identical for the objective examinations (size = 2 degrees of visual angle, luminance = 1000 Asb, duration = 200 ms), except for the frequency of stimulation which is chosen as 1 Hz with VER and .5 Hz with pupillary responses. The VER are averaged over 64 stimulations whereas 10 stimulations are sufficient for the pupillary reflex.

RESULTS

Case 1. A.M. was a 25 years old normal patient. Fig. 1 shows pupillary reactions elicited by stimuli of different retinal positions. P20,45 indicates a stimulus 20 degrees away from the retina, on a meridan line with an angle of 45 degrees relative to the horizontal. This same notation will be used throughout this paper. Responses were still obtained as far as 60 degrees away from the fovea.

Fig. 2 shows visual evoked responses at different retinal locations. The response obtained with foveal stimulation becomes considerably altered for stimuli more than 12 degrees of eccentricity. Further away, different waveforms are recorded which do not have a clearly established significance.

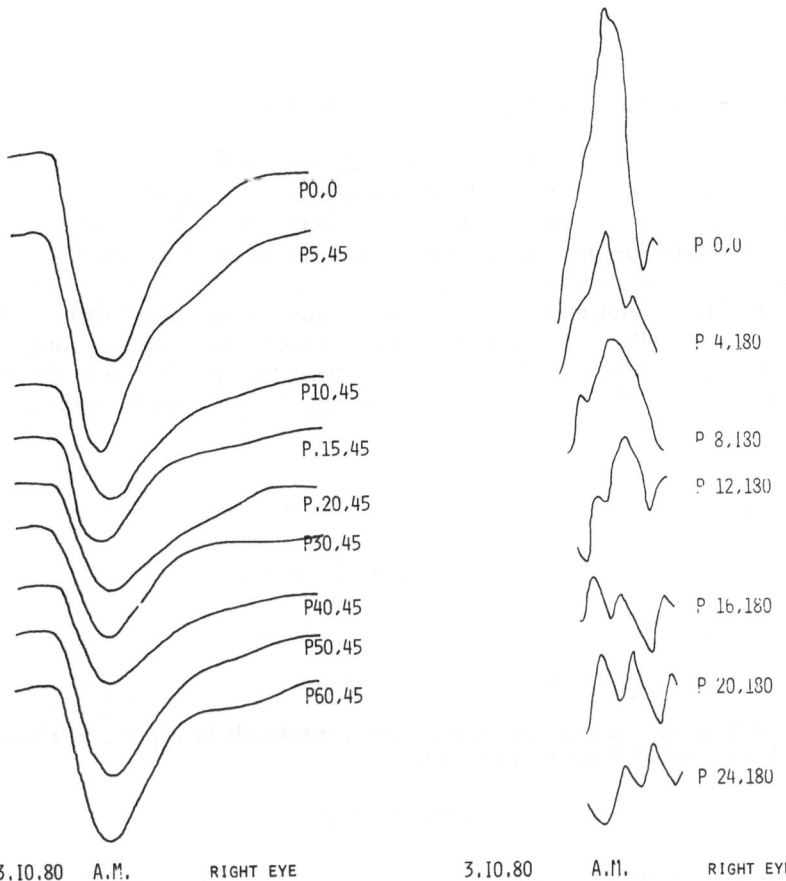

Fig. 1. Pupillary responses at different retinal locations.

Fig. 2. VER at different locations.

265

Case 2. M.J. was a 35 years old man with right homonymous hemianopsia. The subjective visual field findings were confirmed by the pupillary responses (Fig. 3). These results demonstrate that stray light within the hemispherical screen or the eye does not play a significant role.

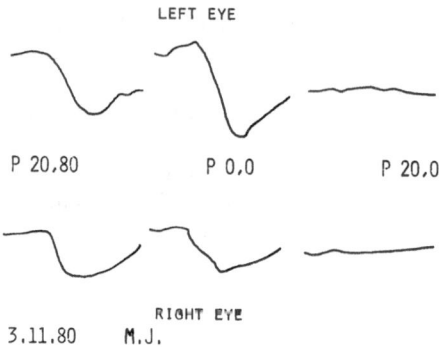

Fig. 3. Pupillary responses in right homonymous hemianopsia.

Case 3. P.M. was a 52 years old man with suspected tobacco-alcohol amblyopia. Visual acuity was 1/20 on both sides. The visual field examination indicated a general contraction of peripheral vision. This finding was in conflict with the behavior of the patient who did not have much difficulty avoiding obstacles when walking. Patient's collaboration was poor. Central VER (Fig. 4) indicated an important alteration in agreement with a central scotoma. Pupillary responses (Fig. 5) with amplitudes increasing toward the periphery were elicited. The central scotoma and the persistance of peripheral vision as well as the absence of other neurological disease were confirmed.

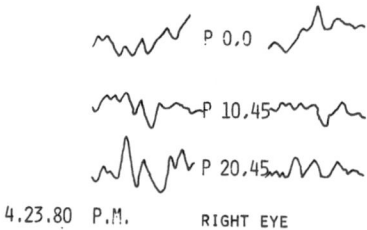

Fig. 4. VER of a patient with tobacco-alcohol amblyopia in response to stimuli of various locations, left and right hemispheres.

CONCLUSIONS

A new instrument for the clinical evaluation of light perception has been presented. This instrument permits subjective and objective examinations in comparable controlled conditions. The first clinical results indicate a good correlation between subjective and objective responses when similar

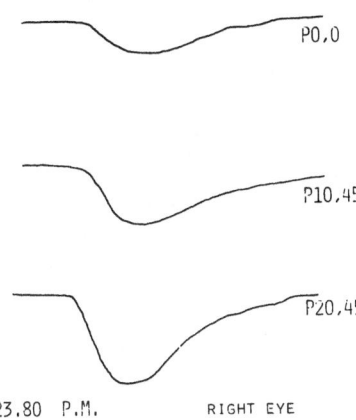

4.23.80 P.M.   RIGHT EYE

Fig. 5. Pupillary responses of a patient with tobacco-alcohol amblyopia in response to stimuli of various locations.

conditions are used. Objective measurements are extremely valuable when patient's collaboration is poor. There is some evidence that the visual evoked responses and pupillary responses provide different types of information about vision. They are concerned with suprathreshold perception and they are involved with different anatomic structures and physiologic mechanisms. More investigation is necessary to establish the significance of the different responses which are now available and to obtain a valuable tool for clinical diagnosis.

REFERENCES

Adachi, E. Perimetry by the human scotopic visual evoked cortical potentials. Acta Soc. Ophthal. Jap. 81: 340–346 (1977).
Hache, J.C., Dubois, P. & Francois, P. Study of clinical interest of the visual evoked responses obtained by focal stimulation following the eye movements. In: 11th ISCERG Symposium (Ed. E. Dodt & J.T. Pearlman). Junk, The Hague, (Doc. Ophthal. Proc. Series Vol. 4) 321–322 (1974).
Harms, H., Aulhorn, E. & Ksinsik, K. Die Ergebnisse pupillomotorischer Perimetrie bei Sehhirnverletzten und die Vorstellungen über den Verlauf der Licht reflexion. Die normale und die gestörte Pupillenbewegung. Symp. Dtsch. Ophthal. Ges. 72–82 (1949).
Hellner, K.A., Hamann, K.U., Jensen, W., Muller-Jensen, A. & Zschoke, S. Visual evoked response and pupillary reaction in the diagnostic approach of homonymous hemianopsia. In: 16th ISCEV Symposium. (Ed. Y. Tazawa). Jap. J. Ophthal. 20: 237–240 (1979).
Henkes, H.E. & Van Lith, G.H. Electroperimetry. Ophthalmologica 169: 151–159 (1974).
Lowenstein, O., Kawabata, H. & Loewenfeld, I.E. The pupil as an indicator of retinal activity. Am. J. Ophthal. 57: 569–596 (1964).
Van Lith, G.H. Perimetry and electrophysiology. In: Second International Visual Field Symposium (Ed. E.L. Greve) Junk, The Hague (Doc. Ophthal. Proc. Series Vol. 14) 169–172 (1977).

Authors' addresses:
J.R. Charlier
Service d'exploration fonctionnelle de la vision
C.H.R. de Lille
Place de Verdun
F-59000 Lille, France

J.C. Hache
Centre de Technologie Biomédicale INSERM
13 à 17 rue Camille Guérin
F-59800 Lille, France

PART FIVE

BINOCULARITY

ELECTROPHYSIOLOGY AND PSYCHOPHYSICS OF MOTION IN DEPTH

D. REGAN

(Halifax, Canada)

ABSTRACT

A number of visual features have been shown to be processed remarkably independently by the visual system, i.e. the visual system contains 'channels' for these features. The features include stereoscopic motion, stereoscopic depth, and changing size. In some individuals with normal perimetric fields, some parts of the visual field are blind to position in depth while other parts are blind to motion in depth. We found psychophysical evidence for binocularly-driven channels tuned to the ratio between the velocities of the left and right retinal images (and, therefore, tuned to the direction of motion in depth). Correspondingly, some neurons in cat visual cortex are sharply tuned to the direction of motion in depth and maintain this tuning over a wide range of absolute speeds and positions in depth. The human visual pathway contains channels that computes changing size almost independently of the stimulus object's sideways motion, its contrast and accompanying changes of brightness. Corresponding neural behaviour has been found in cat visual cortex. Stereoscopic motion and changing size stimuli can both produce a sensation of motion in depth (and if opposed may cancel). For everyday judgements of motion in depth (e.g. driving or flying), the visual system seems to use whichever of these two inputs is most effective, and that depends on the specific visual situation (Regan, Beverley & Cynader 1979).

INTRODUCTION

In order to survive for more than a few days, an automobile driver must be able to judge the future positions of objects with unfailing accuracy. Such predictions are based on estimates of current positions and velocities of objects in the external world and of his velocity with respect to the external world, most of which information is obtained visually. This review discusses research on how the visual system computes these positions and velocities from retinal image data. Our approach to this problem has been based on the notion that the visual system processes certain abstract visual features rather independently of all other visual parameters (In psychophysical jargon, the visual system contains sets of 'channels' for these abstract features). One advantage of such independence in visual processing is that a given visual feature, for example motion in depth, could be accurately computed in the complex everyday world when many visual stimuli are usually present at the same time. We envisage that the total number of sets of channels will prove not to be large. In the research described below we have endeavoured to identify which visual features are processed in channels, and which are not, and we have studied the properties of some channels involved in judgements of motion in depth.

STEREOSCOPIC PERCEPTION OF POSITION-IN-DEPTH
AND OF MOTION-IN-DEPTH

Psychophysics

Recent evidence supports the idea that there are separate stereoscopic channels for position in depth and for motion in depth. Beverley and Regan (1973) pointed out that the relative velocities of the left and right retinal images provide a precise cue to the direction of motion in depth (Fig. 1).

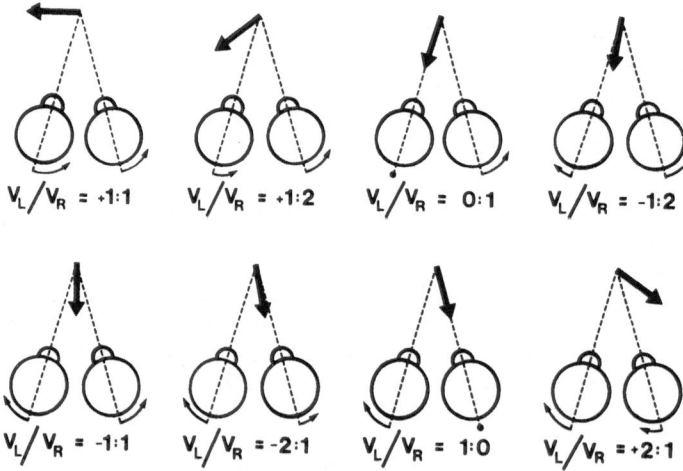

Fig. 1. The ratio between the velocities of the left (V_L) and right (V_R) retinal images provides an unambiguous cue to the direction of motion in depth. Positive values of V_L/V_R mean that the retinal images move in the same direction, while negative values indicate opposed motion.

Their evidence that the human visual pathway uses this cue was obtained psychophysically. They found that, after inspecting an image oscillating in depth, visual sensitivity to motion in depth was depressed. The important point was that only a narrow range of directions of motion in depth was affected. They proposed that there are four sets of stereoscopic motion-in-

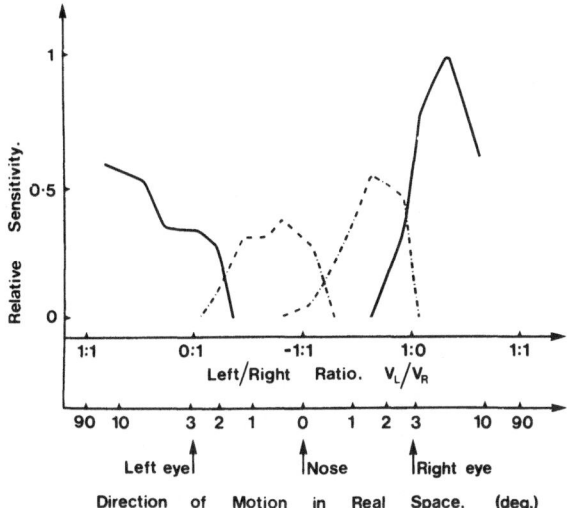

Fig. 2. Sensitivity curves for stereoscopic motion channels in the human visual system. These channels are selectively tuned to the ratio V_L/V_R (see Fig. 1). Values of V_L/V_R are plotted as abscissa, with corresponding directions in space indicated. Note that the narrow cone of directions passing between the eyes is exaggerated in this plot, so that the two centre channels are very sharply selective to the direction of motion in depth.

depth channels, tuned to different directions in depth. Fig. 2 shows the sensitivity curves of these channels for one human subject.

Richards & Regan (1973) reported a different sort of evidence that there is separate visual processing of binocular disparity and of the relative velocities of the left and right retinal images. They found subjects whose visual field contained regions that were 'blind' to disparity, yet were sensitive to motion in depth, while other regions of the visual field were blind to motion in depth, yet sensitive to disparity.

Single-unit studies

Recording from area 18 and from the 17/18 border in cat visual cortex, Cynader & Regan (1978, 1980) found single neurons that were selectively sensitive to the ratio between left and right retinal image velocities. In other words, these neurons were tuned to the direction of motion in depth.* All the psychophysical motion-in-depth channels in man shown in Fig. 2 had their equivalent neurons in cat visual cortex. Some of the most sharply-tuned neurons fired best when the retinal images moved in opposite directions, and thus responded to a range of directions spanning no more than 1° to 2°. Many of these neurons maintained their directional tuning over at least a four-fold range of speeds (Fig. 3A). A second class of neurons fired best for trajectories that missed the head. These were tuned to a broader

*Note that these motion-in-depth neurons cannot be described as being selectively sensitive to the rate of change of disparity, i.e. to the difference between the left and right image velocities (Regan & Cynader 1980).

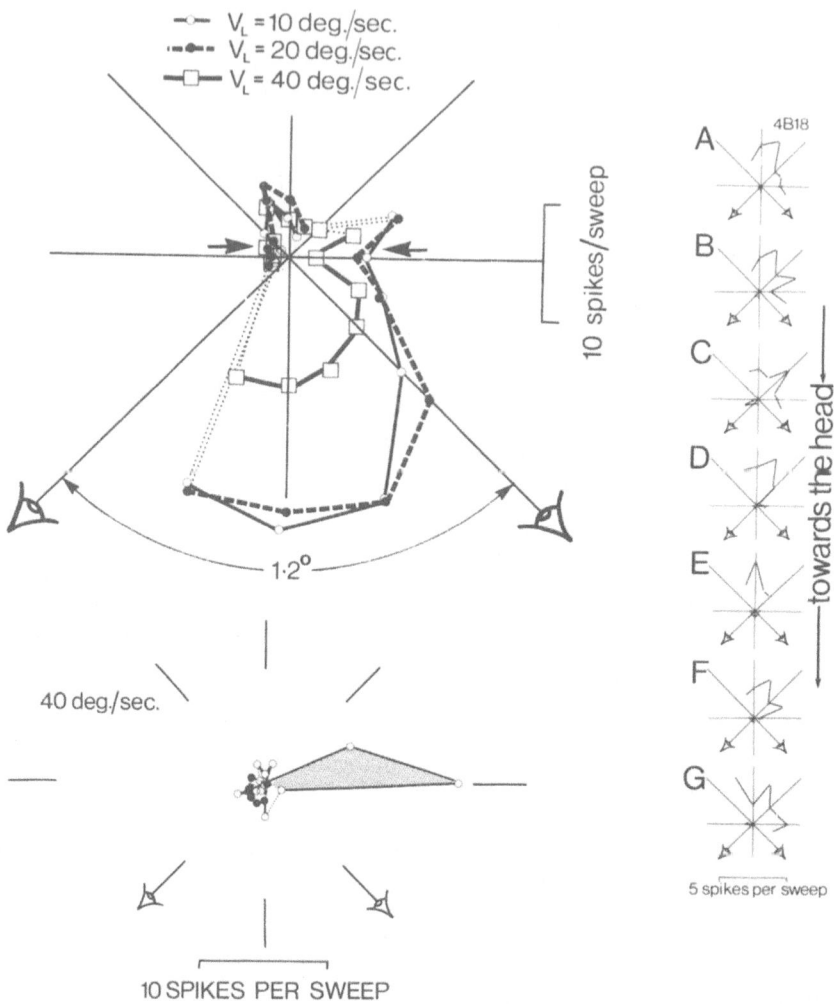

Fig. 3. Spikes recorded from single neurons in cat visual cortex (plotted radially) as a function of the direction of motion in depth (plotted as azimuthal angle).

A – This unit maintains its very selective tuning to the direction of motion in depth over a 4:1 speed range. Note that firing is almost restricted to a range of directions little wider than 1°. This directional tuning is achieved by interocular inhibition as shown by the arrows.

B – This unit fired appreciably only when the target moved closely parallel to the frontoparallel plane in a left-right direction and when vision was binocular. Closed circles show firing when the two eyes were stimulated separately and open circles show firing when binocular vision was used. The dotted area indicates the very strong interocular facilitation observed for binocular vision.

C – Each polar plot was recorded at a different disparity ranging from 6° in front of the frontoparallel plane to 6° behind at 2° intervals. This unit maintained its tuning to approximately the same range of directions of motion in depth over a wide range of positional disparities.

range of directions than the 'hitting the head' class of neurons. A third class of neurons showed strong interocular facilitation (up to 100-fold) when motion was accurately parallel to the frontoparallel plane (Fig. 3B). This class of neurons also can be regarded as being very selective to the direction of motion in depth.

This third class of neurons was comparatively sharply tuned to disparity, i.e. to position in depth. In this they differed from many neurons in the first two classes, some of which maintained their tuning to motion in depth over a range of disparities as large as $12°$ (Fig. 3C). Other neurons of this type systematically changed their tuning as a function of disparity, for example, favouring motion towards the frontoparallel plane whether the object were nearer or farther than the frontoparallel plane.

Evoked potentials

Evoked potential studies bridging the inter-species gap between our psychophysical studies in man and animal single-unit experiments were carried out before these other studies were started. Regan & Spekreijse (1970) used Julesz patterns to obtain evoked potentials to stereoscopic motion in depth. Regan & Beverley (1973) later found that different evoked potentials were produced by different directions of motion in depth, anticipating the conclusions of subsequent psychophysical and single-unit studies.

More recently, Lehmann & Julesz (1978) succeeded in recording stereoscopic evoked potentials using dynamic noise patterns that were displayed on a large-screen television. This technique can be used to test stereoscopic visual function in young infants, and may prove to be useful in the study and management of amblyopia.

MONOCULAR AND BINOCULAR PROCESSING OF CHANGING-SIZE

Since the channels described above are sensitive to the relative velocity of the retinal images, they can only be driven binocularly. A second stimulus for motion in depth is, however, effective monocularly as well as binocularly. This is the stimulus of changing-size.

Fig. 4 shows experimental evidence that the processing of changing-size information cannot be explained entirely in terms of responses to motion. Subjects viewed a pair of bright squares on a dimmer background. We used the following two stimulus oscillations: inphase oscillations, in which opposite edges of a square moved in the same direction at any instant; antiphase oscillations, in which opposite edges of a square moved in opposite directions at any instant. Subjects first measured the smallest oscillation amplitude that could just be detected for an inphase test oscillation and for an antiphase test oscillation. Then they inspected a strong antiphase oscillation for 20 min and measured the two thresholds again. The antiphase threshold was much elevated, but the inphase threshold was comparatively little affected. When the experiment was repeated with an inphase adapting

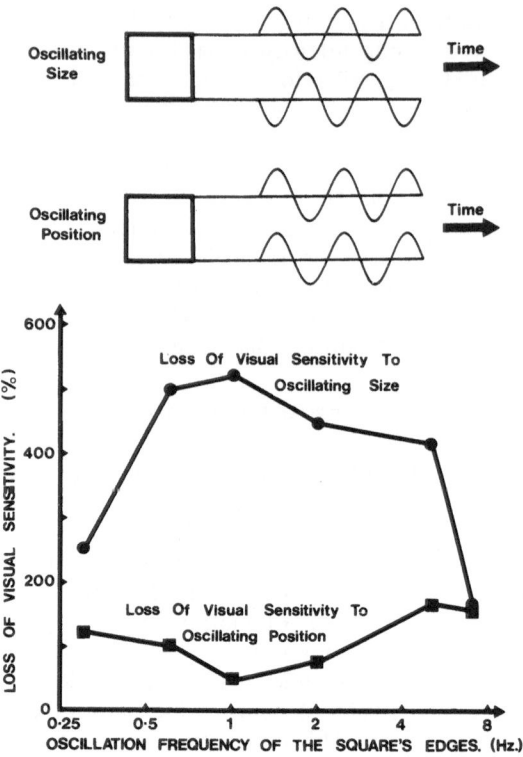

Fig. 4. Selective threshold elevations for changing size. The two test stimuli are shown at the top. Ordinates plot loss of visual sensitivity to oscillation caused by inspecting a strong 2 Hz size oscillation. Changing-size sensitivity fell considerably, but sensitivity to oscillating position was little affected. Note that the only difference between the two test stimuli is in the relationship between the motion of opposite edges of the square.

oscillation, threshold elevations were small for both test stimuli (Regan & Beverley 1978).

This differential effect was still observed when the adapting stimulus was a bright square on a dark ground and the test stimulus was a dark square on a bright ground.

A weakness of these early experiments is that they were limited to two directions of motion, namely motion parallel to the frontoparallel plane (i.e. inphase oscillations), and motion along a line through the eye (i.e. antiphase oscillations). A more recent experiment extended the conclusions to a range of adapting trajectories. The rationale of this later experiment is illustrated in Fig. 5A. On separate days, subjects adapted to 11 different trajectories. Each adapting oscillation had the same velocity along a line through the eye, i.e. the same antiphase component, but each adapting oscillation had a different

276

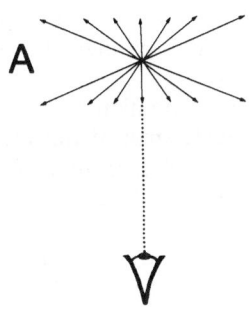

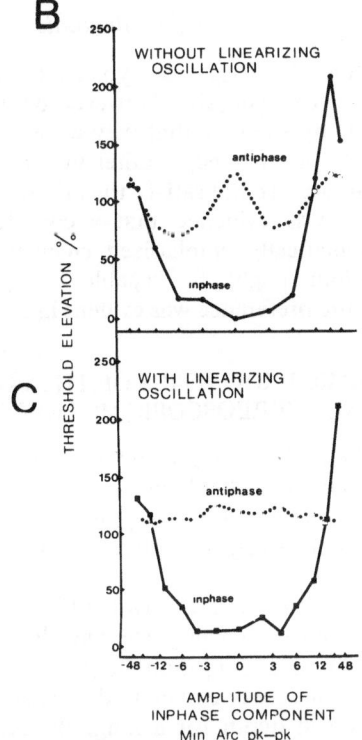

Fig. 5. A – Experimental rationale. All trajectories had the same antiphase oscillation component of 6 min arc pk-pk, but different amplitudes of inphase component were added.
B – Threshold elevations produced by adapting to the 11 trajectories in A. Antiphase test oscillations are dotted, while the continuous line plots inphase test oscillations.
C – An 8 Hz 'jitter' oscillation was added to the 2 Hz adapting oscillation of B.

velocity parallel to the frontoparallel plane (i.e. a different inphase component of oscillation). If the changing-size channel responded to the antiphase component and was unaffected by the inphase component, then all 11 adapting oscillations should produce the same threshold elevation for the antiphase test stimulus.

Fig. 5B shows that this prediction was upheld to an accuracy of about ± 30% over a very wide span of trajectories. (The abscissa in Fig. 5B plots inphase components ranging from zero to ± 8 times the amplitude of the antiphase component.) Further evidence suggested that, in everyday vision, the prediction probably holds to considerably better than ± 30% due to the effect of eye movement. The experiment of Fig. 5B was repeated with a rapid 'jitter' oscillation added to the adapting stimulus. As shown in Fig. 5C, the effect of this 'jitter' was to reduce the influence of an inphase component upon the antiphase threshold elevation so that the influence was less than measurement errors (± 5%) (Regan & Beverley 1980).

Single-unit studies

All 101 units studied by Regan & Cynader (1979) in area 18 of cat visual cortex responded to changing-size. However, control experiments eliminated most of these units by showing that they were responding to changes in light flux or to motion of a single edge rather than to changing size. Nevertheless, a very few units in area 18 did satisfy the criteria for changing-size responses. In addition, there was evidence that a considerable proportion of units slightly, but systematically emphasized changing-size information, so that population behaviour might be capable of signalling changing-size even though no systematic preference was evident in simple spike counts.

DYNAMIC PROPERTIES OF THE CHANGING-SIZE AND STEREOSCOPIC MOTION CHANNELS

Fig. 6 plots thresholds for just-detectable motion in depth produced by two different visual inputs, namely changing-size (continuous line), and changing-disparity (bold broken line). The two plots are clearly different. In particular, changing-size grows relatively less effective at oscillation frequencies below about 1 Hz.

Fig. 6 also plots thresholds for two different sensations produced by a single input. The input is changing-size, and the two sensations are changing-size (fine dotted line), and motion in depth (continuous line). The chief difference between the two curves is that changing-size is ineffective as a stimulus for motion in depth for a range of frequencies above about 3 Hz over which it is still effective in producing a sensation of changing-size.

TWO STIMULI FOR MOTION-IN-DEPTH: COMPARATIVE EFFECTIVENESSS OF CHANGING-DISPARITY AND CHANGING-SIZE

Fig. 7 illustrates that when an object moves directly toward the head, the two retinal images move away from each other and also grow larger. As discussed above, either of these two visual inputs by itself is capable of causing a sensation of motion in depth. In the real visual world the situation is almost

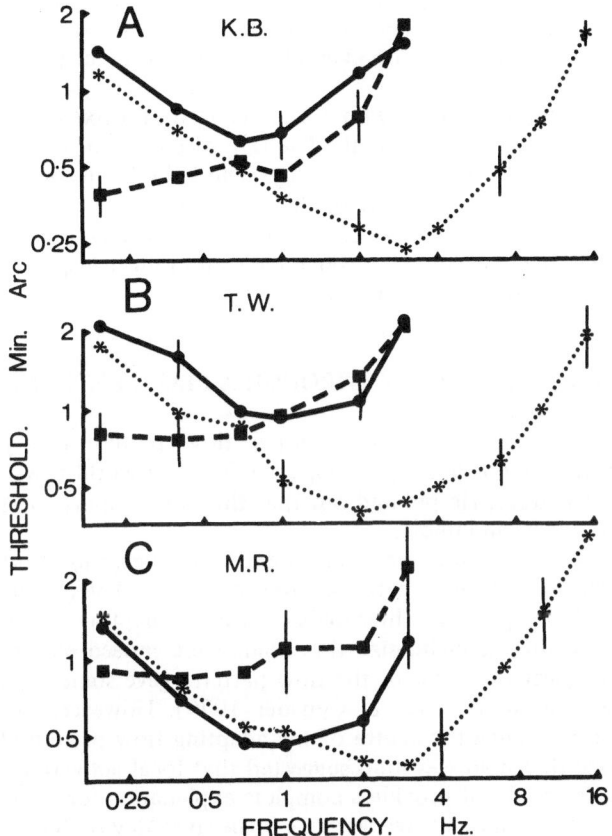

Fig. 6. Threshold versus oscillation frequency curves for changing-size stimulation producing motion-in-depth sensation (continuous line), changing-size stimulation producing changing-size sensation (fine dotted line) and changing-disparity stimulation producing motion-in-depth sensation (bold broken line). From Vis. Res. 19: 1331 (1979).

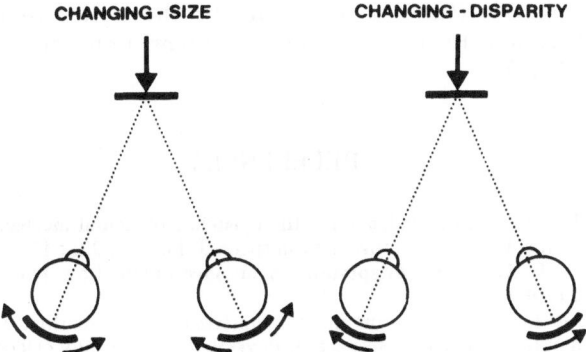

Fig. 7. When a real-world nonrotating object moves closer, the retinal images grow larger and move apart. From Vis. Res. 19: 1331 (1979).

always as shown in Fig. 7, but in order to measure the relative effectiveness of the two inputs, we created artificial stimuli in which the two inputs of Fig. 7 were antagonistic (for example, as an object came closer it grew smaller).

Subjects viewed a square whose size changed at a fixed rate, so that the square appeared to move in depth. The rate of change of disparity was then adjusted by the subject so as to exactly cancel the impression of motion in depth produced by the fixed rate of change of size. In this way it was possible to show that the relative effectiveness of the changing-disparity inputs was increased by faster speeds, narrower targets and longer inspection times, but was not affected by the viewing distance.

MOTION OF THE SUBJECT THROUGH A FIXED EXTERNAL WORLD

Gibson (1950) discussed how a visual flow pattern can produce the impression that one is moving through the external world towards the focus of the flow pattern. He pointed out that this is an important visual cue for automobile drivers and pilots.

Testing the suggestion that changing-size channels might be involved in visual sensitivity to flow patterns, Regan & Beverley (1979b) measured elevations of changing-size thresholds caused by adapting to a flow pattern. Their finding that changing-size thresholds were indeed elevated, but only for locations near the focus of the flow pattern, gave some support to those suggestions (Regan, Beverley & Cynader 1979). However, the subsequent finding that removing the centre of the adapting flow pattern abolished the changing-size threshold elevation suggested that local activation of changing-size channels could not provide a complete explanation for a subject's ability to judge the location of a flow pattern's focus (Beverley & Regan 1980).

ACKNOWLEDGEMENTS

This research was supported by the Natural Science and Engineering Research Council of Canada (Grant A-0323) and by the United States Air Force Office of Scientific Research, Air Force Systems Command, USAF (Grant AFOSR-78-3711).

REFERENCES

Beverley, K.I. & Regan, D. Evidence for the existence of neural mechanisms selectively sensitive to the direction of movement in space. J. Physiol. 235: 17–29 (1973).
Beverley, K.I. & Regan, D. Adaptation to an incomplete flow pattern. Perception. submitted (1980).
Cynader, M. & Regan, D. Neurons in cat parastriate cortex sensitive to the direction of motion in three-dimensional space. J. Physiol. 274: 549–569 (1978).
Cynader, M. & Regan, D. Neurons in cat visual area 18 tuned to the direction of motion in depth: effect of positional disparity. submitted (1980).

280

Gibson, J.J. The perception of the visual world. Baltimore: Houghton Mifflin (1950).

Lehmann, D. & Julesz, B. Lateralized cortical potentials evoked in humans by dynamic random noise stereograms. Vis. Res. 18: 1265–1272 (1978).

Regan, D. & Beverley, K.I. Electrophysiological evidence for the existence of neurons selectively sensitive to the direction of movement in depth. Nature 246: 504–506 (1973).

Regan, D. & Beverley, K.I. Looming detectors in the human visual pathway. Vis. Res. 18: 415–421 (1978).

Regan, D. & Beverley, K.I. Binocular and monocular stimuli for motion-in-depth: changing-disparity and changing-size inputs feed the same motion-in-depth stage. Vision Res. 19: 1331–1342 (1979a).

Regan, D. & Beverley, K.I. Visually guided locomotion: psychophysical evidence for a neural mechanism sensitive to flow patterns. Science 205: 311–313 (1979b).

Regan, D. & Beverley, K.I. Independence of visual responses to changing size and sideways motion for different directions of motion in depth. J. opt. Soc. Am., submitted (1980).

Regan, D., Beverley, K.I. & Cynader, M. The visual perception of motion in depth. Sci. Am. 241: 136–151 (1979).

Regan, D. & Cynader, M. Neurons in area 18 of cat visual cortex selectively sensitive to changing size: nonlinear interactions between the responses to two edges. Vis. Res. 19: 699–711 (1979).

Regan, D. & Cynader, M. Neurons in cat visual area 18 tuned to the direction of motion in depth: effect of stimulus speed. submitted (1980).

Regan, D. & Spekreijse, H. Electrophysiological correlate of binocular depth perception in man. Nature 255: 92–94 (1970).

Richards, W. & Regan, D. A stereo field map with implications for disparity processing. Invest. Ophthalmol. & Vis. Sci. 12: 904–909 (1973).

Authors' address:
Department of Physiology and Biophysics
Gerard Hall, Halifax Infirmary
5303 Morris Street
Dalhousie University
Halifax, Nova Scotia B3J1B6
Canada

INTEROCULAR SUPPRESSION IN VISUALLY EVOKED CORTICAL POTENTIALS (VECP)

M. MATSUHASHI & Y. OGUCHI

(Tokyo, Japan)

ABSTRACT

Using the rotating polaroid method with additional polaroid lenses in front of each eye orthogonally oriented, each eye is stimulated alternately under binocular conditions. By this method, the right eye originated waves and the left eye originated waves can be separated in the binocular visually evoked cortical potentials (VECP). In this investigation the ratio of the average right eye and left eye amplitudes were calculated and denoted as the Laterality Index. Values were calculated in only one response trace, the procedure which minimizes the experimental error when amplitudes are compared.

In the normal subjects, the average of both eye originated waves were almost equal in amplitude and the Laterality Index was 101.8 ± 15.1%. Reduction in the amplitude of non-fixating eye originated waves in the binocular VECP was recognized in cases with defective binocular vision and the Laterality Index was 57.3 ± 8.4% (significant difference p < 0.001). This reduction is an objective indication of interocular suppression.

INTRODUCTION

In analyzing the visually evoked cortical potentials (VECP), the amplitudes are rather unstable parameters compared with the latencies. The comparison of amplitudes among several response traces obtained under different conditions can involve errors caused by large scattering of the amplitude values. Therefore, the comparison of amplitudes of waves within a single trace is the condition which minimizes the experimental error.

Lennerstrand (1978) examined the effect of binocular vision on VECP, but he compared the amplitude of the binocular VECP with that of the monocular VECP. Siegfried et al. (1979) described a technique for recording the monocular VECP under conditions of binocular stimulation. The authors adopted this method and were able to separate the right eye originated waves and the left eye ones in a single response trace from binocular stimulation. Consequently, the comparison of amplitudes of waves in one trace could be made.

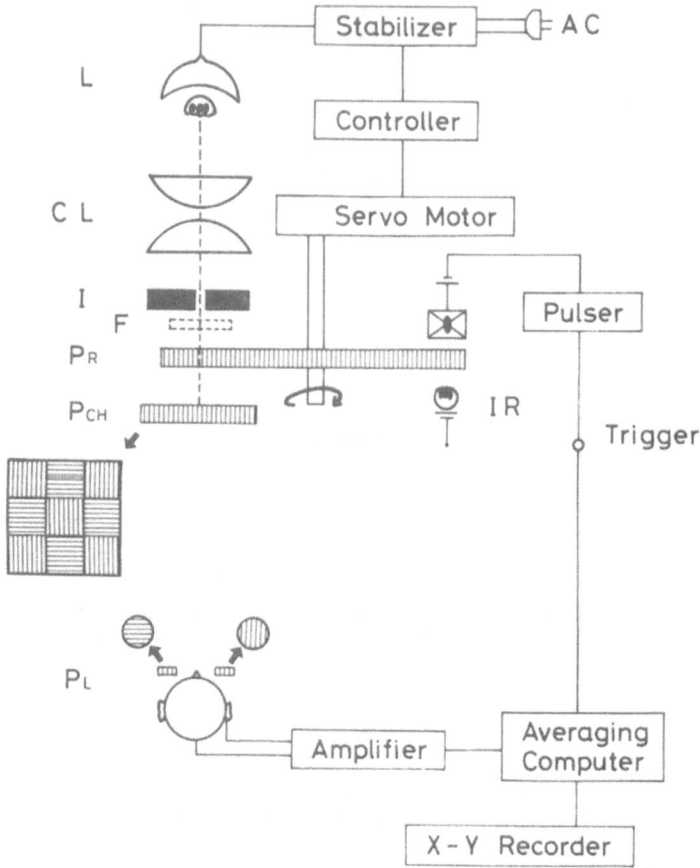

Fig. 1. Apparatus for stimulating and recording. L indicates halogen light source; CL: condenser lenses; I: iris; F: location where filters can be inserted.; P_R: rotating polaroid disc; P_{CH}: polaroid checkerboard target field. The Fresnel lens is attached behind the polaroids. The iris and the Fresnel lens minimize the decrease of luminance in the periphery.; P_L: polaroid lenses orthogonally oriented before each eye; IR: infrared light emitting diode for trigger source.

The light passes through three polaroid filters, P_R, P_{CH} and P_L, before reaching to the eye.

In binocular viewing, the contribution of the right eye and the left eye should differ in cases with defective binocular vision but not in normal subjects. In this paper the analysis of the comparison of amplitudes between both eye originated waves in the binocular VECP is reported.

METHODS

The stimulator was similar to the conventional rotating polaroid pattern-reversal stimulator. A checkerboard pattern composed of orthogonally

284

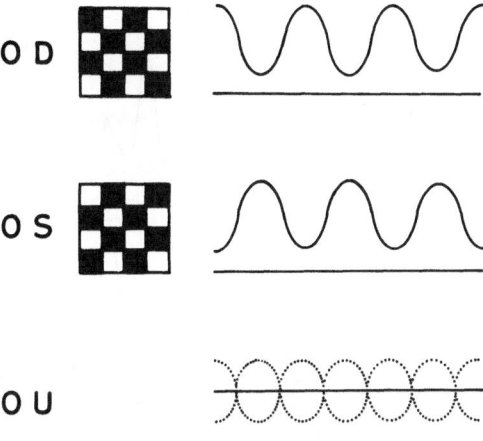

O D

O S

O U

Fig. 2. Schematic of the stimulus. When viewed monocularly, half of the checks look constantly black. The rest of the checks vary in luminance sinusoidally. When the other eye is used, those checks illuminated for the fellow eye look black and the rest vary in luminance with the phase changed by a half period. When viewed binocularly with normal binocularity, the black checks are fused. The illuminated checks are fused also and appear to be fixed in luminance; the right and the left eye appear to be darkened alternately.

oriented polaroid checks was placed 3.45 m from the examinee. At this distance the total field subtended a visual angle of 3° 20' and the individual checks, 20'. The stimulus screen was back illuminated through the rotating polaroid disc, and was viewed by the subject through polaroid lenses placed perpendicularly to each other (Fig. 1).

Sinusoidal contrast changes were obtained when viewed monocularly. When viewed binocularly with normal binocularity, the checkerboard target field appeared to have a constant luminance; when viewed with the right or the left eye the target field appeared to be alternately darkened (Fig. 2).

The VECPs were recorded with monopolar derivations, the active electrode placed 5% above the inion. The signals were amplified (Nihon Kohden VC-9) and fed to an averaging computer (Nihon Kohden ATAC 201). The

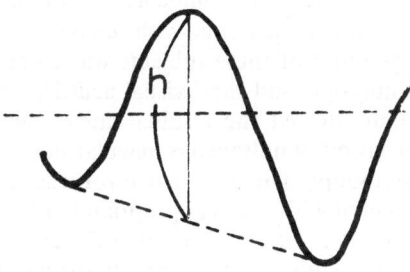

Fig. 3. Method of measuring the amplitude of waves. The errors produced by fluctuations of the baseline are minimized.

285

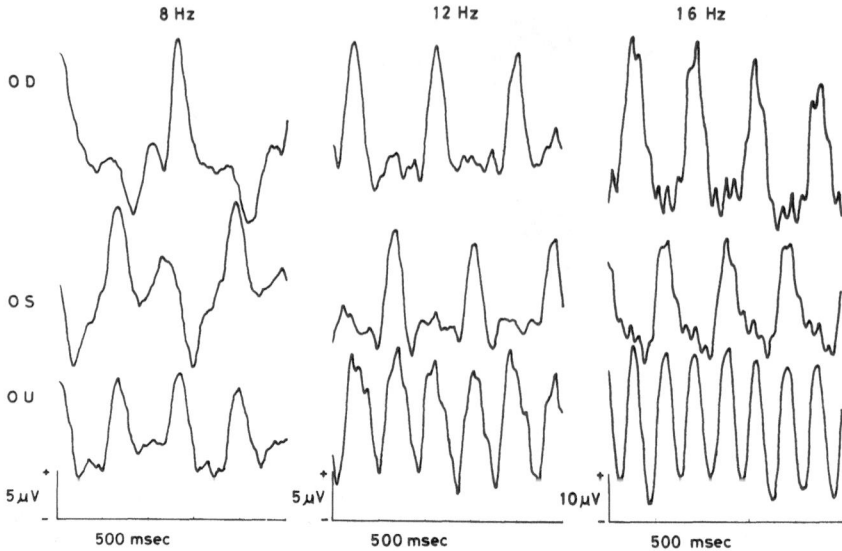

Fig. 4. Sample records of a normal subject. This subject had the largest amplitude VECPs of all the examinees. OD and OS are the monocular VECPs. OU is the binocular VECP. Note that in the binocular VECP, the waves coincide with those in the monocular VECPs. Accordingly, the waves are separated into odd and even numbers and called the right eye originated waves and the left eye originated waves. In normal subjects, the average of the dominant eye originated waves and the non-dominant ones are almost equivalent. Laterality Indices are 101.4% in 8 Hz, 103.7% in 12 Hz and 99.9% in 16 Hz.

number of sweeps accumulated was 128 and the sampling period was 500 msec. The stimulus frequencies were 8, 12 and 16 Hz. The method of measuring the amplitude of waves is shown in Fig. 3.

MATERIALS AND METHODS

Subjects. Five cases with defective binocular vision including four female and one male post-operative patients with infantile esotropia participated in this study. The age range of these subjects was from 19 to 23 years. They had no history of amblyopia and their visual acuities were normal. The post-operative eye positions showed the residual angle ranging from 10$^\Delta$ to 20$^\Delta$. As for the binocular vision, simultaneous macular perception was not present with the major amblyoscope. The refractive error was corrected and the angle of deviation was corrected with prism appropriately placed before each eye.

The control group consisted of 17 female subjects from 18 to 26 years of age with normal visual acuity and normal binocular vision. The angle of stereopsis for each normal subject, ascertained with the Titmus test, was at least 40 seconds of arc. Eye postion and ocular movements were also normal.

286

16 Hz

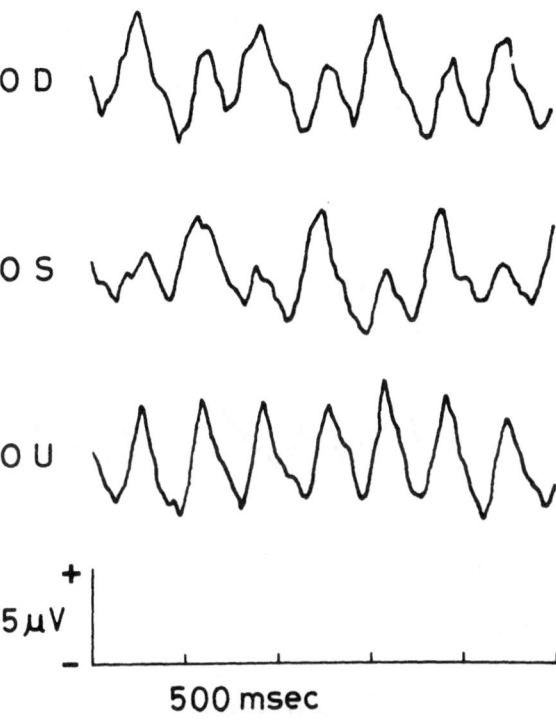

O D

O S

O U

+
5 μV
-

500 msec

Fig. 5. Sample records of a normal subject. Second harmonics are found in the mono-cular VECPs. The Laterality Index, calculated in the same manner, is 99.8%.

RESULTS

The binocular VECP showed the same number of waves as the stimulation frequencies and the monocular VECPs showed half the number (Fig. 4). The waves in the binocular VECP coinciding with the right monocular VECP were called the right eye originated waves, and the same for the left. The binocular VECP, the right eye originated waves and the left eye originated waves appeared alternately. The monocular originated waves were separated into odd and even numbers and the averages of the amplitudes were calculated. The ratio of the right and left eye (the dominant eye i.e. the eye producing the greatest amplitude response, for the normal subjects or the fixating eye amplitude for the cases was used as the denominator) responses were calculated, expressed as a percentage and denoted as the Laterality Index.

Some subjects showed second harmonics present in the monocular VECPs (Fig. 5). In these instances the Laterality Index was calculated in the same manner.

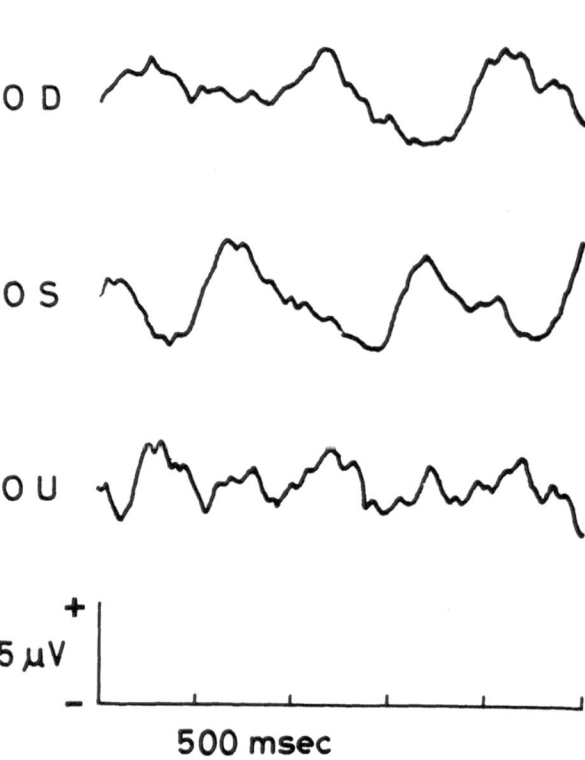

1 2 Hz

O D

O S

O U

+

5 μV

−

500 msec

Fig. 6. Sample records of a case with defective binocular vision and right eye fixation. The reduction of the left eye originated waves is recognized in the binocular VECP. The Laterality Index is 63.0%.

In the control group, the right eye originated waves and the left were almost equal in amplitude. Across all conditions and subjects the average (± 1 standard deviation) Laterality Index was 101.8 ± 15.1% (Table 1).

Fig. 6 illustrates a case with defective binocular vision (right eye fixation). There was no large difference in amplitude between the two monocular VECPs, but concerning the binocular VECP, the right eye originated waves were larger than the left ones. The Laterality Index was 63.% in this case. Table 2 shows the results of the cases with defective binocular vision. The average (± 1 standard deviation) Laterality index was 57.3 ± 8.4%. A significant difference ($p < 0.001$, t-test) was obtained between this index and that from normal subjects. The reduction in amplitude of the non-fixating eye originated waves under the binocular condition was recognized in all cases.

Some cases could fixate with either eye under the binocular condition and in these instances, the side of the amplitude reduction was reversed (Fig. 7).

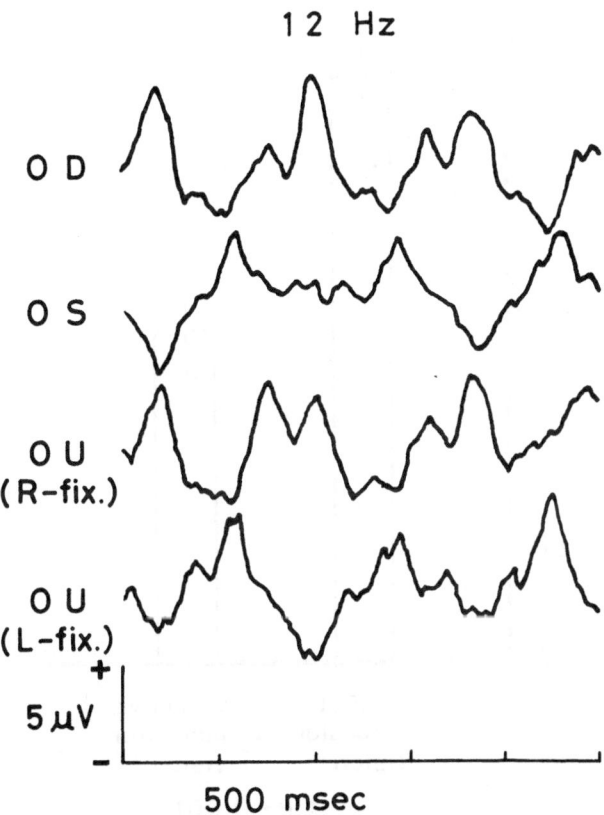

12 Hz

O D

O S

O U
(R-fix.)

O U
(L-fix.)

+

5 μV

-

500 msec

Fig. 7. Sample records of a case with defective binocular vision. This case prefers right eye fixation but can keep fixating with the left eye with effort. OU(R-fix.) is the usual binocular VECP; OU(L-fix.) is the binocular VECP with the fixating left eye. The number of waves in the binocular VECPs is reduced by half of the stimulus frequency and is the same number as in the monocular VECPs. The Laterality Index is not calculated in these instances. Note that the side of the amplitude reduction is reversed between both of the binocular VECPs.

Some cases showed the number of waves in the binocular VECP reduced by half of normals and the same as in the monocular VECPs (Fig. 7). The Laterality Index was not calculated in these cases.

Fig. 8 illustrates the results of the mean Laterality Index across all conditions and subjects for the cases and the controls. The Laterality Index of the cases was 57.3% and showed a significant difference from that of the controls.

DISCUSSION

Previous findings have shown that in normal subjects the amplitude of the binocular VECP is larger than the monocular VECP. The lack of binocular

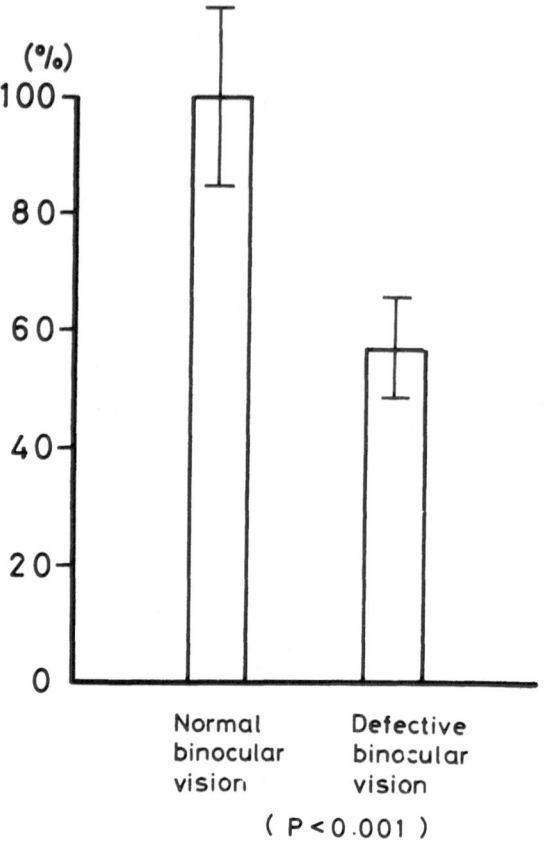

Fig. 8. Mean Laterality Indexes. The results of the average (± 1 standard deviation) are 101.8 ± 15.1% in the normal subjects and 57.3 ± 8.4% in the cases with defective binocular vision.

summation has been examined in cases with defective binocular vision (Amigo 1978). However, in these studies, the amplitudes of different response traces, the monocular VECPs and the binocular VECPs, were compared. The difficulty with this method is that when attention during one trace varies from another, erroneous binocularity estimate may be calculated.

When dichoptic stimulation was used and retinal rivalry was facilitated, a reduction of VECP amplitudes was found by Lancing (1964) and Lawwill & Biersdorf (1968); on the other hand, Riggs & Whittle (1967), Martin (1970), and Harter et al. (1976) showed no reduction.

Harter et al. (1977) demonstrated the size-specific interocular suppression of VECP, but independent stimulation of the right and left eye was used. Therefore it was different from natural binocular conditions.

Lennerstrand (1978) showed the interocular suppression of VECP for dichoptic stimulation. The stimulus frequencies used were 10 Hz in the right eye and 7 Hz in the left eye, and he compared the binocular VECPs with the monocular VECPs. Again this was a comparison of different response traces.

Table 1. Laterality index in the normal subjects

Subject No.	Age	Sex	Dominant eye	Laterality index 8 Hz	12 Hz	16 Hz
1	18	F	R	88.1	84.6	138.8
2	18	F	R	81.6	97.1	–
3	18	F	R	86.0	117.5	114.3
4	19	F	R	–	108.0	–
5	19	F	R	125.9	101.2	83.5
6	19	F	L	–	94.8	100.5
7	19	F	R	–	98.2	–
8	19	F	R	–	111.4	157.8
9	19	F	R	–	104.4	97.8
10	20	F	L	105.6	102.4	103.0
11	20	F	R	–	96.4	89.9
12	20	F	L	101.4	103.7	99.9
13	20	F	R	–	105.3	99.8
14	21	F	R	82.8	90.5	100.0
15	21	F	R	–	105.4	93.3
16	23	F	R	–	88.3	121.1
17	26	F	R	–	97.8	90.5

Mean ± standard deviation: 101.8 ± 15.1

– indicates the monocular and the binocular VECPs could not be recorded clearly.

It is sometimes experienced that the amplitude of VECP varies from time to time and the scattering of the amplitude values is vary large even though the examinee is encouraged to keep attention throughout the examination.

In this study the authors compared the amplitude of the waves in only one response trace. Therefore, the results are not influenced by varying levels of attention. A good trace could be selected according to the reproducibility, that is, the repetitious pattern of sinusoidal waves in the steady-state response. In this manner, the amplitudes were compared under conditions which minimize the experimental error.

The reduction of the amplitude of the non-fixating eye originated waves in the binocular condition in the cases with defective binocular vision is recognized in this study. The dominancy does not influence the amplitude of both eye originated waves as in the normal subjects. It can be supposed that the normal binocular interaction in visual cortex neurons affects the amplitude of both eye originated waves equally. Therefore, this reduction might be caused by abnormal binocular interaction or interocular suppression. It is uncertain what kind of interocular relation exists in cases with abnormal or no fusion. The relation between the suppression observed clinically or by psychophysical tests and the reduction of non-fixating eye originated waves in the binocular VECP should be further investigated.

Table 2. Laterality index in the cases with defective binocular vision.

Case No.	Age	Sex	Preoperative diagnosis	Eye position	Fixating eye		Laterality index		
							8 Hz	12 Hz	16 Hz
1	19	F	inf. ET	10 > XT	R	L/R	52.8	59.4	*
						(L-fix. R/L)	52.5	60.5	*
2	20	M	ET	10 > XT	R	L/R	–	72.2	–
3	22	F	inf. ET	20 > LHT	R	L/R	48.0	38.0	66.2
						(L-fix. R/L)	64.8	54.2	–
4	22	F	inf. ET	12 > XT	R	L/R	–	63.0	–
5	23	F	inf. ET	14 > LHT	R	L/R	–	*	56.3
						(L-fix. R/L)	–	*	56.6

Mean ± standard deviation: 57.3 ± 8.4

– indicates the monocular and the binocular VECPs could not be recorded clearly.;

*: the number of waves in the binocular VECP was reduced by half, the same as in the monocular VECPs.;

inf. ET: infantile esotropia; XT: exotropia; LHT: left hypertropia.

SUMMARY

1. In the binocular VECP the right eye originated waves and the left ones were separated. The ratio of the average amplitudes was calculated and denoted as the Laterality Index.

2. In normal subjects, the dominant eye originated waves and the non-dominant ones were almost equal in amplitude. The Laterality Index was 101.8 ± 15.1%.

3. In the cases with normal visual acuity but defective binocular vision, the nonfixating eye originated waves showed reduction in amplitude in the binocular VECP. The Laterality Index was 57.3 ± 8.4% showing a siggnificant difference.

ACKNOWLEDGEMENT

The authors wish to express our appreciation to Prof. Yasuo Uemura, Keio University, for his helpful discussion and valuable comments on the manuscript.

REFERENCES

Amigo, G., Fiorentini, A., Pirchio, M. & Spinelli, D. Binocular vision tested with visual evoked potentials in children and infants. Invest. Ophthalmol. Vis. Sci. 17: 910–915 (1978).

Harter, M.R., Towle, V.L. & Musso, M.F. Size specificity and interocular suppression: monocular evoked potentials and reaction times. Vis. Res. 16: 1111–1117 (1976).

Harter, M.R., Towle, V.L., Zakrzewski, M. & Moyer, S.M. An objective indicant of binocular vision in humans: size-specific interocular suppression of visual evoked potentials. Electroenceph. clin. Neurophysiol. 43: 825–836 (1977).

Lancing, R.W. Electroencephalographic correlates of binocular rivalry in man. Science 146: 1325–1327 (1964).

Lawwill, T. & Biersdorf, W.R. Binocular rivalry and visual evoked responses. Invest. Ophthalmol. Vis. Sci. 7: 378–385 (1968).

Lennerstrand, G. Binocular interaction studied with visual evoked responses (VER) in humans with normal or impaired binocular vision. Acta Ophthal. 56: 628–637 (1978).

Martin, J.I. Effects of binocular fusion and binocular rivalry on cortically evoked potentials. Electroenceph. clin. Neurophysiol. 28: 190–201 (1970).

Riggs, L.A. & Whittle, P. Human occipital and retinal potentials evoked by subjectively faded visual stimuli. Vis. Res. 7: 441–451 (1967).

Siegfried, J., May, J. & Cummings, R. A technique for recording monocular VEPs under conditions of binocular stimulation. In: 16th ISCEV Symposium, Morioka (1978) (Ed. Y. Tazawa). Jap. J. Ophthal. 1979.

Authors' address:
Department of Ophthalmology
School of Medicine
Keio University
35 Shininomachi, Shinjuku-ku
Tokyo 160
Japan

THE BINOCULAR VER

The effect of interocular luminance differences

G.L. TRICK, W.W. DAWSON & J.R. COMPTON

(*Big Rapids, Mich./Gainesville, Florida, U.S.A.*)

ABSTRACT

Although the visual evoked response (VER) is frequently used to assess binocularity, the contribution of the monocular components to the binocular VER is poorly understood. In a typical binocular situation, both eyes view the same stimulus pattern and the amplitude of the binocular VER is approximately 1.4 times larger than the amplitude of either monocular response. This parallels psychophysical reports of binocular brightness and contrast summation. We have examined checkerboard (14' checks) pattern-reversal (3.75 Hz) VERs evoked from observers with normal binocularity using conditions in which interocular luminance differences (from 0.0 to 2.0 log units) were established. We found that for luminance differences up to 0.6 log units, the amplitude of the binocular VER did not vary significantly. Larger luminance differences resulted in decreased amplitudes with luminance differences between 1.3 and 2.0 log units resulting in amplitudes significantly smaller than the amplitude of *either* monocular VER. These results imply some type of inhibitory binocular interaction. Furthermore, observers with anomalous binocularity exhibited deviations from this normal pattern.

INTRODUCTION

The mechanisms underlying normal binocular vision are poorly understood. While it is obvious that the visual system is capable of integrating information from the two eyes into a singular binocular impression, the manner in which this is accomplished remains obscure. Furthermore, it is unclear what changes in the functioning of these mechanisms can be associated with abnormal binocular vision.

One strategy which has been employed to examine the interactions involved in binocular vision is to record pattern-reversal VERs for each eye individually and then for both eyes simultaneously. This approach has been utilized by a number of investigators (Srebro 1978; Wanger & Nilsson 1978) with the general agreement that the amplitude of the binocular pattern-reversal VER is greater than the amplitude of either corresponding monocular response, but frequently less than the sum of the monocular responses. Although this result seems to hold for a large group of individuals with normal binocularity, the results for individuals with binocular anomalies (such as amblyopia or strabismus) have been ambiguous (Srebro 1978; Wanger & Nilsson 1978; Arden, Barnard & Mushin 1974).

An alternative approach is to examine binocularity using both similar and dissimilar patterns for the two eyes. This approach has been employed extensively in psychophysical experimentation (Trick & Guth 1980; Blake & Rush 1980; for example), but its application to VER research has been limited (Lennerstrand 1978; Harter 1977; Cobb, Morton & Ettlinger 1967). However, such a procedure has the advantage of allowing a more thorough manipulation of the variables which could influence binocular vision.

This line of reasoning has led us to consider the influence of interocular luminance differences on the binocular pattern-reversal VER. We have found that sufficiently large interocular luminance differences result in binocular VERs of an amplitude significantly less than the amplitude of either corresponding monocular response. In addition, preliminary results indicate that these effects vary considerably in cases of anomalous binocular vision.

MATERIALS AND METHODS

Using a commercially available signal averaging computer (Nicolet CA-1000), visual evoked responses were differentially recorded between an active electrode (Ag-AgCl), attached with conductive electrode paste 2 cm above the inion on the mid-sagittal plane, and linked reference electrodes (also Ag-AgCl) clipped to the earlobes. A forehead electrode grounded the subject. Signals were amplified by a low noise differential amplifier and were actively filtered, cut off frequencies (-3 db points) at 0.1 and 100 Hz. The filtered signal was then fed to the averaging computer which summed either 100 or 200 responses.

A black and white checkerboard pattern, generated on a television screen by a Nicolet visual stimulator (NIC-1006), was used to evoke the pattern-reversal responses. At the 1 meter viewing distance, the television screen provided a 16.5° by 12.6° pattern, with each check subtending 14′ of arc. The mean luminance of the pattern was 26 cd/m², with a 74% contrast. The black and white checks were alternated at 3.75 Hz. A dark spot in the center of the screen served as a fixation point.

Each experimental session included a standard binocular (OU) condition along with right eye (OD) and left eye (OS) monocular conditions. In addition, all sessions included a series of conditions in which one eye viewed the pattern through various neutral density filters (ranging from 0.3 to 2.0 log units) while the other eye viewed the unattenuated pattern. A series of control conditions, in which the checkerboard pattern was monocularly viewed through the same series of neutral density filters, was included in the experimental conditions for five subjects.

All of the volunteer subjects were fully informed of the nature of the

Table 1. Visual characteristics of the subjects with abnormal binocular vision.

Subject	Age	Sex	Corrected visual acuity		Cover test	Bagolini	Stereoacuity	Diagnosis
			OD	OS				
D.W.	23	M	20/60	20/15	— —	— — —	$200''^{a}$	Non-strabismic amblyope
D.F.	23	F	20/20	20/15	$10 \triangle RET^{b}$	OD Suppression (NCR)	$800''$	Small angle strabismic with NCR
L.M.	20	F	20/20	20/20	$RHET^{c}$	Harmonious (ARC)	$800''$	Small angle strabismic with ARC

[a]Stereoacuity varied with distance
[b]Right Esotropia
[c]Right HyperEsotropia ($10 \triangle$ Vertical, $8 \triangle$ Horizontal)

297

procedure, gave their informed consent and received a complete optometric examination. The ten subjects (ages 21–28) classified as visually normal were emmetropic or corrected to emmetropia, had equal acuity in both eyes, were essentially orthophoric, and exhibited good stereoacuity. In addition, three patients with binocular abnormalities were examined. The clinical data for these patients is presented in Table 1.

RESULTS AND DISCUSSION

VER amplitude and latency were determined for each experimental condition. VER amplitude was defined as the difference in voltage between the first major negative potential (N_1) and the next major positive potential (P_2) in the averaged waveform. VER latency was defined as the time from the onset of the pattern-reversal to the peak of the P_2 potential.

Since the data for all of the normal subjects revealed the same general trends, mean VER amplitude and latency were used as summary measures. Consider first the monocular (either OD or OS) and binocular (OU) conditions in which no attenuation was involved (Fig. 1). The mean binocular

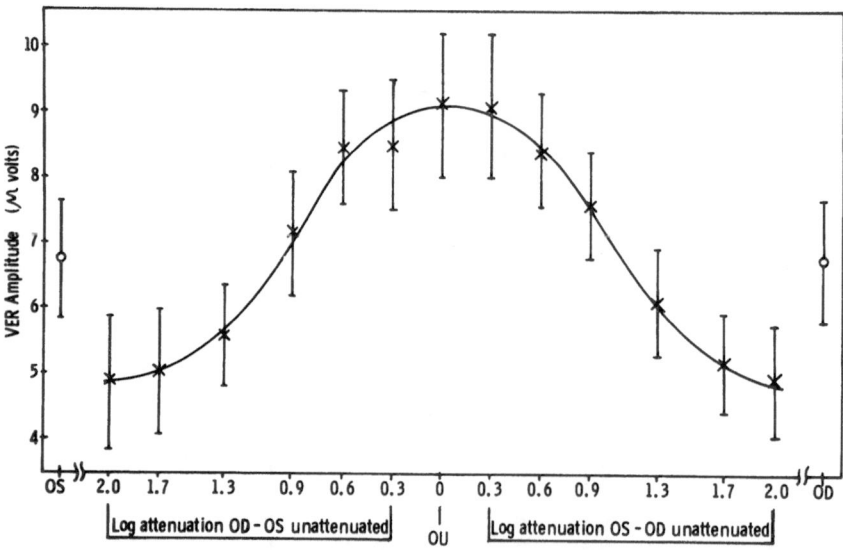

Fig. 1. A comparison of the mean VER amplitude (for ten normals) for all the binocular conditions (X's), as well as for the right (OD) and left eye (OS) conditions (open circles). The error bars represent the standard errors around the mean values given. The smooth curve plotted represents a best fit (by eye) to the data.

amplitude exceeded the mean monocular amplitude (for either eye) by a factor of about 1.375. This is in good agreement with the $\sqrt{2}$ factor reported in other binocular VER experiments (Srebro 1978; Wanger & Nilsson 1978), as well as in psychophysical reports of contrast sensitivity and visual acuity (Home 1978; Campbell & Green 1965), brightness and detection (Fry & Bartley 1933; Cook 1934), and temporal resolution (Blake & Rush 1980; Cavonius 1979).

In addition to the $\sqrt{2}$ factor, another trend was apparent for the binocular conditions in which the stimulus to one eye was attenuated (Fig. 1). Although small amounts of attenuation (0.6 log units or less) had little effect upon the amplitude of the evoked response, increasing attenuation resulted in a significant decrease in the amplitude of the binocular response. When the interocular luminance difference was greater than 0.9 log units, the amplitude of the evoked response was less than the amplitude of either monocular response. In fact, the data for each of the ten normals reveals a significantly lower amplitude response for the conditions with the greatest attenuation (1.7 and 2.0 log units) than for either unattenuated monocular condition.

For these same conditions, analysis of VER latency revealed no significant changes (Fig. 2). This was not surprising since in all conditions at least one unattenuated eye contributed to the response, and this contribution apparently occurred at approximately the same point in time regardless of the condition of the other eye.

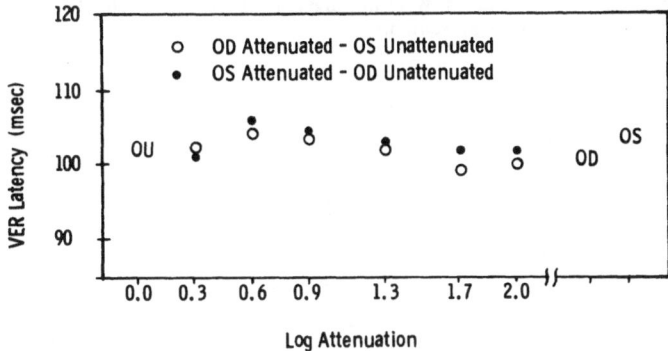

Fig. 2. The mean VER latency (for ten normals) for each of the binocular conditions and for the right (OD) and left (OS) eye alone conditions.

Given the changes noted in the binocular response when the stimulus to one eye was attenuated, we felt that a comparison of corresponding monocular and binocular conditions might more clearly depict the influence of attenuation on VER amplitude and latency. Therefore, monocular conditions, using the same set of neutral density filters, were included in the experimental sessions for five of the normal subjects. As expected (Kinney 1977; Vaughn, Costa & Gilden 1966), increasing attenuation had no significant effect on the amplitude of the monocular VER (Fig. 3), but increased the latency of the monocular response (Fig. 4). This is in sharp contrast to the binocular conditions in which attenuation of the stimulus to one eye resulted in a significant decrease in the amplitude of the response

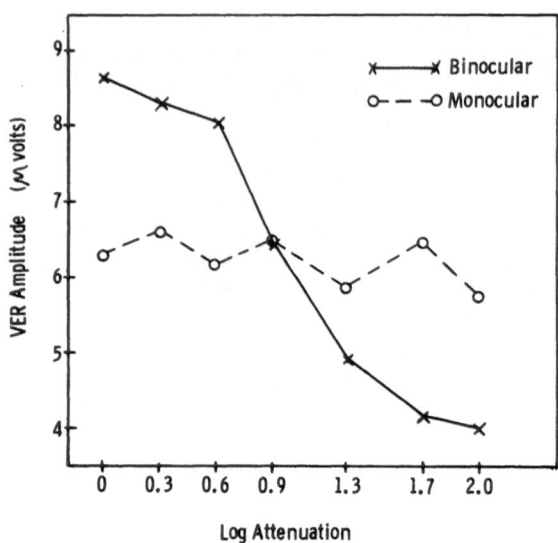

Fig. 3. A comparison of the effect of attenuation of the stimulus on both monocular and binocular viewing conditions for five normals. For the binocular data both OD attenuation and OS attenuation were averaged, while in the monocular data the average of OD and OS conditions is presented.

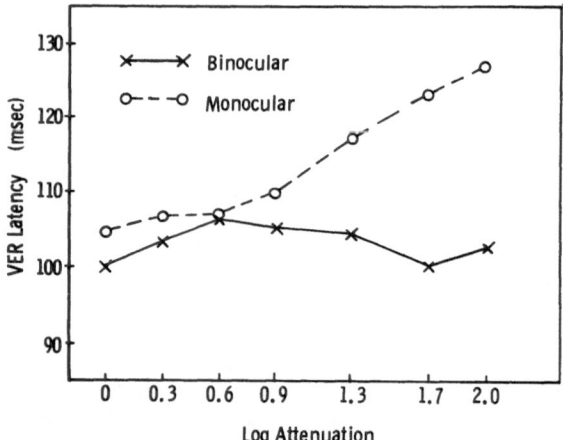

Fig. 4. A comparison of the latency data for both monocular and binocular conditions.

(Fig. 3), but no obvious change in latency (Fig. 4). Furthermore, a comparison of the influence of attenuation on monocular and binocular response amplitudes demonstrates that an averaging of the monocular responses can not account for the binocular results.

These results are quite similar to the psychophysical findings on the

300

binocular interactions mediating brightness (Levelt 1965; Fry & Bartley 1933), contrast sensitivity (Blake & Levinson 1977; Abadi 1976), and temporal resolution (Cavonius 1979; Blake & Rush 1980). The psychophysical results indicate that summation occurs when the stimuli to the two eyes are fairly similar, but large differences between the stimuli result in an interaction which reduces the binocular response to a level below the monocular (Blake & Fox 1973). In the psychophysical literature this interaction has often been referred to as binocular 'inhibition'. The results of the present investigation suggest a similar interaction in the binocular VER.

A close examination of the latency data suggests an explanation for these results. The increased latency of the monocular response to the attenuated stimulus implies that attenuation of the stimulus to one eye during binocular viewing could result in a constructive or destructive interference between the monocular components of the response. In this manner, the phase difference between the monocular components could produce the type of effects described above.

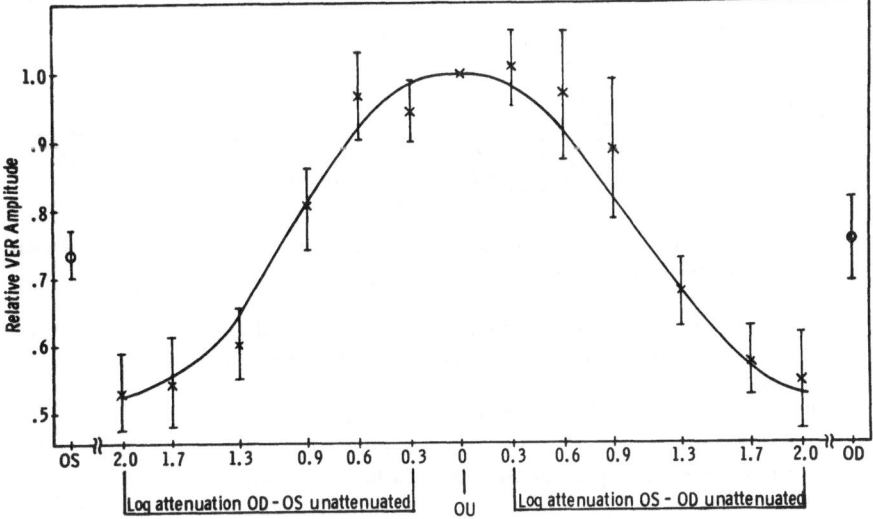

Fig. 5. The normalized VER amplitude data are presented here. The normalization was accomplished by dividing each subject's data by the OU amplitude. The mean of the normalized values for each experimental condition was then obtained. The error bars represent the standard errors for the normalized values.

In order to make comparisons between the normal subjects and individuals with abnormal binocularity, the normal data was normalized relative to the OU condition (Fig. 5). This procedure minimizes the influence of variability due to the intersubject amplitude differences unrelated to the experimental manipulations, thus yielding a more reliable comparison.

The three subjects with binocular anomalies received the same experimental treatment as the normals except each subject served in two experimental sessions. The data for each session was then normalized, and the

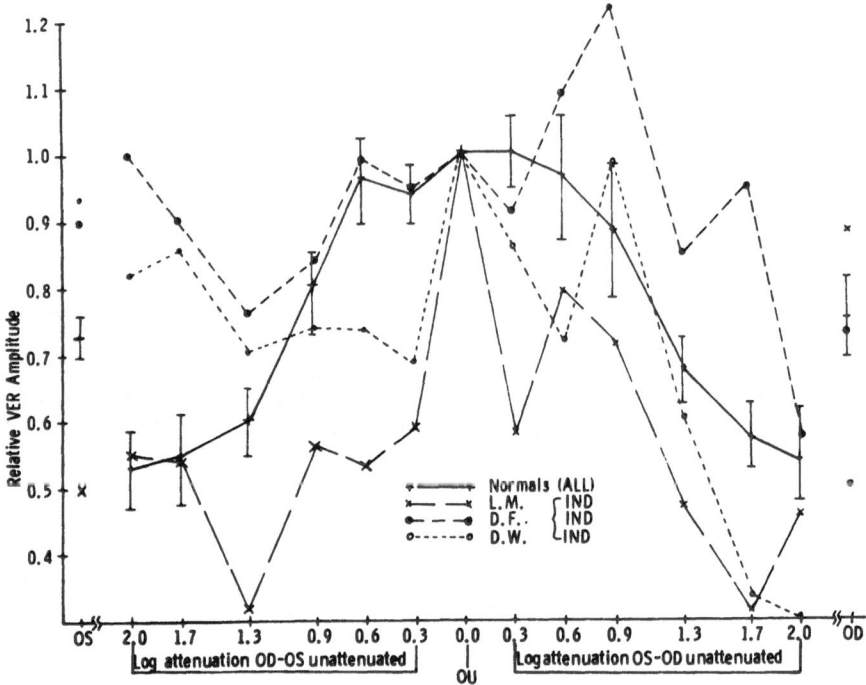

Fig. 6. A comparison of the normalized normal data with the data for the subjects with anomalous binocularity. See text for details.

average of the two sessions taken. The results for all three of these subjects (Fig. 6) deviate from the normal trend. For the amblyope there was a marked asymmetry in the function, but the largest interocular luminance differences still reduced the amplitude of the binocular responses to a level below the monocular amplitudes. On the other hand, for the two strabismics, the most consistent difference was greater amplitude for the monocular response from OD than the binocular VER amplitude for the largest corresponding interocular luminance differences.

CONCLUSIONS

Under the conditions of the present study the amplitude of the binocular VER was found to be approximately 1.4 ($\sqrt{2}$) times larger than the amplitude of either corresponding monocular response. Similar results have been reported elsewhere (Wanger & Nilsson 1978; Srebro 1978), although, it has been suggested that the amount of binocular interaction varies with contrast level (Srebro 1978). However, the previously reported reduction in the degree of interaction for contrasts greater than 30% (Srebro 1978) is contrary to the results of Wanger & Nilsson (obtained with a 98% contrast checkerboard pattern) as well as the present data. It is conceivable that this discrepancy is a result of the different temporal frequencies used in the three studies (6.3 Hz, 1.4 Hz and 3.75 Hz for Srebro, Wanger & Nilsson, and the present study respectively). This possibility suggests a spatio-temporal interaction which has yet to be examined in detail.

The variation in VER amplitude as a function of the interocular luminance difference is indirectly substantiated by the psychophysical literature on binocular interactions. We postulate that these interactions are due to phase differences induced by attenuating the stimulus to one eye, and a resultant waveform interference. It is unclear whether this interaction is mediated by the activity of binocular cortical cells, or by separate groups of monocular cells, although the distribution of binocular neurons in the monkey visual cortex (Hubel & Wiesel 1968) would tend to support the latter alternative.

The results for the amblyopic and strabismic subjects can not be considered conclusive. Although the results suggest some interesting differences between these subjects and normals, the results need to be verified on a larger population. Yet, these results do make it clear that there is a further need to investigate the influence of spatial and temporal variables on the binocular VER of patients with amblyopia and strabismus.

REFERENCES

Abadi, R.V. Induction masking – A study of some inhibitory interactions during dichoptic viewing. Vis. Res. 16: 269–275 (1976).

Arden, G.B., Barnard, W.M. & Mushin, A.S. Visually evoked responses in amblyopia. Br. J. Ophthal. 58: 183–192 (1974).

Blake, R. & Fox, R. The psychophysical inquiry into binocular summation. Perception and Psychophysics 14: 161–185 (1973).

Blake, R. & Levinson, E. Spatial properties of binocular neurones in the human visual system. Exp. Brain Res. 27: 221–232 (1977).

Blake, R. & Rush, C. Temporal properties of binocular mechanisms in the human visual system. Exp. Brain Res. 38: 333–340 (1980).

Campbell, F.W. & Green, D.G. Monocular versus binocular visual acuity. Nature 208: 191–192 (1965).

Cavonius, C.R. Binocular interactions in flicker. Quarterly J. Exp. Psych. 31: 273–280 (1979).

Cobb, W.A., Morton, W.B. & Ettlinger, G. Cerebral potentials evoked by pattern reversal and their suppression in visual rivalry. Nature 216: 1123–1125 (1967).

Cook, T.W. Binocular and monocular relations in foveal dark adaptation. Psychological Monographs 45: 1–85 (1934).

Fry, G.A. & Bartley, S.H. The brillance of an object seen binocularly. Am. J. Ophthalmol. 16: 687–693 (1933).

Harter, M.R. Binocular interaction: evoked potentials to dichoptic stimulation. In: Visual evoked potentials in man: new developments. (Ed. J.E. Desmedt) Clarendon Press, Oxford. 208–233 (1977).

Home, R. Binocular summation: A study of contrast sensitivity, visual acuity, and recognition. Vis. Res. 18: 579–585 (1978).

Hubel, D.H. & Wiesel, T.N. Receptive fields and functional architecture of monkey striate cortex. J. Neurophysiol. 195: 215–243 (1968).

Kinney, J.A.S. Transient visually evoked potential. J. Opt. Soc. Am. 67: 1465–1474 (1977).

Lennerstrand, G. Some observations on visual evoked responses (VER) to dichoptic stimulation. Acta Ophthal. 56: 638–647 (1978).

Levelt, W.J.M. On binocular rivalry, Monograph, Institute for Perception, Soesterburg, The Netherlands 33–55 (1965).

Srebro, R. The visual evoked response: Binocular facilitation and failure when binocular vision is disturbed. Arch. Ophthal. 96: 839–844 (1978).

Trick, G.L. & Guth, S.L. The effect of wavelength on binocular summation. Vis. Res. In Press (1980).

Vaughan, H.G., Costa, L.D. & Gilden, L. The functional relation of visual evoked response and reaction time to stimulus intensity. Vis. Res. 6: 645–656 (1966).

Wanger, P. & Nilsson, B.Y. Visual evoked responses to pattern-reversal stimulation in patients with amblyopia and/or defective binocular functions. Acta Ophthal. 56: 617–627 (1978).

Authors' addresses:
G.L. Trick & J.R. Compton
College of Optometry
Ferris State College
Big Rapids, Michigan 49307, U.S.A.

W.W. Dawson
Department of Ophthalmology
University of Florida
Gainesville, Florida, U.S.A.

MONOCULARLY EVOKED CORTICAL POTENTIALS TO SIMULTANEOUS STIMULATION OF CENTRAL AND PERIPHERAL HUMAN RETINA WITH DIFFERENT PATTERNS

C. TEPING & A. GRONEBERG

(Frankfurt/M., Bad Nauheim & München, F.R.G.)

ABSTRACT

In order to determine the relative contribution of different parts of the retina to the visually evoked cortical potential (VECP) the eye was exposed to separate, $90°$ phase-displaced checkerboard stimulation of central ($4°$ in diameter) and peripheral ($14° \times 18°$, center occluded) parts of the human retina. With high contrast central stimuli of 18 minutes of arc the VECP was always greater than the response to peripheral stimuli between 4 and 390 min of arc. With high contrast peripheral stimulation of 96 min of arc the central response to stimuli of 18 min of arc was suppressed only if the stimulus to the central field was less than 10 per cent contrast, if the check size of the central stimulus was smaller than 6 min of arc, or if central vision was blurred to less than 0.25 visual acuity. Simultaneous phase-shifted stimuli of the central (18 min of arc) and the peripheral (96 min of arc) parts of the retina led always to a predominance of the central retina. This was not seen when the VECPs in response to separate stimulation of the central and peripheral parts of the retina were added with the aid of a computer.

INTRODUCTION

Visually evoked cortical potentials (VECPs) are recorded either with flash stimulation (luminance response) or with pattern reversal stimuli (contrast response). For more detailed studies the use of contrast responses is superior since it permits separation of the responses of the more central parts of the retina, using check patterned stimuli ranging in size from approximately 5 to 25 min of arc, from the more peripheral parts, using check sizes from approximately 60 to 90 min of arc. The above check sizes of pattern yield the highest VECP amplitudes for central and peripheral vision as shown by occluding the peripheral and the central retinal fields (Harter 1970) and by presenting small test fields of different eccentricities (Groneberg 1980). The assumption was made that the above check sizes of pattern correspond to the modal size of the retinal receptive field centers at different retinal eccentricities (Wiesel & Hubel 1966).

The recording of VECP contrast responses has also some bearing for clinical purposes since it allows cortical responses from distinct retinal areas to be evoked. For this purpose, mostly half-field or quadrant stimulation is used with and without occluding the foveal region of the retina (Arden 1977). In cases of monocular field defects phase changes and extinction of quadrant VECPs were found and were helpful for diagnostic purposes (Cappin & Nissim 1975). In such investigations some difficulties of evaluation arise, when the different retinal fields are stimulated successively. Even with careful control of the stimulus parameters the VECP amplitudes to successive presentation to various retinal fields show considerable variation. Nevertheless Regan & Cartwright (1970) developed a method of simultaneous VECP recording during retinal half-field stimulation by using slightly different frequencies for each field.

The following investigation follows similar lines by presenting simultaneously, $90°$ phase-displaced pattern stimuli to the central ($4°$) and peripheral ($14° \times 18°$, center occluded) retinal field.

METHODS AND MATERIALS

The stimulus set-up consisted of two TV monitors and two independent pattern generators providing checkerboard pattern-reversal stimuli $90°$ out of phase (Cobb, Morton & Ettlinger 1967) at a rate of 7 reversals per second One TV screen stimulated the peripheral ($14° \times 18°$, center occluded) visual field; stimulation of the central visual field ($4°$ in diameter) was provided by a circular mirror placed in the center of the test field, onto which the screen of the second TV was projected (Fig. 1). At a distance of 1.5 m the the subject fixed monocularly the center of the mirror. The check size of pattern was varied between 2 min of arc (15 c/d) to 6.5 degrees (0.08 c/d); the pattern contrast could be widely adjusted without changing the mean luminance of the screen (0.9 log ft. − lambert or 27.2 cd/m^2). The VECP was recorded by means of a standard gold disk electrode from the midline of the scalp, 3 cm above the inion, the reference and ground electrodes were placed at the earlobes. The output of the pre-amplifier (filter frequency cut-offs 1 Hz and 30 Hz) was led to a signal averager; 128 or 256 sweeps were accumulated and recorded on an X-Y plotter. Amplitudes of potential (negativity downward) were measured by peak-to-trough method.

Ten healthy subjects (aged 16–30 years) with normal visual acuity and normal visual fields took part in the experiment.

RESULTS

Separate exposure of the $4°$ central field (check size 9 min of arc, Fig. 2A) and of the $14° \times 18°$ (center occluded) peripheral field (check size 96 min of arc, Fig. 2B) led to VECPs of about equal amplitude. Simultaneous $90°$ phase-displaced stimulation of the central and peripheral field showed a clear dominance of the response of the central retinal field (Fig. 2C) which

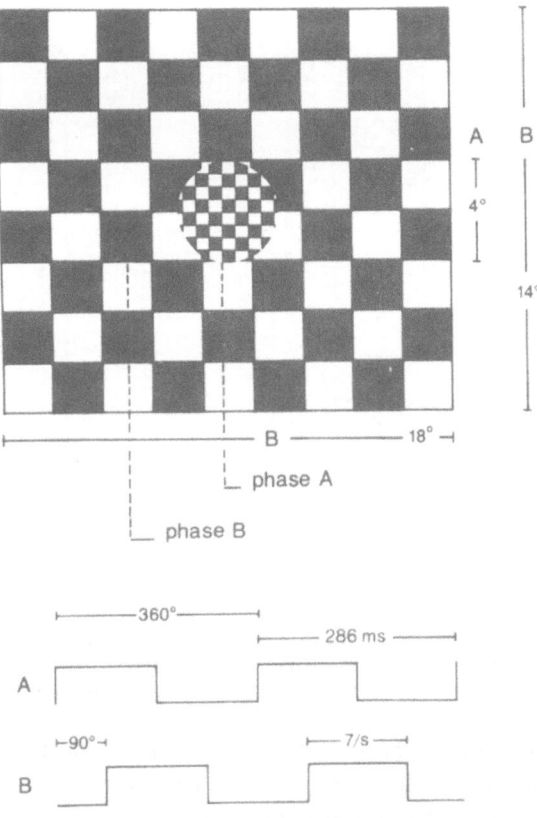

Fig. 1. Schematic description of the stimulus set up. Central (4° in diameter) and peripheral (14° × 18°) parts of the retina were stimulated simultaneously with 90° phase-displaced checkerboard patterns of different size.

indicates a suppression of the visual response of the peripheral retinal field. Under the experimental conditions presently chosen the amount of suppression was about 50% as determined by the height of the VECP amplitude when the center was blank (Fig. 2E). Algebraic adding of the separately recorded responses (Fig. 2A and B) by means of a computer did not lead to any recognizable dominance (Fig. 2D). This clearly indicates that neural interaction in the visual pathway is responsible for the changes observed and not recording conditions.

In a series of experiments the relative contribution of the central and peripheral retina was investigated more closely by changing the parameters (check size, contrast, blurring) of the stimulus. Varying the check size of the peripheral stimulus from 4 to 390 min of arc (7.5 to 0.08 c/d) led to an increase of amplitude of the response (Fig. 3, solid circles). However, the central response to checks of 18 min of arc (1.7 c/d) was only slightly diminished and preserved dominance (open circles).

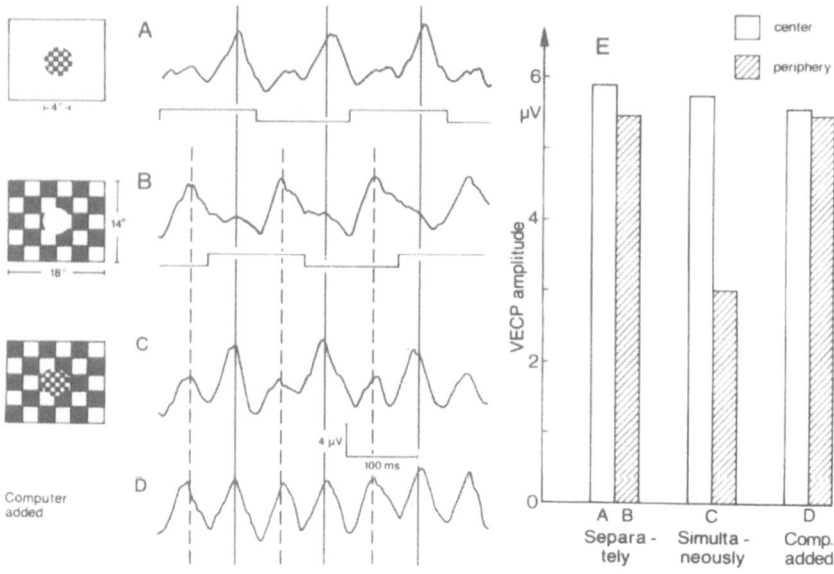

Fig 2. Monocular VECPs (n = 128) to 90° phase-displaced checkerboard stimulation of the central (continuous lines) and peripheral (dashed lines) retina. The VECP wave forms for one subject are presented in A–C; the VECP mean amplitude for five subjects are presented in E.

A: Stimulation of the center (check size 9 min corresponding to 3.3 c/d)

B: Stimulation of peripheral parts (check size 96 min corresponding to 0.31 c/d)

C: Simultaneous stimulation of center and periphery

D: Computer adding of records A and B

Dominance of the peripheral retina as determined by VECP amplitude, however, was seen for smaller check sizes (Fig. 4), or lower contrast (Fig. 5) of the central stimulus, i.e., when the central parts of the retina were operating under less than optimal conditions. Dominance of the peripheral response was also seen when vision was blurred by inserting spherical plus lenses for both central and peripheral vision (Fig. 6), i.e., when the sharpness of pattern contrast was equally diminished for the patterned stimulus presented both to the central and peripheral parts of the retina.

From these experiments we conclude that dominance of the peripheral retina only occurs if the check size of the central stimulus is decreased to less than 6 min of arc or if the contrast between the darker and brighter checks of the central stimulus pattern is decreased to less than about 10 per cent, providing the peripheral stimulus is set at its optimum (large check sizes, high levels of contrast). From the blurring experiment dominance of peripheral vision can be expected in case of myopic, otherwise normal eyes if the refractive error exceeds 1.75 diopters corresponding to 0.25 visual acuity.

308

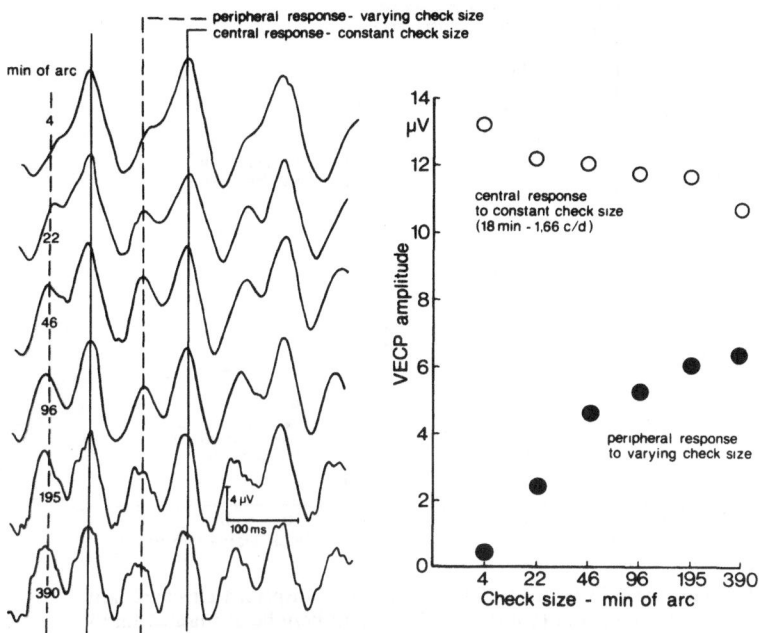

Fig. 3. Monocular VECPs (n = 256) to 90° phase-displaced checkerboard stimulation of the central (continuous lines) and peripheral (dashed lines) retina. Check size variation in the peripheral test field from 4 to 390 min (7.5 and 0.08 c/d), central stimulation of constant check size (18 min, corresponding to 1.66 c/d). Contrast appr. 100%.
Left: VECP wave forms of one subject
Right: VECP mean amplitudes of three subjects

DISCUSSION

The present experiments show that the central and peripheral parts of the retina do not contribute independently to the visual evoked cortical potential. Optimal stimulus conditions for central and peripheral vision led always to a strong dominance of the central retina at the visual cortex. This dominance could only be overcome with less than optimal adjustment of the central stimulus such as small check sizes and/or low levels of contrast which induced a distinct amplitude increase or even dominance of the peripheral retina in response to a constant stimulus. Dominance of the peripheral response was also seen when central and peripheral vision was blurred by inserting spherical plus lenses. Thus VECP recording in response to 90° phase-displaced pattern stimulation of central and peripheral parts of the retina provides evidence for mutual inhibitory interaction and release between central and peripheral vision.

So far the present experiments do not provide evidence as to whether the suppression occurs at the retinal or at the cortical level. However, with dichoptic stimulation a similar interaction was seen between the center of

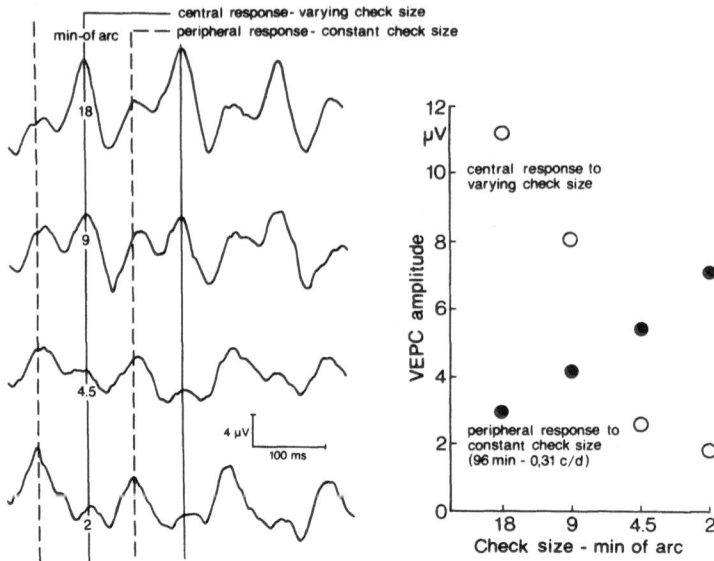

Fig. 4. Monocular VECPs (n = 256) to 90° phase-displaced checkerboard stimulation of the central (continuous lines) and peripheral (dashed lines) retina. Check size variation in the central retinal field from 18 to 2 min (1.66 to 15 c/d); peripheral stimulation of constant check size (96 min corresponding to 0.31 c/d). Contrast appr. 100%.
Left: VECP wave forms of one subject
Right: VECP mean amplitudes of five subjects

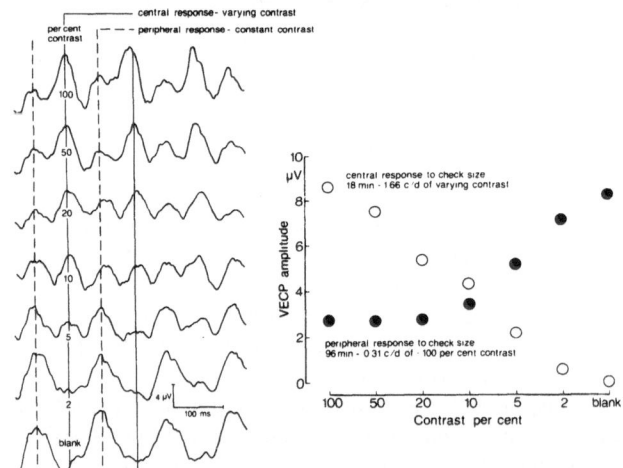

Fig. 5. Monocular VECPs (n = 256) to 90° phase-displaced checkerboard stimulation of the central (continuous lines) and peripheral (dashed lines) retina to checks of constant size; center − 18 min, periphery − 96 min. Contrast in the central retinal field varying from appr. 100% to zero, contrast in the peripheral test field constant appr. 100%.
Left: VECP wave forms of one subject
Right: VECP mean amplitudes of seven subjects

310

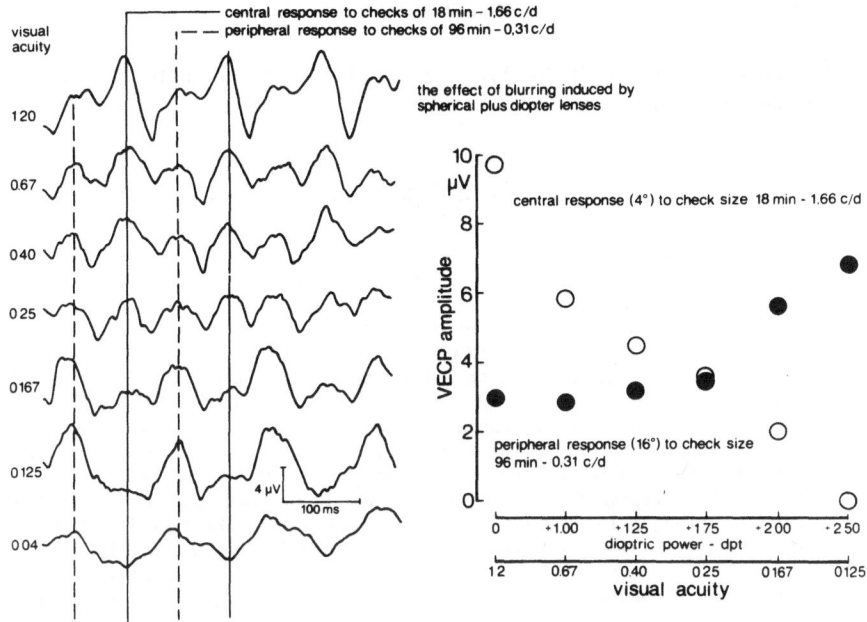

Fig. 6. Monocular VECPs (n = 256) to 90° phase-displaced checkerboard stimulation of the central (continuous lines) and peripheral (dashed lines) retina to checks of constant size; center – 18 min, periphery – 96 min. Changes of response are due to blurring by inserting spherical plus lenses of different dioptric power leading to losses of visual acuity. Contrast appr. 100%.
Left: VECP wave forms of one subject
Right: VECP mean amplitudes of five subjects

one eye and the periphery of the fellow eye (Groneberg & Teping 1981). The disinhibition of VECP amplitude for peripheral vision of one eye occurred with centrally applied pattern stimuli of the other eye at check sizes smaller than 7.5 min of arc or at stimulus contrast at and below 5 per cent. These observations closely correspond to the results of the present investigations using the central and peripheral parts of the same eye and provide evidence that the suppression occurs at the cortical level.

Independent evidence pointing into the same direction comes from clinical disturbances of central vision. According to Spekreijse et al. (1972) the fovea of the amblyopic eye contributes little to the pattern VECP and its response is made up mainly of parafoveal components. In contrast, the electroretinogram of the amblyopic eye elicited by checkerboard stimuli is essential normal (Groneberg 1980). Pattern VECPs of the normal eye similar to those of the amblyopic eye can be obtained after blurring of vision by inserting spherical plus lenses (Groneberg & Teping 1980), shown in the present investigation to disinhibit the peripheral components during simultaneous stimulation of the central and peripheral retina.

ACKNOWLEDGEMENT

The authors wish to thank Prof. Dr. E. Dodt for his helpful advice and reading the paper.

REFERENCES

Arden, G.B., Faulkner, D.J. & Mair, C. A versatile television pattern generator for visual evoked potentials. In: Visual evoked potentials in man: new developments. (Ed. J.E. Desmedt) Clarendon Press, Oxford. 90–109 (1977).

Cappin, J.M. & Nissim, S. Visual evoked responses in the assessment of field defects in glaucoma. Arch. Ophthal. 93: 9–18 (1975).

Cobb, W.A., Morton, H.B. & Ettlinger, G. Cerebral potentials evoked by pattern reversal and their suppression in visual rivalry. Nature 216: 1123–1125 (1967).

Groneberg, A. Simultaneously recorded retinal and cortical potentials elicited by checkerboard stimuli. In: 17th ISCEV Symposium. (Ed. E. Schmöger & J. Kelsey). Junk, The Hague. (Doc. Ophthal. Proc. Series Vol. 23). 255–262 (1980).

Groneberg, A. & Teping, C. Pattern evoked cortical potentials to simultaneous stimulation of both eyes. In: 18th ISCEV Symposium. (Ed. H. Spekreijse & P.A. Apkarian) Junk, The Hague. (Doc. Ophthal. Proc. Series Vol. 27) This volume (1981).

Groneberg, A. & Teping, C. Topodiagnostik von Sehstörungen durch Ableitung retinaler und kortikaler Antworten auf Umkehr-Kontrastmuster. Ber. Dtsch. Ophthalmol. Ges. 77: 409–415 (1980).

Harter, M.R. Evoked cortical responses to checkerboard patterns: Effects of check size as a function of retinal eccentricity. Vis. Res. 10: 1365–1376 (1970).

Regan, D. & Cartwright, R.F. A method of measuring the potentials evoked by simultaneous stimulation of different retinal regions. Electroenceph. clin. Neurophysiol. 28: 314–319 (1970).

Spekreijse, H., Khoe, L.H. & Van der Tweel, L.H. A case of amblyopia: electrophysiology and psychophysics of luminance and contrast. In: The visual system Neurophysiology, biophysics and their clinical applications. (Ed. G.B. Arden). Plenum Press, New York. (Recent Advances in Exp. Biol. and Med. Vol. 24). 141–156 (1972).

Wiesel, T.N. & Hubel, D.H. Spatial and chromatic interactions in the lateral geniculate body of the rhesus monkey. J. Neurophysiol. 29: 1115–1156 (1966).

Authors' address:
C. Teping
Abt. f. Augenheilkunde
Medizin. Fakultät
Rhein.-Westf. Techn. Hochschule
Goethestr. 27/29
D-5100 Aachen, F.R.G.

A. Groneberg
Augenklinik der T.U.
Ismaingenstr. 20
D-8000 München, F.R.G.

PATTERN EVOKED CORTICAL POTENTIALS
TO SIMULTANEOUS STIMULATION OF BOTH EYES

A. GRONEBERG & C. TEPING

(*Frankfurt, Bad Nauheim & München, F.R.G.*)

ABSTRACT

In order to determine the relative contribution of each eye to the binocular
VECP the right and the left eye of healthy subjects were separately exposed
to simultaneous, 90° phase-displaced checkerboard stimuli. With identical
stimulation of either eye no dominance of phases in the VECP in response
to the right or the left eye was seen. However, a decrease of check size to one
eye resulted in a predominance of the response elicited by stimulation of the
other eye. A similar effect was seen for changes of contrast if the modulation
depth of the checkerboard stimulus presented to one eye was less than 20
per cent of that presented to the other eye. Dominance of one eye by
presenting stimuli of different check size was reversed if the stimulus contrast
was decreased to a very low level (5 per cent). Similarly to findings with
monocular stimulation of central and peripheral parts of the retina (Teping
& Groneberg 1981), predominance of the central retina was suppressed by
presenting large checks of high contrast to the peripheral retina of the other
eye if the contrast of the central stimulus was low (10 per cent).

INTRODUCTION

Visually evoked cortical potentials (VECPs) have been used to study the
relative contribution of either eye to binocular vision. Under *dioptic* viewing
conditions, i.e., with virtually identical images projected on corresponding
retinal areas of both eyes, binocularly elicited VECPs were bigger in amplitude than those evoked monocularly. The amount of summation was
generally less than two-fold and was found to depend on the type of stimulus
used (Perry & Childers 1968; Cigánek 1970; Arden, Barnard & Mushin 1974;
Harter 1977; Abe 1978). It was the greatest for pattern stimuli of 10–20 min
of arc (Harter, Seiple & Salmon 1973). Under *dichoptic* viewing conditions,
i.e., with dissimilar pattern stimulation of the two eyes, the amplitude of
VECP was smaller as compared to that with monocular stimulation (Cigánek
1971; Harter, Seiple & Salmon 1973; Abe 1979). Presenting pattern stimuli

to each eye at different rates of reversal, the interocular suppression became larger as the stimuli were made similar and was highest for identical stimulus patterns (Lennerstrand 1978a, b).

Applying congruent patterns in a 90° out-of-phase mode of stimulation to either eye, it was found to be possible to detect in the VECP the so-called dominant eye (Cobb, Morton & Ettlinger 1967). Using a similar method of stimulation, the present investigation is concerned with the determination of the relative contribution of each eye to the VECP under different stimulus (check size and contrast) and viewing conditions (central and peripheral areas).

MATERIAL AND METHODS

The stimulus set-up was composed of two TV monitors, displaced to the viewer in a 90° visual angle. While the left eye was staring directly at the screen of TV I, the right eye looked at the screen of TV II via a mirror (Fig. 1). Correspondence of the two eyes was achieved by a small bar in

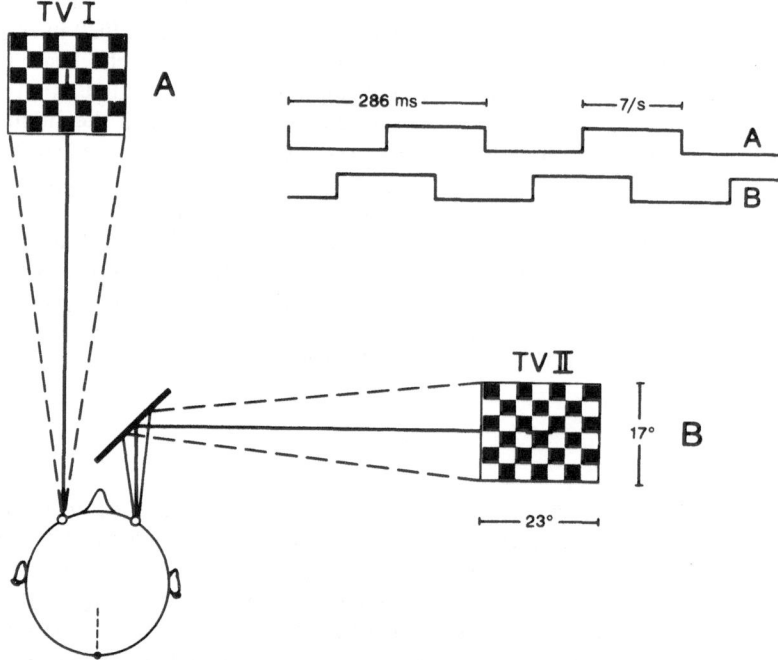

Fig. 1. Stimulus set-up for separate exposure of the left (A) and the right eye (B) to checkerboard reversal, 90° phase-displaced. Fusion of the two eyes is obtained by superimposing a vertical and horizontal bar on the TV monitors I and II.

the center of each screen, one (TV I) horizontal and the other (TV II) vertical. When the two images were properly superimposed, a cross was observed by the viewer.

Checkerboard pattern reversal stimuli were produced by two modified pattern generators (Medelec system) which were time displaced by a 90° phase shift (Fig. 1, upper right). Reversal rate was 7 per second and the total luminance of each screen was about 1.0 log ft.-lambert. The check size could be varied stepwise between 6 and 60 min of arc. The subjects were tested in a seated position at a distance of 90 cm to the target, the size of the test field being 17° × 23°. The contrast ratio between the light and the dark checks could be changed between approximately 100 per cent and zero without changing the mean luminance. The VECP was recorded with standard gold disc electrodes 3 cm above the inion, the reference electrode placed on the earlobe. The output of the pre-amplifier was fed into a signal averager (NIC 1072). Low and high frequency cutoffs were 1 and 30 Hz. After accumulation of 128 sweeps, each trial was plotted on a X-Y plotter. Amplitudes were measured from the peak to the trough of the major deflection.

A total of nine subjects between 16 and 42 years of age took part in the investigation. Acuity for both eyes of all subjects was normal; stereopsis was tested with TNO and Titmus and found to be normal. Attention was paid that VECP amplitudes, monocularly evoked from the right and left eye, were of the same magnitude, shape, and latency.

RESULTS

Large field stimulation. Highest interocular depression of VECP amplitude was observed with phase-displaced stimulation of congruent pattern. Referring to the monocularly evoked height of potential (Figs. 2A & 2B), the amplitude with dichoptic stimulation was reduced to about one quarter, under congruent pattern stimulus conditions (Fig. 2C). Computer adding of the monocularly elicited cortical potentials resulted in a frequency-doubled response showing a small reduction in amplitude (Fig. 2E). A nearly identical series of potentials of slightly higher amplitude was obtained with dioptic, in-phase stimulation at a reversal rate of 14/s (Fig. 2D), i.e., with the same number of reversals as with dichoptic phase-displaced stimulation of 7/s.

Starting with congruent 45 min checks for the left and the right eye (Fig. 3A) the check size for the right eye was decreased to 6 min of arc, keeping the check size for the left eye constant at 45 min of arc. This caused a nearly threefold increase of VECP amplitude in response to the checkerboard stimulus of the left eye whereas the VECP in response to stimulation of the right eye exhibited a loss of amplitude to very low values (Figs. 3 B–D). The dominance of the left eye obtained in this way was higher as compared to that seen after computer adding of the monocularly evoked cortical potentials (not seen in the figure).

Further experiments studied the effect of monocular variation of contrast on ocular dominance during 90° phase-displaced stimulation with congruent (Fig. 4) and dissimilar (Fig. 5) checkerboard patterns.

Presenting congruent checkerboard stimuli of 30 min of arc to both eyes,

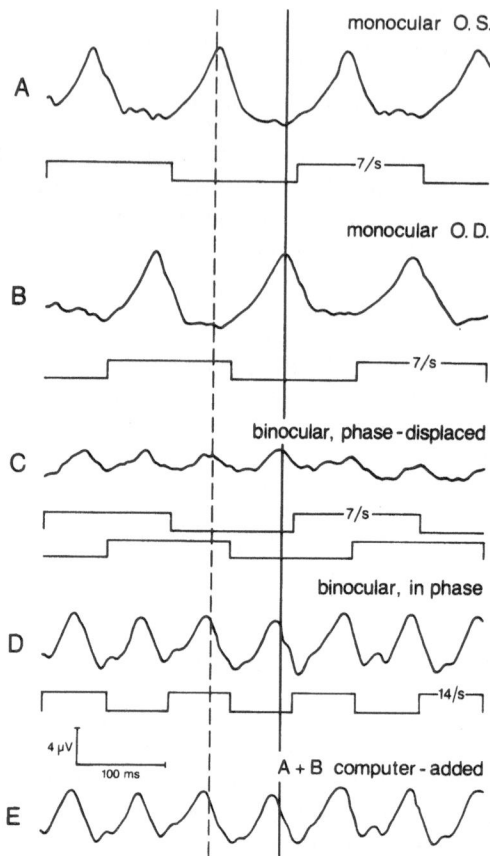

Fig. 2. VECP wave forms (n = 128) in response to 90° phase-displaced checkerboard stimuli (reversal rate 7/s, contrast approx. 100 per cent, check size 30 min, size of the test field 17° × 23°).

A and B: Monocularly viewed by the right and left eye.

C: Responses during simultaneous stimulation of both eyes.

D: Binocular in-phase stimulation, reversal rate 14/s.

E: Monocularly evoked responses A and B added by the computer.

dominance of the right eye in the VECP was noted when the contrast between the darker and brighter checks presented to the left eye was lowered from 50 to 20 per cent (Fig. 4C). Maximum amplitude was obtained when the stimulus contrast to the left eye was reduced to 5 per cent. Further lowering of pattern contrast did not lead to a further increase of the cortical potential in response to pattern stimuli applied to the right eye.

Under conditions where applications of dissimilar check sizes had led to an ocular dominance (cf. Fig. 3), lowering of pattern contrast, applied to the dominant eye, decreased its VECP amplitude at a constant level above

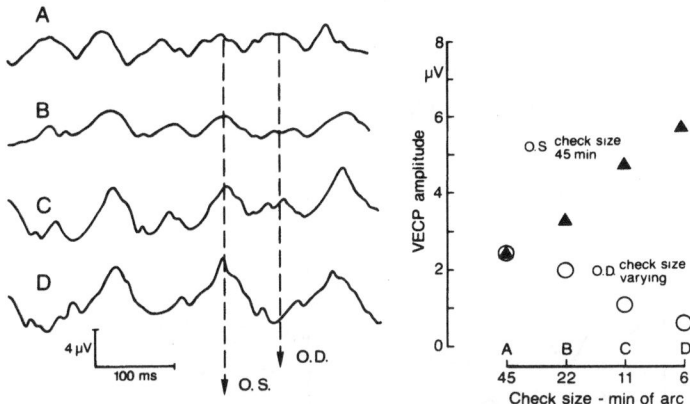

Fig. 3. VECPs (n = 128) in response to 90° phase-displaced checkerboard stimuli, separately presented to the right and the left eye (reversal rate 7/s, contrast approx. 100 per cent, size of test field 17° × 23°). Starting with congruent pattern of 45 min checks for the right and left eye (A) the check size for the right eye was decreased stepwise (B – 22 min, C – 11 min, D – 6 min) while the check size for the left eye was kept constant. The graph at the right represents averaged data of three subjects.

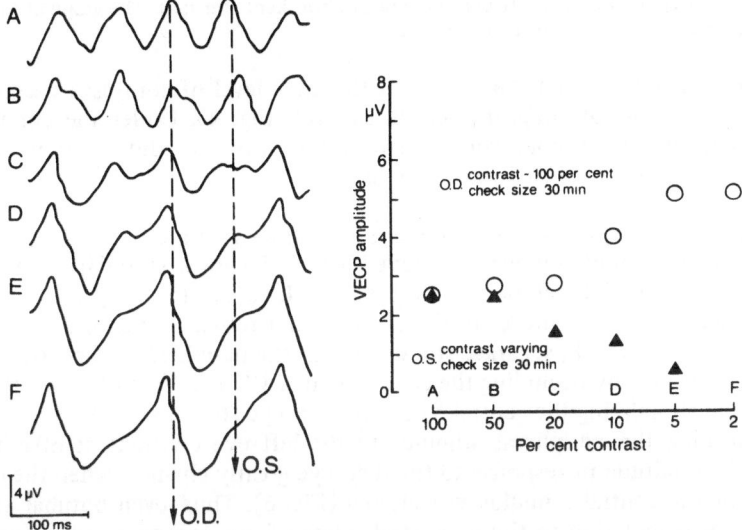

Fig. 4. VECPs (n = 128) in response to 90° phase-displaced checkerboard stimuli separately presented to the right and the left eye (reversal rate 7/s, check size 30 min, field size 17° × 23°). Starting with approx. 100 per cent contrast for the right and the left eye (A) the level of contrast for the left eye was diminished stepwise (B - 50 per cent; C - 20 per cent; D – 10 per cent; E – 5 per cent; F – 2 per cent), while the contrast for the right eye was kept constant at about 100 per cent. The graph at the right represents averaged data of three subjects.

317

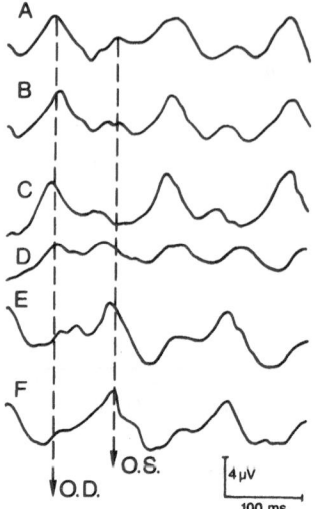
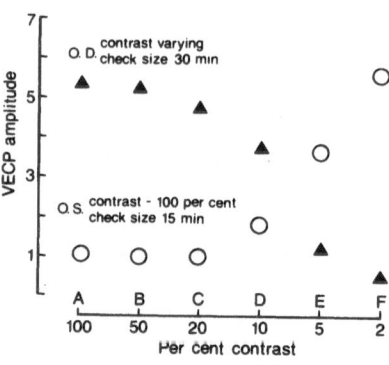

Fig. 5. VECPs (n = 128) in response to 90° phase-displaced checkerboard stimuli separately presented to the right and the left eye (reversal rate 7/s, size of test field 17° × 23°, check size to the right eye 30 min, check size to the left eye 15 min). Starting with approx. 100 per cent contrast for both eyes (A) the contrast for the right eye was diminished stepwise (B— 50 per cent; C – 20 per cent; D – 10 per cent; E – 5 per cent; F – 2 per cent). For the left eye the contrast was kept constant. The graph at the right represents averaged data of three subjects.

20 per cent (Fig. 5C). This is about the same level of contrast as seen with pattern stimuli of congruent check size (cf. Fig. 4). Under the conditions chosen, change of dominance between the two eyes did occur when the contrast was lowered to 5 per cent (Fig. 5E).

Central and peripheral field stimulation. In the experiments described above large field stimulation was employed which includes stimulation of both central and peripheral parts of the retina. In order to study more closely the contribution of the central and peripheral retina to dichoptic vision by means of the VECP, separate stimulation of the peripheral and central retina was performed by occluding the central 5° in a 17° × 23° test field of the left eye and stimulating the central 5° of the right eye (Fig. 6 and 7).

Keeping the peripheral stimulus to the left eye constant at 60 min the VECP amplitude in response to the right eye greatly changed when the check size of the central stimulus was altered (Fig. 6). Thus, even optimal adjustment of stimulation to the peripheral retina of one eye does not disturb the well known variation of VECP amplitude with check size ('spatial tuning') for centrally applied stimuli to the other eye. However, with further decreasing check sizes centrally applied to the right eye, the VECP elicited by large checks to the peripheral retina of the left eye increased and became dominant when the check size of the centrally presented stimulus diminished to 7.5 min of arc.

318

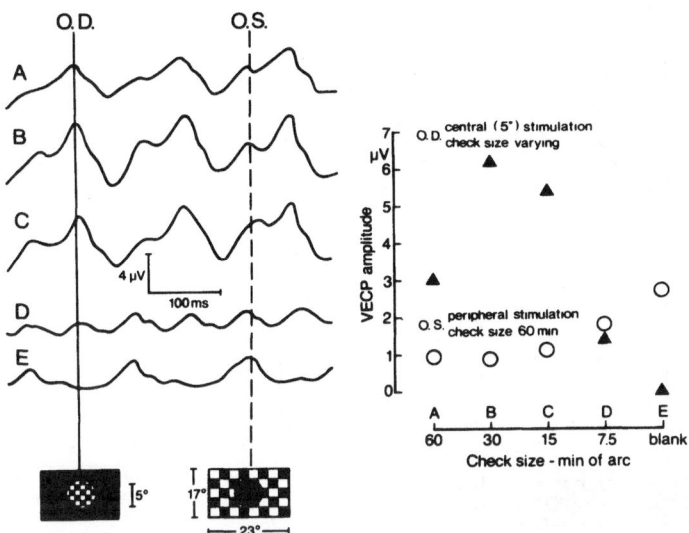

Fig. 6. VECPs (n = 128) in response to 90° phase-displaced checkerboard stimuli, separately presented to the right and the left eye. Reversal rate 7/s. The right eye was centrally stimulated in a 5° test field, while the left eye was stimulated in a 17° × 23° test field, centrally (5°) occluded. The check size in the peripheral field was kept constant (60 min); the check size in the central 5° field was reduced from 60 min (A) to 30 min (B), 15 min (C) and 7.5 min (D). In E only the peripheral stimulus was given. Contrast was approx. 100 per cent. The graph at the right represents averaged data of three subjects.

Similar results were obtained with changes of pattern contrast of the centrally applied stimulus (Fig. 7). With a pattern stimulus of 60 min check size presented at full contrast to the peripheral retina of the left eye, the VECP amplitude to a pattern stimulus of 30 min check size, applied to the central retina of the right eye, did not change before the contrast ratio of the central stimulus was lowered to less than 20 per cent. Balance of VECP amplitudes for central and peripheral dichoptic stimulation was obtained when the contrast of the centrally applied checkerboard stimulus was decreased to 5 per cent (Fig. 7E). Further lowering of contrast made the peripheral retina of the other eye dominant.

DISCUSSION

In agreement with Lennerstrand (1978a, b) the present study indicates strong interaction at the cortical level when identical stimuli are presented dichoptically to both eyes. The interocular suppression could be explained best by the 'occlusion model' of Harter (1977). In this model, the input from one eye activates elements in the central channel so that only few elements are left to respond to the input from the other eye. This model

319

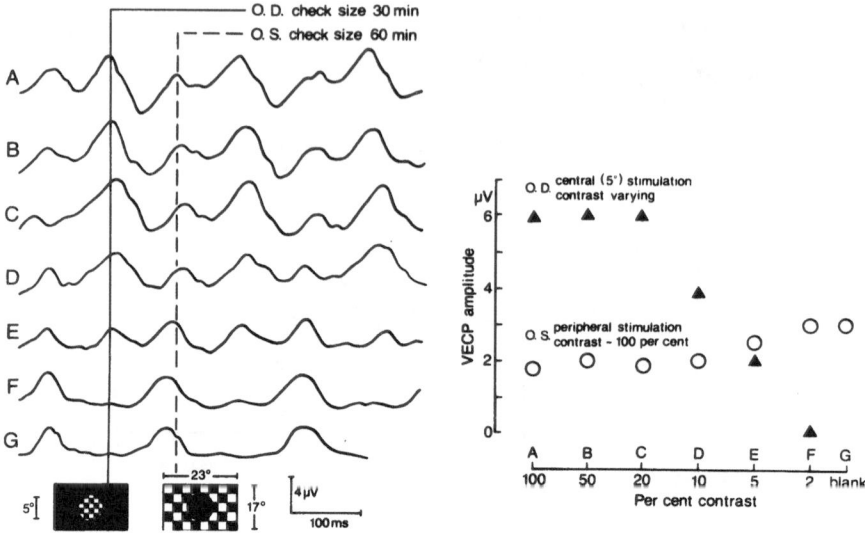

Fig. 7. VECPs (n = 128) in response to 90° phase-displaced checkerboard stimuli, separately presented to the right and the left eye. Reversal rate 7/s. The right eye was centrally stimulated with 30 min checks in a 5° test field, the left eye was peripherally stimulated with 60 min checks in a 17° × 23° test field, centrally (5°) occluded. The contrast of the centrally viewed test field was diminished from approx. 100 per cent (A) to zero (G) in steps of 50 per cent (B), 20 per cent (C), 10 per cent (D), 5 per cent (E), 2 per cent (F). The graph at the right represents averaged data of three subjects.

also aids in the understanding of why lower inputs from one eye, in correspondence to under-optimal adjustment of the stimulus, cause rising amplitudes of the fellow eye in response to a constant stimulus. Since the recovery of interocular suppression is complete not before 500 ms after the off-set of the suppressing stimulus (Harter 1977), the input of the fellow eye arrives at the visual brain cells within the recovering time, i.e., when they are not fully available.

The interocular depression of peripheral inputs of one eye, exerted by the inputs of the retinal center of the fellow eye, roughly corresponds to the observations of Teping and Groneberg (1981) using the central and peripheral parts of the same eye. Under both conditions of stimulation dominance of the peripheral retina is seen only at a lower level of adjustment of the central stimulus.

ACKNOWLEDGEMENT

We are grateful to Prof. Dr. E. Dodt for the helpful advice and reading the manuscript.

320

REFERENCES

Abe, H. Checkerboard pattern reversal VECP in response to monocular and binocular stimulation in normals and amblyopes. Ber. Dtsch. Ophthalmol. Ges. 75: 522–527 (1978).

Abe, H. Suppression visuell evozierter kortikaler Potentiale (VECP) bei binokularer Darbietung von Kontrastreizen. Ber. Dtsch. Ophthalmol. Ges. 76: 445–452 (1979).

Arden, G.B., Barnard, W.M. & Mushin, A.S. Visually evoked responses in amblyopia. Br. J. Ophthal. 58: 183–192 (1974).

Cigánek, L. Binocular addition of the visually evoked response with different stimulus intensities in man. Vis. Res. 10: 479–487 (1970).

Cigánek, L. Binocular addition of the visual response evoked by dichoptic patterned stimuli. Vis. Res. 11: 1289–1297 (1971).

Cobb, W.A., Morton, H.B. & Ettlinger, G. Cerebral potentials evoked by pattern reversal and their suppression in visual rivalry. Nature 216: 1123–1125 (1967).

Harter, M.R. Binocular interaction: Evoked potentials to dichoptic stimulation. In: Visual evoked potentials in man: new developments (Ed. J.E. Desmedt) Clarendon press, Oxford. 208–233 (1977).

Harter, M.R., Seiple, W.H. & Salmon, L. Binocular summation of visually evoked responses to pattern stimuli in humans. Vis. Res. 13: 1433–1446 (1973).

Lennerstrand, G. Some observations on visual evoked responses (VER) to dichoptic stimulation. Acta Ophthal. 56: 638–647 (1978a).

Lennerstrand, G. Binocular interaction studied with visual evoked responses (VER) in humans with normal and impaired binocular vision. Acta Ophthal. 56: 628–637 (1978b).

Perry, N.W. & Childers, D.G. Cortical potentials in normal and amblyopic binocular vision. In: 6th ISCERG Symposium. (Ed. E. Schmöger) VEB G. Thieme, Leipzig. 151–161 (1968).

Teping, C. & Groneberg, A. Monocularly evoked cortical potentials to simultaneous stimulation of central and peripheral human retina with different patterns. Doc. Ophthal. Proc. Series. 27: 305–312 (1981).

Authors' address:
Dr. A. Groneberg
Augenklinik der Technischen Universität
Ismaingenstr. 20
D-8000 München, F.R.G.

C. Teping
Abt. f. Augenheilkunde
Medizin Fakultät
Rhein-Westf. Techn. Hochschule
Goethestr. 27/29
D-5100 Aachen, F.R.G.

BINOCULAR FACILITATION IN THE VEP OF NORMAL OBSERVERS AND STRABISMIC AMBLYOPES

P.A. APKARIAN & C.W. TYLER

(San Francisco, Calif., U.S.A.)

ABSTRACT

Electrophysiological correlates of normal and abnormal binocular function were investigated by studying the binocular interactions from monocular and binocular visual evoked potentials (VEPs) over a wide range of stimulus conditions. The steady-state visual evoked potentials were recorded with synchronous narrow-band filtering techniques using sinusoidal grating stimuli which were temporally modulated in counterphase.

The degree of binocular interaction in normal as well as in abnormal observers was found to be highly dependent upon several stimulus determinants including spatial and temporal frequency. Detailed sampling and testing across stimulus conditions revealed that the range of binocular interactions in normal observers extends from zero summation to pronounced facilitation. The binocular interactions of strabismic amblyopes show complex response characteristics typical in many respects to those of normal observers, including marked facilitation. The results suggest that some degree of binocular function is preserved in the cortex of patients with strabismic amblyopia.

INTRODUCTION

Visual evoked potential (VEP) investigations of binocular interactions typically yield partial summation of the binocular response in relation to the monocular responses (Harter, Seiple & Salmon 1973; Perry, Childers & McCoy 1968; White & Bonelli 1970), although the range of binocular interactions reported in the literature is from zero summation (Inoue 1966) to small amounts of facilitation (Cigánek 1970; Srebro 1978). Despite conflicting reports as to the degree and type of binocular interactions which exist, it has been suggested that either the presence of zero summation (Amigo, Fiorentini, Pirchio & Spinelli 1978; Fiorentini, Maffei, Pirchio & Spinelli 1978) or the absence of facilitation (Srebro 1978) may be used to differentiate normal from abnormal binocular function. However, the results of a recent and detailed study of binocular interactions in the VEP of normal observers (Apkarian, Nakayama & Tyler 1980) show that the degree of interaction is highly specific, dependent upon several stimulus determinants including spatial frequency, temporal frequency and contrast. Furthermore, optimization techniques which relied upon fine spatiotemporal frequency tuning procedures allowed the identification of regions of zero summation as well as marked facilitation within the VEP response profiles of a given observer.

The complicated nature of binocular interactions in the VEP of normal observers suggests that similar optimization techniques are necessary for the electrophysiological assessment of binocularity in the VEP of observers with abnormal binocular function. In the present study, we investigated the monocular and binocular response profiles of several strabismic amblyopes. Our results indicate that while some strabismic amblyopes show binocular inhibition, under appropriate conditions the full range of binocular interactions, including facilitation can be obtained. The similar binocular response characteristics of normal and amblyopic observers suggest a strong cautionary note when attempting to use the degree of binocular interaction for assessing binocular abnormality.

METHODS AND MATERIALS

Stimulus

In order to study binocular interactions comprehensively in clinical patients, a method which can rapidly assess the responses over a wide range of stimulus parameters is essential. For this reason we employed the electronic spatial frequency sweep technique that we have recently described (Tyler, Apkarian, Levi & Nakayama 1979). Briefly, the stimulus, a vertical sinusoidal grating presented on a cathode ray tube (CRT) display, is counterphase-modulated in contrast at a fixed rate (temporal frequency) while continuously varying in spatial frequency. Under this condition, a patient perceives flickering bars continually increasing or decreasing in size. For the studies presented here, spatial frequency was swept in 20 seconds from 0.2 to 20 cycles per degree. The space average luminance of the Hewlett-Packard CRT display (Model 1332A, P31 Phosphor) was $46 \, cd/m^2$; contrast, defined according to the standard Michelson definition (Michelson 1927), was 80%. All light measures were made with a Spectra Pritchard photometer (Model 1980A).

Recording

The observers, resting comfortably in a supine position, viewed an over-head front-surface mirror image of a $15° \times 20°$ CRT display which appeared at a distance of 37 cm. Background EEG activity and observer vigilance were monitored continuously.

A bipolar electrode configuration (3 cm above the inion on the midline, and 3 cm above and lateral) with the ear serving as ground was used to record the EEG. The EEG was amplified and filtered at the temporal frequency of pattern reversal, by means of a synchronous narrow-band filtering technique. The amplified EEG was pre-filtered through a Krohn-Hite (Model 330M) 24 db/octave bandpass filter with cut-off frequencies set at 0.1 log unit above and below the pattern reversal rate, thus eliminating harmonics of the response frequency. The pre-filtered signals were then passed through a synchronous constant narrow bandwidth (0.6 Hz) commutating filter, with the center frequency phase-locked to that of the stimulus pattern reversal rate.

The filter output was full-wave rectified and smoothed, thus ensuring that the amplitude was unaffected by phase shifts in the response. The rectified signal was fed to the Y-axis of an X-Y plotter, while the X position was controlled by the same ramp that controlled the spatial frequency of the stimulus. In 20 seconds, we were able to obtain a plot of VEP amplitude as a function of the spatial frequency of the alternating pattern. At least two plots were taken in every condition to determine response variability. In order to give equal weight to each octave of spatial frequency across the range of bar sizes, the spatial frequency of the gratings was swept logarithmically. This approach also provides enhanced resolution at lower spatial frequencies.

Observers

Paid volunteers participated in these experiments; data are presented here from 7 observers ranging in age from 11 to 37 years. Five observers were unilateral amblyopes, while two observers AH and HS had normal monocular Snellen acuities of 20/20 + and normal binocular vision. All of the amblyopic observers were constant unilateral strabismics, and one, SL, was also anisometropic. Pertinent visual characteristics are presented for each observer in Fig. 5. All observers were free of pathology and were carefully corrected for refractive error prior to testing. Prisms were worn to ensure bifoveal stimulation during testing, and presentation of the stimuli was randomized between the right eye (OD), left eye (OS) and binocular (OU) viewing. During monocular trials, the untested eye was occluded with an opaque patch.

Analysis

The degree of binocular interaction is represented in the form of an interaction index $OU/((OD + OS)/2)$ in which the binocular response is divided by the mean monocular response. The expression $(OD + OS)/2$ is the mean of the two mean monocular amplitudes ($\overline{M}$) and OU is the mean binocular amplitude (B). Binocular interaction indices from inhibition to facilitation are defined as follows:

$B < \overline{M}$ — inhibition

$B = \overline{M}$ — zero summation

$$\overline{M} < B < 2\overline{M} \quad - \text{partial summation}$$

$$B = 2\overline{M} \qquad - \text{summation}$$

$$B > 2\overline{M} \qquad - \text{facilitation}$$

One consideration relevant to the method of computing the degree of binocular interaction is the situation of unequal monocular responses. It is important to consider how the binocular interaction index is affected by unequal monocular response amplitudes. We first note that this is largely of theoretical interest since the monocular amplitudes are roughly equal in the regions of facilitation reported. Let us consider the worst theoretical case in which the amplitude from the amblyopic eye is zero. Now the mean monocular response is half the value of the response from the nonamblyopic eye, giving an index value of 2, or perfect summation. Values greater than 2 would still represent valid cases of binocular facilitation, but values less than 2 would require different definitions from those given above, since they would constitute cases of interocular inhibition. Since we are mainly interested in the question of facilitation, the binocular index as defined is still an accurate reflection of this condition, but in general, care must be exercised in its use with unequal responses from the two eyes when the value of the binocular interaction ratio falls below 2.

RESULTS AND DISCUSSION

Normal binocular interactions

Fig. 1 is an example of the spatial frequency tuning functions and binocular interactions obtained for normal observers AH (left) and HS (right). The responses for the right (OD) and left (OS) eyes are characteristically quite similar in shape and amplitude. Note also that both the monocular and binocular tuning functions may show more than one response peak. The multiple peaks occurring at different spatial frequencies presumably correspond to some neural specificity for particular bar sizes in the mechanisms generating the pattern VEP.

It should be pointed out that the detailed localization of peak positions and the resulting pattern of binocular interactions differ in both spatial and temporal frequency for different observers. The interindividual variability requries tailored stimulus conditions for each observer when attempting to record a given degree of binocular interaction, e.g. facilitation. However, once a region of binocular interaction has been identified by careful stimulus tuning procedures, general response characteristics across observers may be noted. For example, careful examination of the binocular response functions for both AH and HS reveals that the form is rather more complex than that of the monocular components and that the binocular peaks can occur at different spatial frequencies from those obtained under monocular conditions. This is shown more clearly by taking the ratio of the measured

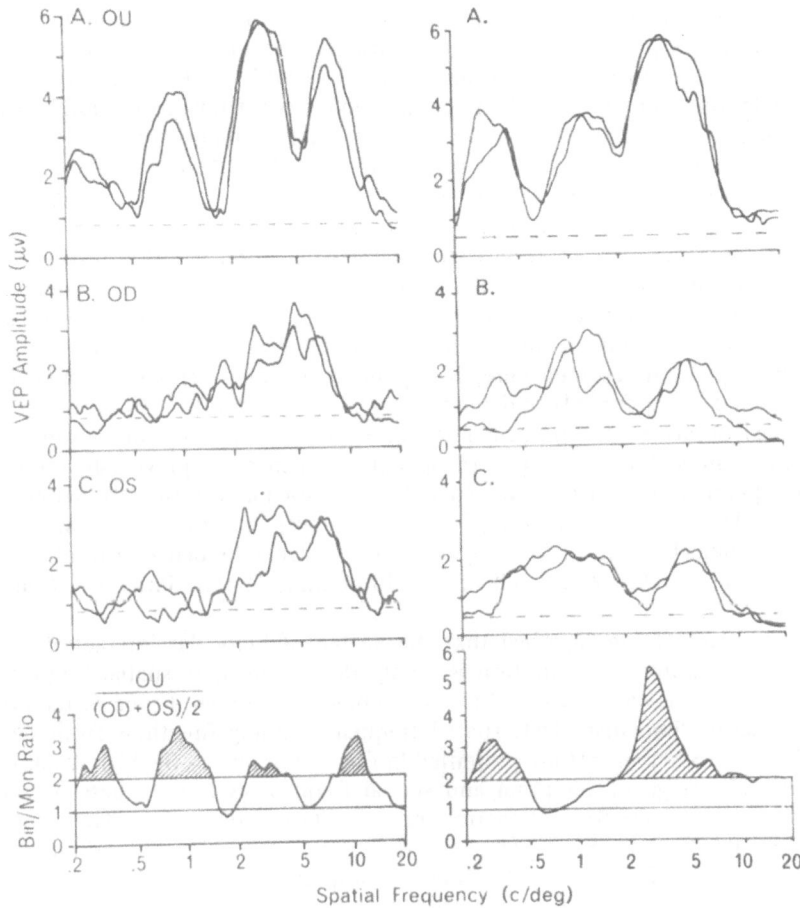

Fig. 1. Spatial frequency tuning functions for normal observers AH (left) at 26 rps and HS (right) at 28 rps for both eyes (A), right eye (B) and left eye (C). The separate traces are superimposed to show repeatability of the responses. The dashed line indicates the recorded physiological noise level. The binocular/monocular interaction ratios as a function of spatial frequency are shown in the lower traces. The amplitude of the binocular response (A) is divided by the mean monocular responses (B) and (C). A ratio of 1 indicates zero summation, 2 indicates perfect summation and > 2 (hatched regions) shows facilitation.

binocular response to the mean of the monocular responses (Fig. 1, lower traces). In these plots, the mean monocular response $(B = \bar{M})$ is represented by the value of 1, the sum of the two monocular responses $(B = 2\bar{M})$ is represented by the value of 2, and values greater than 2 (shaded regions) represent binocular facilitation $(B > 2\bar{M})$. It is clear that at some spatial frequencies there is extensive binocular facilitation, reaching values of more than three and a half times the mean monocular response for observer AH

327

and more than 5 and a half times for HS. Note also that this facilitation occurs in regions where there is an absence of a corresponding peak monocular response. At other spatial frequencies the binocular response is around the summed monocular responses, which we refer to as full summation, while at still other spatial frequencies it falls to the level of the mean monocular response which we refer to as zero summation.

In agreement with several authors (Campbell & Maffei 1970; Cigánek 1970; Harter, Seiple & Salmon 1973; Wanger & Nilsson 1978) we find that the binocular response is usually greater than either monocular response. There are, however, exceptions to this generalization in normal, as well as in abnormal observers. There are several conditions for which zero summation in a normal observer can occur in the absence of perceived binocular rivalry. The most frequent of these are spatial frequency regions where trough responses occur, as seen here, for spatial frequency responses around 0.5, 1.5 and 5 c/deg for AH and between 0.5 and 1 c/deg for HS. Although in normal observers, the binocular response may equal zero summation (over more than a 3 octave range of spatial frequencies as previously reported by Apkarian et al. 1981), it generally does not fall significantly below this level. The zero summation observed, however, places severe limitations on its clinical use as a screening index for abnormal binocular vision (Amigo, Fiorentini, Pirchio & Spinelli 1978; Fiorentini, Maffei, Pirchio & Spinelli 1978).

The data of Fig. 1 reveal that the degree of binocular interaction from zero summation to facilitation is highly dependent upon spatial frequency. Figs. 2, 3 and 4 are presented as an example of the high degree of temporal specificity. Binocular (OU) spatial frequency tuning functions from 12 to 72 rps for observer AH are presented in Fig. 2. Because of the high resolution and wide range of temporal and spatial frequencies tested, these data are summarized in the form of spatiotemporal (STF) contour maps. The summed monocular (OD + OS) responses are shown in Fig. 3, the resultant binocular to monocular OU/((OD + OS)/2) interaction ratios in Fig. 4.

The typical features of the VEP as a function of spatial and temporal frequency are evident for both the binocular and monocular STF maps. The narrow temporal frequency tuning observed can show a dramatic response amplitude attenuation with less than a 10% change in temporal frequency. For example, the narrow peak at 48 rps for approximately 4 c/deg drops more than 50% from 48 to 52 rps (The width of the temporal tuning is actually narrower than it appears due to expansion of the temporal frequency axis by a factor of 4 to facilitate presentation of the data). In addition to the narrow and multiple temporal frequency tuning, narrow and multiple spatial frequency tuning is also shown.

For the monocular STF map (Fig. 3) a number of peak spatial and temporal frequency responses can be seen throughout. It is important to note that the regions of facilitation $(B > 2\overline{M})$ seen in Fig. 4 (hatched regions) generally occur at the temporal and spatial frequencies for which there is a corresponding absence of peak monocular responses. This lack of correspondence between binocular facilitation and monocular peak responses (described previously in Fig. 1) further corroborates the notion that binocular

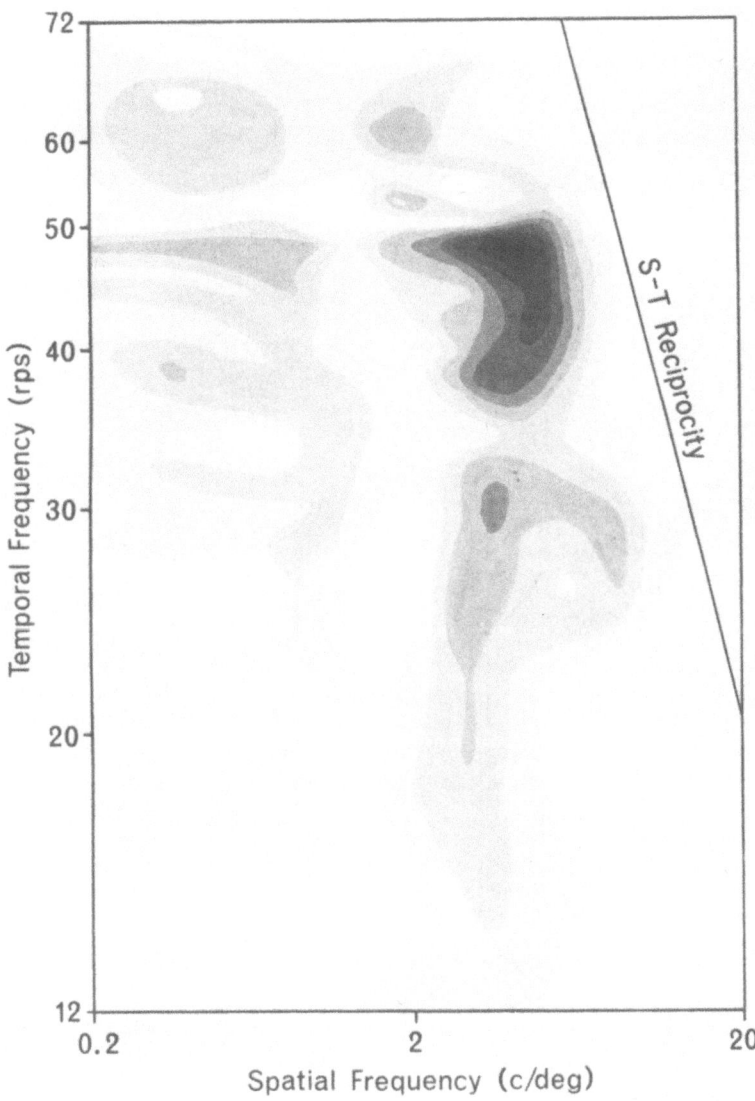

Fig. 2. Contour map derived from separate binocular spatial frequency tunings (digitized in 0.25 octave steps) as a function of temporal frequency for observer AH. The spatial frequency tuning functions were recorded in 3 rps steps across the temporal frequency domain except between 24 and 36 rps where additional tunings in 1 to 2 rps steps were obtained. Note that the temporal frequency ordinate is expanded by a factor of 4 relative to the abscissa, so the oblique line (having a slope of -4) represents spatio-temporal reciprocity. Amplitude is indicated by shades of grey with darker regions representing higher amplitudes.

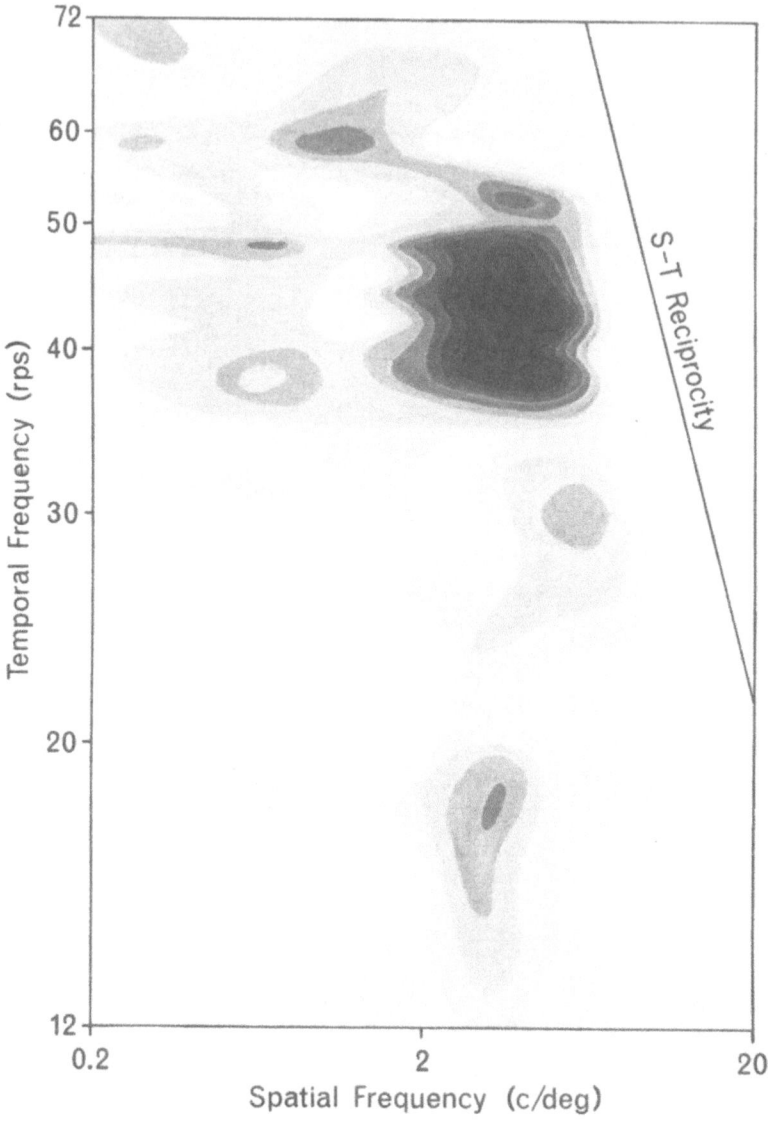

Fig. 3. Spatiotemporal contour map of the summed monocular spatial and temporal frequency tunings. Details are the same as in Fig. 2, except that equivalent shades of grey represent twice the signal amplitude.

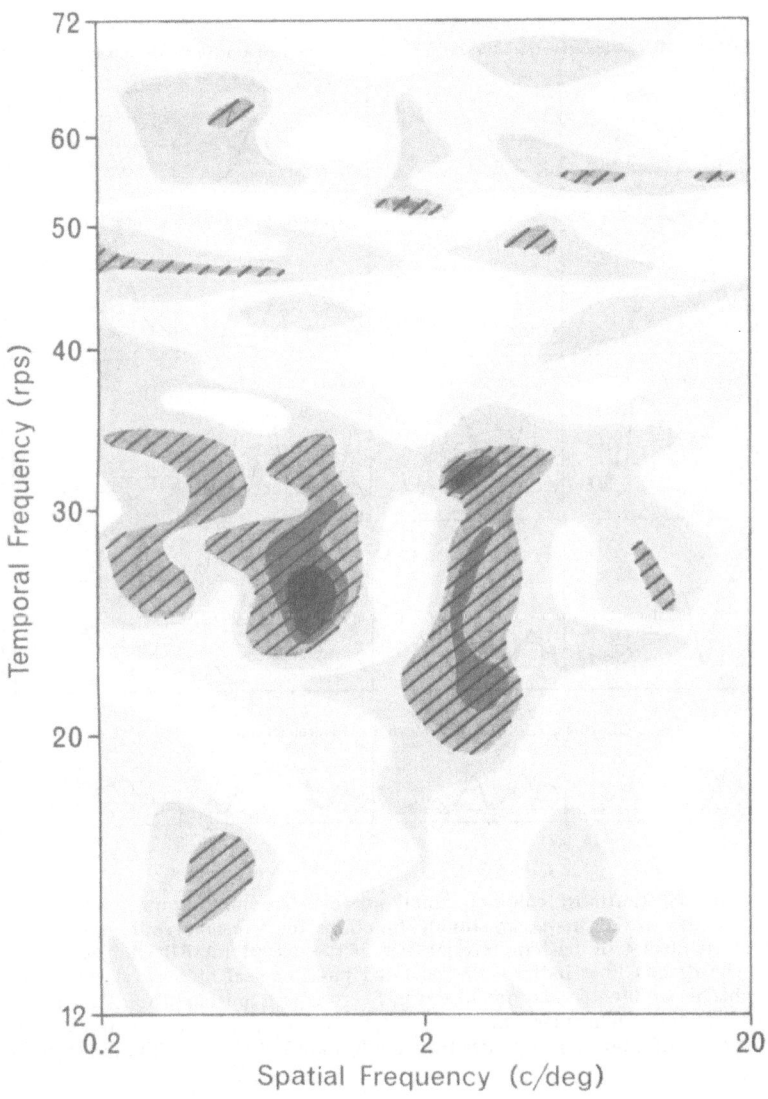

Fig. 4. Spatiotemporal contour map of binocular interaction ratios derived from the binocular and monocular response profiles of Figs. 2 & 3. Shades of grey represent binocular to monocular ratio values. Hatched areas represent facilitation. For other details see Fig. 2.

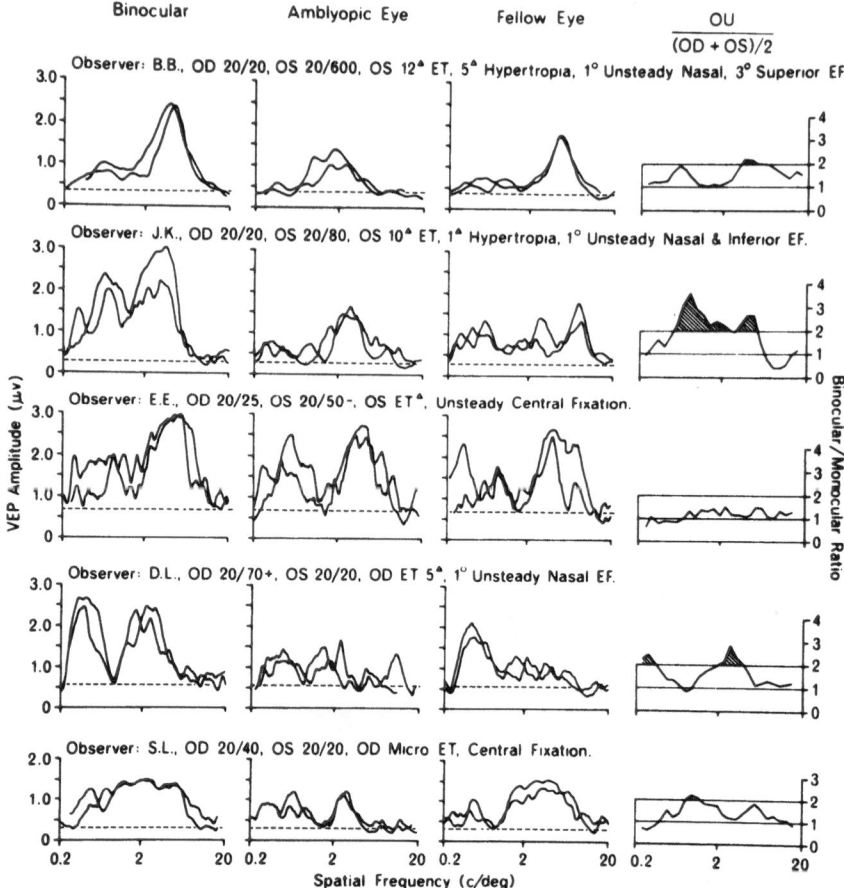

Binocular	Amblyopic Eye	Fellow Eye	$\dfrac{OU}{(OD + OS)/2}$

Fig. 5. Binocular (leftmost column), amblyopic eye (second column), and fellow eye (third column) spatial frequency tuning functions for five amblyopic observers. The temporal frequency of pattern reversal was 24 rps except for BB who was tested at 20 rps. The dashed lines indicate the recorded physiological noise level. All observers had strabismic amblyopia and one observer, SL, was also anisometropic (bottom row). The corresponding binocular interaction ratios are plotted in the rightmost column. Note the range of binocular responses from inhibition $(B < \overline{M})$ to facilitation $(B > 2\overline{M})$.

mechanisms respond independently of the underlying monocular responses. The four most robust and reliable regions of binocular facilitation for this observer occur between approximately 14 and 18 rps at 0.3 to 0.6 c/deg and between approximately 20 and 34 rps at 0.2 to 0.6, at 0.4 to 1.4, and at 1.6 to 4 c/deg. In the observers tested thus far, facilitation is typically most predominant in the low to medium temporal and lower spatial frequency regions as seen here.

Binocular interactions in strabismic amblyopia

It might be expected that the pattern of binocular interactions in strabismic amblyopia would differ significantly from those of normals; however, this is not the case. Fig. 5 shows the responses obtained from five strabismic amblyopes with differing degrees of amblyopia. The visual acuities, angle of deviation and type and degree of fixation are presented above each raw trace. In the leftmost column are the binocular spatial frequency tunings; the amblyopic eye and fellow eye tunings are presented in the second and third columns and the calculated binocular interaction ratios are presented in the rightmost column. It is of interest to note the repeatability of these traces, particularly as three of the observers (EE, DL, SL) were completely naive to visual experimentation. The range of binocular interactions is summarized in the binocular to monocular ratio plots and varies from binocular inhibition ($B < \bar{M}$) to marked facilitation ($B > 2\bar{M}$). As with normal observers, the binocular interactions are highly dependent upon spatial frequency. In addition, marked facilitation ($B > 2\bar{M}$) is found at several points in the traces and the general range of binocular interactions, with the exception of inhibition (e.g. JK, second row, higher spatial frequency region) is very similar to that found in normals.

Although the binocular responses of the amblyopes tested are similar in many respects to those found in normals, marked anomalies are more evident when comparing the monocular VEP traces. The monocular VEPs of our amblyopic observers show significant differences between the two eyes. These differences usually appear as a downward shift in peak spatial frequency responses of the amblyopic eye relative to the normal eye. Similar changes have been reported by Sokol & Shaterian (1976). This appears to correspond to the downward shift in peak spatial frequency seen in the psychophysical contrast sensitivity functions of amblyopes at threshold and suprathreshold levels (Levi & Harwerth 1977; Levi, Harwerth & Manny 1979). Thus, as may be seen in the data of BB and JK, for example, the amblyopic eye may actually show a larger response than the non-amblyopic eye at low spatial frequencies.

A second consistent difference between the two eyes of amblyopic observers is seen in the cutoff spatial frequency (i.e., the highest spatial frequency beyond which no significant response can be obtained). This cutoff spatial frequency is always lower in the amblyopic eye than in the non-amblyopic eye of the same observer, presumably reflecting the reduced acuity characteristic of the amblyopic eye. This is consistent with the findings of many investigations, which suggest that, in general, monocular comparison of VEP elicited by small checks or stripes is a sensitive indicant of acuity loss (Sokol & Bloom 1973; Spekreijse, Khoe & Van der Tweel 1972; Tyler, Apkarian, Levi & Nakayama 1979). The abnormal responses and the corresponding apparently normal binocular interactions further suggest, as in normal observers, an independence between the underlying monocular and binocular neural mechanisms.

The data of Fig. 5 reveal that the binocular interactions of strabismic amblyopes show complex response characteristics typical of normal observers including facilitation. These results suggest that cortical binocular function is preserved to a substantial degree in certain amblyopic observers. The fact that even severe amblyopes may demonstrate binocular facilitation under the appropriate conditions limits its use as an index for differentiating between normal and disturbed binocular vision as does the presence of zero summation in normal observers.

CONCLUSIONS

The results of investigating normal and abnormal binocular function in the visual evoked potential suggest:

1) Binocular interactions are highly dependent upon several stimulus determinants including spatial and temporal frequency.

2) Binocular facilitation can be recorded under appropriate stimulus conditions in the visual evoked potential of both normal observers and strabismic amblyopes.

3) The spatial frequency tuning functions of strabismic amblyopes which show complex binocular interactions similar in many respects to the binocular interactions of normal observers suggest that some binocular function may be preserved in the cortex of patients with disturbed binocularity.

4) The zero summation recorded in normal observers and the facilitation recorded in strabismic amblyopes places severe limitations on their use as screening indices in differentiating normal from abnormal binocular function.

REFERENCES

Amigo, G., Fiorentini, A., Pirchio, M. & Spinelli, D. Binocular vision tested with visual evoked potentials in children and infants. Invest. Ophthalmol. Vis. Sci. 17: 910–915 (1978).

Apkarian, P., Nakayama, K. & Tyler, C.W. Binocularity in the human visual evoked potential: facilitation, summation and suppression. Electroenceph. clin. Neurophysiol. 51: 32–48 (1981).

Campbell, F.W. & Maffei, L. Electrophysiological evidence for the existence of orientation and size detectors in the human visual system. J. Physiol. (Lond.), 207: 635–652 (1970).

Cigánek, L. Binocular addition of the visually evoked response with different stimulus intensities in man. Vis. Res. 10: 479–487 (1970).

Fiorentini, A., Maffei, L., Pirchio, M. & Spinelli, D. An electrophysiological correlate of perceptual suppression in anisometropia. Vis. Res. 18: 1617–1621 (1978).

Harter, M.R., Seiple, W.H. & Salmon, L. Binocular summation of visually evoked responses to pattern stimuli in humans. Vis. Res. 13: 1433–1446 (1973).

Inoue, J. Visual evoked potentials by monocular and binocular double flashes. Jap. J. Ophthal. (Suppl.) 10: 362–368 (1966).

Levi, D.M. & Harwerth, R.S. Spatio-temporal interactions in anisometropic and strabismic amblyopia. Invest. Ophthalmol. Vis. Sci. 16: 90–95 (1977).

Levi, D.M., Harwerth, R.S. & Manny, R.E. Suprathreshold spatial frequency detection and binocular interaction in strabismic and anisometropic amblyopia. Invest. Ophthalmol. Vis. Sci. 18: 714–725 (1979).

Michelson, A.A. Studies in optics. University of Chicago Press, Chicago (1927).

Perry, N.W., Childers, D.G. & McCoy, J.G. Binocular addition of the visual evoked response at different cortical locations. Vis. Res. 8: 567–573 (1968).

Sokol, S. & Bloom, B. Visually evoked cortical responses of amblyopes to a spatially alternating stimulus. Invest. Ophthalmol. Vis. Sci. 12: 936–939 (1973).

Sokol, S. & Shaterian, E. The pattern evoked cortical potential in amblyopia as an index of visual function. In Orthoptics, Past, Present, Future, Transactions of Third International Orthoptics Congress, Miami (ed. S. Moore, J. Mein & L. Stockbridge) 59–67 (1976).

Spekreijse, H., Khoe, L.H. & Van der Tweel, L.H. A case of amblyopia; electrophysiology and psychophysics of luminance and contrast. In: The Visual System (Ed. G.B. Arden), Plenum Press, New York 141–156 (1972).

Srebro, R. The visually evoked response: Binocular facilitation and failure when binocular vision is disturbed. Arch. Ophthalmol. 96: 839–844 (1978).

Tyler, C.W., Apkarian, P., Levi, D.M. & Nakayama, K. Rapid assessment of visual function: an electronic sweep technique for the pattern VEP. Invest. Ophthalmol. Vis. Sci. 18: 703–713 (1979).

Wanger, P. & Nilsson, B. Visual evoked responses to pattern-reversal stimulation in patients with amblyopia and/or defective binocular functions. Acta Ophthal. 56: 617–627 (1978).

White, C.T. & Bonelli, L. Binocular summation in the evoked potential as a function of image quality. Am. J. Optom. & Arch. Am. Acad. Optom. 47: 304–309 (1970).

Authors' address:
P.A. Apkarian
The Netherlands Ophthalmic Research Institute
P.O. Box 6411
1005 EK Amsterdam, The Netherlands

C.W. Tyler
Smith-Kettlewell Institute of Visual Sciences
San Francisco, Calif., U.S.A.

A COMPARISON OF DIFFERENT VEP METHODS FOR THE ASSESSMENT OF BINOCULAR VISION

P. JACOBSSON & G. LENNERSTRAND

(*Linköping, Sweden*)

ABSTRACT

In order to determine how accurately four different VEP methods, previously described, correlated with stereoscopic acuity, eighteen subjects were tested with all methods. Ten subjects had normal binocular vision and eight had impaired binocular vision. Their stereoscopic acuity was determined with psychophysical methods. A VEP method suggested to evaluate the state of binocular interaction in the striate cortex showed the best correlation with stereopsis. VEP methods thought to reflect neural summation in the striate cortex seemed less useful in this respect. However, none of the VEP procedures seemed reliable enough for an electrophysiological method to separate the individuals with binocularity from those with defective binocular vision.

INTRODUCTION

Humans with normal binocular vision can distinguish patterns at lower contrast in dioptic binocular viewing than when they use one eye alone (Campbell & Green 1965). Individuals with disrupted binocularity, on the other hand, often fail to demonstrate the binocular improvement of contrast sensitivity, but perform equally well under monocular and binocular conditions (Lema & Blake 1977). A close correlation has been reported between the electrophysiological responses in VEP and the apparent intensity of the contrast stimulation (Franzén & Berkley 1975). In accordance with these findings, subjects with normal binocular functions show larger VEPs to binocular than to monocular stimulation (Campbell & Maffei 1970), while in patients with binocular defects the binocular and monocular responses were found to be about the same (Amigo, Fiorentini, Pirchio & Spinelli 1978; Srebro 1978; Wanger & Nilsson 1978).

Psychophysical experiments with dichoptic presentation of stimuli have demonstrated interocular transfer in individuals with normal binocularity

(Blake & Levinson 1977), but not in subjects with impaired binocular vision (Lema & Blake 1977). These findings may explain the VEP interaction between the two eyes to dichoptic stimulation seen in subjects with normal binocularity, and the much weaker binocular VEP interaction in patients with defects of binocular vision (Lennerstrand 1978). In this case dichoptic presentation implied that the VEP stimuli were of different temporal characteristics, but had the same spatial properties, luminance and contrast.

Based on these principles several clinical VEP methods have been developed for assessment of binocular functions. The aim of the present study has been to compare four of them and evaluate their ability to detect and quantify binocular deficiences. Subjects with bifoveal single vision or with varying degrees of binocular defects, due to small angle squint and/or anisometropia, have been tested with all four methods. The VEP results have been correlated to the stereoscopic acuity of the subjects.

MATERIALS AND METHODS

Test subjects. Eighteen subjects have been tested. Ten of them had normal vision and binocular functions, and the other eight were patients with small angle squint (less than 5°) and/or anisometropia. All patients had Snellen visual acuities of 0.6 or better in both eyes.

Binocular testing. As a measure on the quality of the binocular functions, the maximal stereoscopic resolution was used. In the normals and some of the patients it was determined with an eidometer constructed by Monjé (1947–48; cited by Enoksson 1964). The eidometer is based on the 'three rod principle', in which the subject has to specify the position of a moving rod in relation to two stationary ones. Stereoscopic resolutions up to about 200 sec of arc could be determined with the eidometer. In the normal subjects the values ranged between 24 and 66 sec of arc. Patients with poorer stereopsis had to be evaluated with the Titmus chart. A stereoblind patient who failed to perceive stereopsis with any of these methods was arbitrarily assigned a resolution of 5000 sec of arc for the statistical analysis. The lowest value found in a patient was 121 sec of arc.

VEP stimulation. In two of the VEP methods the stimulator was a transparent screen made of 5 x 5 mm squares of polarizing material (see also Arden, Barnard & Mushin 1974). The viewing distance was 57 cm. At this distance one square corresponded to a visual angle of 30' of arc and the whole screen to 14°. The contrast of the checker-board pattern was 97% and the mean luminance 2.5 cd/m². For dioptic stimulation the pattern was viewed binocularly through a rotating disc of polarizing material, eliciting steady-state VEPs at a reversing rate of 10 Hz.

For dichoptic polaroid stimulation the pattern was viewed through two polarizing discs, one for each eye, as described by Arden et al. (1974) and Lennerstrand (1978). The discs rotated at different speeds, inducing steady-state VEPs of 10 Hz in the right and 7 Hz in the left eye.

In the third method, similar to the one used by Wanger & Nilsson (1978), a black-and-white reversing checker-board pattern was generated on a 22 inch TV-screen with a pattern generator (Medelec). At a viewing distance of 165 cm the check size corresponded to a visual angle of 23′, the field size 19°. The contrast was approximately 60% and the mean luminance of the pattern 50 cd/m². Transient responses were elicited at a reversal rate of 2 Hz.

As a fourth method VEPs were generated by a reversing grating pattern generated on an oscilloscope, as described by Amigo et al. (1978). The viewing distance was 75 cm and the screen subtended a visual angle of 4.5 × 6°. The mean luminance was 120 cd/m². The contrast was set to 25%. The gratings were of sinusoidal luminance profile with a spatial frequency of 3 cycles/degree. A reversal rate of 16 Hz was used.

VEP recording technique. The recordings were bipolar and made with Ag-AgCl electrodes positioned 2.5 cm above the inion and on the vertex. With the dichoptic polaroid stimulation VEPs were recorded on two channels, one for each eye. The signals were amplified in Medelec AA 6 Mk III amplifiers and fed into two averagers (Medelec AV6). The averagers were triggered by the polaroid discs and the VEPs from each eye were processed in separate averagers, each phase-locked to the movements on one disc. In the other methods, using dioptic stimulation, only one set of amplifier and averager was needed. The measurements on the VEPs to the different modes of stimulation are described below.

RESULTS

Dichoptic polaroid stimulation. The VEP to stimulation of each eye was recorded separately even during binocular viewing. In subjects with normal binocular vision, the amplitude of the steady-state VEP for each eye to binocular stimulation was much lower than the monocular response, as shown in Fig. 1 for subject AK. In patients with binocular defects this reduction was less pronounced. This is shown in Fig. 2 for subject BMB with small angle squint but normal visual acuity of both eyes. The binocular/monocular amplitude ratio was calculated for each eye and the highest value in each subject has been plotted in Fig. 6A against stereoscopic acuity. The correlation coefficient was 0.68, (a coefficient of 1 representing perfect correlation between VEP ratio and stereopsis).

Dioptic polaroid stimulation. VEPs of monocular and binocular stimulation for patient BMB are shown in Fig. 3. The amplitude ratio for the binocular response and the highest monocular response was calculated. The values have been plotted in Fig. 6B against stereoacuity. Since it was presumed that normal binocular functions should lead to a high binocular/monocular ratio and vice versa, a negative correlation was expected. However, the correlation was positive with a coefficient of 0.30 indicating a rather poor correlation between the VEP parameter and stereopsis.

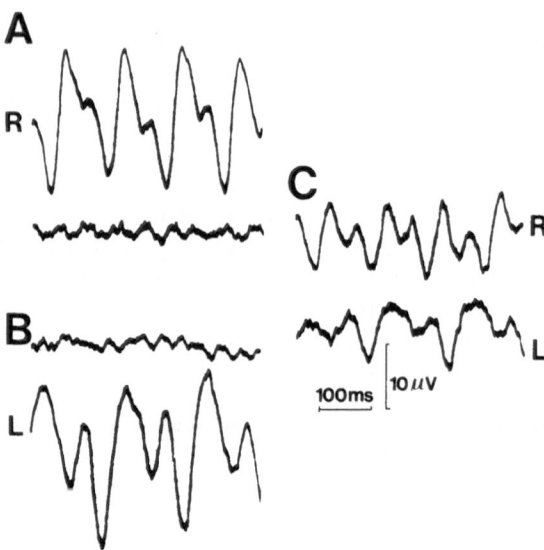

Fig. 1. Steady-state VEPs to dichoptic polaroid stimulation in subject AK with normal binocular vision.
A. Monocular stimulation of the right eye at 10 reversals per sec (upper trace marked R) with left eye occluded (lower trace).
B. Monocular stimulation of left eye at 7 reversals per sec (lower trace; marked L) with right eye occluded.
C. Binocular stimulation with responses elicited from the right eye on the upper trace (marked R) and the left eye on the lower trace (marked L).

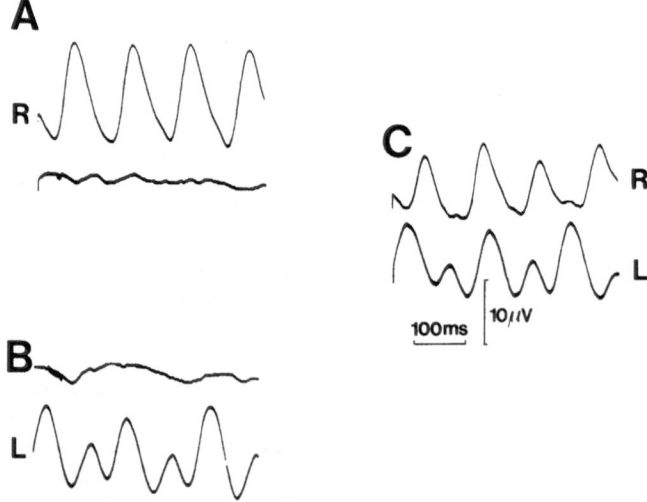

Fig. 2. Steady-state VEPs to dichoptic polaroid stimulation in subject BMB with small angle squint and poor binocular vision (stereoacuity 300 sec of arc) but normal visual acuity of both eyes. Monocular stimulation of right eye in A, left eye in B and binocular stimulation in C. Labelling as in Fig. 1.

340

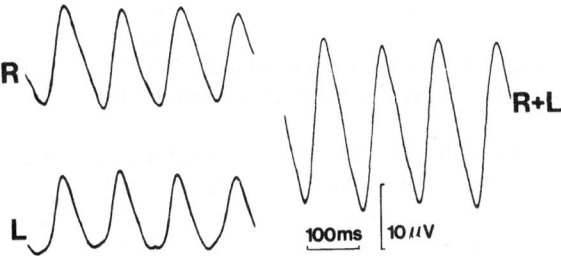

Fig. 3. Steady state VEPs to dioptic polaroid stimulation of subject BMB with the responses to monocular stimulation of the right eye in upper left panel (marked R), to monocular stimulation of left eye in lower left panel (marked L) and to binocular stimulation in right panel (marked R + L).

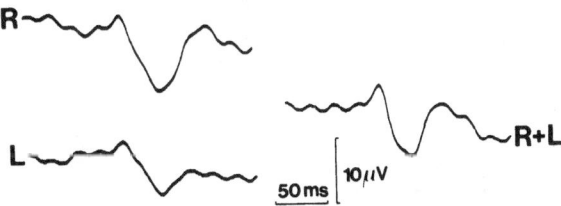

Fig. 4. Transient VEPs to TV checker-board stimulation of subject BMB. Responses of right eye (R) and left eye (L) shown to the left and responses to binocular stimulation (R + L) to the right.

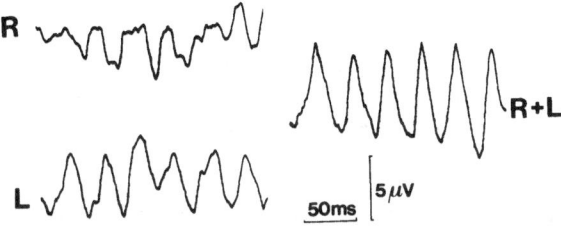

Fig. 5. Steady-state VEPs to grating stimulation of subject AK. Responses to monocular right (R) and left eye (L) stimulation, and to binocular stimulation (R + L).

TV checker-board stimulation. The results obtained with this type of dioptic stimulation in patient BMB with small angle squint are shown in Fig. 4. The binocular/monocular VEP ratio of the eye with the largest monocular VEP has been plotted against stereoacuity in Fig. 6C for the whole group of subjects studied. A negative correlation was expected also with this method. However, the correlation coefficient was 0.22.

Wanger & Nilsson (1978) have suggested additional VEP criteria for this test to indicate normal binocular functions namely that the amplitude difference between the eyes was less than 27% and that the latency difference was less than 5 ms. We applied these to our results, but found that only 3 of our subjects with normal binocularity fullfilled all criteria of normal VEP. Three of the 8 patients also showed normal VEP reactions.

Grating stimulation. Reversing grating pattern on an oscilloscope induced VEPs shown in Fig. 5 for the normal subject AK. The amplitude ratio between the dioptically obtained binocular response and the largest monocular response has been plotted in Fig. 6D against stereoscopic acuity for all subjects in the group. The correlation coefficient was − 0.44 for this VEP method.

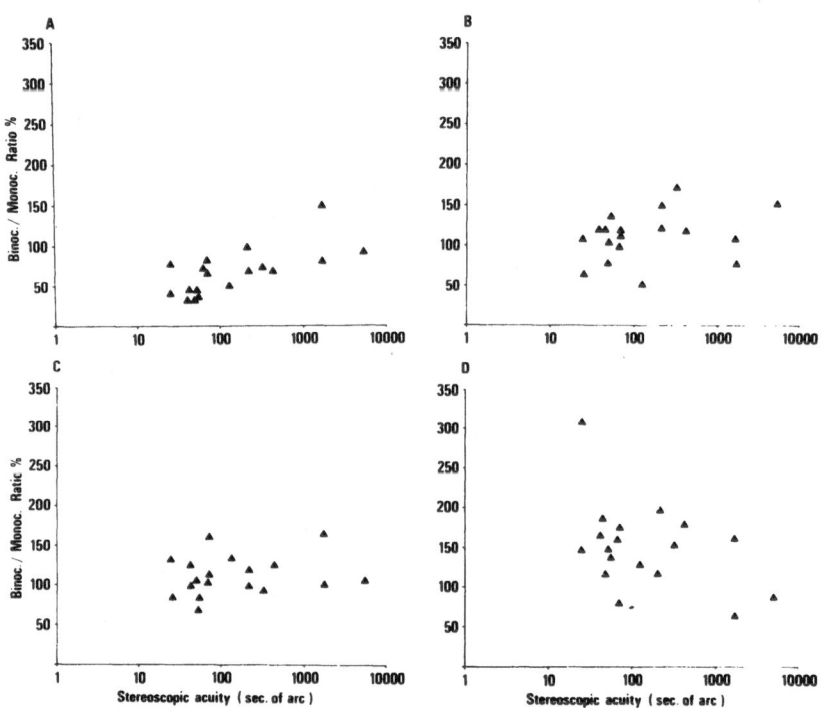

Fig. 6. Graphic representation of binocular/monocular VEP ratios, obtained for different VEP methods. The value for each subject has been plotted against maximal stereoscopic resolution in seconds of arc on a log scale.

A. Dichoptic polaroid stimulation. VEP ratio for the eye with the highest value plotted for each subject. The correlation coefficient between values for VEP ratio and the logarithm of the stereoscopic acuity is 0.68.

B. Dioptic polaroid stimulation. VEP ratio for the eye with the largest monocular response plotted for each subject Correlation coefficient is 0.30.

C. TV checker-board stimulation. VEP ratio representation as in B. Correlation coefficient is 0.22.

D. Grating stimulation. VEP ratio representation as in B. Correlation coefficient is − 0.44.

DISCUSSION

None of the four VEP methods used can be considered suitable for quantitative assessment of binocular vision. Correlation coefficients for comparisons between VEP reactions and the logarithm of the stereoscopic acuity were below 0.7 for all methods. The best correlation was obtained with dichoptically presented checker-board patterns inducing binocular interaction. However, as seen from the diagrams of Fig. 6, none of the methods could reliably discriminate between normal and abnormal binocular functions, but there was a considerable overlap between the groups.

The VEP reactions to dioptic pattern stimulation in normal subjects have been suggested to reflect neuronal summation in striate neurons of signals from the two eyes. In patients with binocular defects less or no summation was predicted. Wanger & Nilsson (1978) found that all of their normal subjects and several of their patients with binocular defects showed a considerable increase in amplitude of the transient VEP to binocular stimulation. Using this and other VEP criteria, they concluded that the method could give potentially valuable information in cases of amblyopia and/or defective binocular vision. However, in our group of subjects we were unable to separate normal from defective binocular vision using the same criteria.

A method based on dioptically elicited steady-state responses to checkerboard patterns showed equally poor correlation to stereoacuity and we agree with Arden et al. (1974), who regard the binocular results obtained with this technique of pattern reversal stimulation as equivocal. A better correlation between stereopsis and VEPs was found for dioptically presented grating patterns.

In the method using dichoptically presented patterns, the VEPs of each eye were compared during binocular and monocular stimulation. The finding of a decrease of VEP amplitude during binocular stimulation in normal subjects would support the idea of interaction in striate cortex neurons between signals from the two eyes (Harter 1977; Lennerstrand 1978). Patients with impaired binocular vision showed less VEP interaction to binocular stimulation. This might be due to a reduced amount of binocularly reacting visual cortex neurons, as demonstrated in experimental studies of squint in animals (Baker, Griggs & von Noorden 1974).

Recent studies by Apkarian et al. (1981; see also this Volume) confirm that VEPs to dioptic stimulation often fail to separate normal and abnormal binocular functions. Apkarian and coworkers demonstrated large variations in binocular VEP summation in the same subject, depending on the contrast, and the temporal and spatial properties of the stimulus. They also found binocular summation and even facilitation in subjects with greatly impaired binocular vision. In view of these findings it is hardly surprising to learn that results from different laboratories, using different techniques of stimulation, can show large variations and that conclusions can be conflicting. We seem to need much better knowledge of basic neurophysiology of VEP and binocular vision before a reliable binocular VEP test for clinical use can be designed.

ACKNOWLEDGEMENT

This investigation was supported by grants from the Swedish Medical Research Council (no 12 x 734), the Research Committee of Östergötlands läns landsting, Konsul Thure Karlssons Foundation and Carmen and Bertil Regner's Foundation.

REFERENCES

Apkarian, P.A., Nakayama, K. & Tyler, C.W. Binocularity in the human visual evoked potential: Facilitation, summation and suppression. Electroenceph. clin. Neurophysiol. 51: 32–40 (1981).

Amigo, G., Fiorentini, A., Pirchio, M. & Spinelli, D. Binocular vision tested with visual evoked potentials in children and infants. Invest. Ophthalmol. Vis. Sci. 17: 910–915 (1978).

Arden, G.B., Barnard, W.M. & Mushin, A.S. Visually evoked responses in amblyopia. Br. J. Ophthal. 58: 183–192 (1974).

Baker, F.H., Grigg, P. & von Noorden, G.K. Effects of visual deprivation and strabismus on the response of neurons in the visual cortex of the monkey, including studies on the striate and prestriate cortex in the normal animal. Brain Res. 66: 185–208 (1974).

Blake, R. & Levinson, E. Spatial properties of binocular neurones in the human visual system. Exp. Brain Res. 27: 221–232 (1977).

Campbell, F.W. & Green, D. Monocular versus binocular visual acuity. Nature 208: 191–192 (1965).

Campbell, F.W. & Maffei, L. Electrophysiological evidence for the existence of orientation and size detectors in the human visual system. J. Physiol. (Lond.) 207: 635–652 (1970).

Enoksson, P. Binocular rivalry and stereoscopic acuity. Acta Ophthal. (Kbh.) 42: 1–14 (1964).

Franzén, O. & Berkley, M. Apparent contrast as a function of modulation depth and spatial frequency: a comparison between perceptual and electrophysiological measures. Vis. Res. 15: 655 660 (1975).

Harter, M.R. Binocular interaction: evoked potentials to dichoptic stimulation. In: Visual evoked potentials in man: new developments (Ed. J.E. Desmedt), Clarendon Press, Oxford. (1977).

Lema, S.A. & Blake, R. Binocular summation in normal and stereoblind humans. Vis. Res. 17: 691–695 (1977).

Lennerstrand, G. Binocular interaction studied with visual evoked responses (VER) in humans with normal or impaired binocular vision. Acta Ophthal. (Kbh). 56: 628–637 (1978).

Srebro, R. The visually evoked response. Binocular facilitation and failure when binocular vision is disturbed. Arch. Ophthal. 96: 839–844 (1978).

Wanger, P. & Nilsson, B.Y. Visual evoked responses to pattern-reversal stimulation in patients with amblyopia and/or defective binocular functions. Acta Ophthal. (Kbh.) 56: 617–627 (1978).

Authors' address:
Department of Ophthalmology
University Hospital
S-581 85 Linköping
- Sweden

PART SIX

CENTRAL ASPECTS

CORTICAL ABNORMALITIES AND
THE VISUAL EVOKED RESPONSE

L.D. BLUMHARDT & A.M. HALLIDAY

(*London, England*)

ABSTRACT

Since the introduction of electronic averaging it has been hoped that EP methods would provide useful techniques for the detection and location of lesions in the cerebral hemispheres. High inter-subject waveform variation of the flash evoked potential obtained by using an unstructured stimulus generated from an Xenon discharge tube, limited the confident recognition of abnormality in the early studies even in cases with such severe cortical damage that hemianopic visual field defects were present.

Multichannel recordings of the pattern VER have also shown considerable inter-subject and inter-hemisphere waveform variability. This appears to correlate with certain major features of the anatomy of the visual cortex. However, the polarity and form of the potentials generated from each visual half-field have consistent relationships with the underlying cortical generators. Activity arising from half-field stimulation is invariably distributed on both sides of the scalp but the potentials recorded on either side of the midline have distinct characteristics. There is no convincing evidence of a significant trans-callosal contribution. The ability to separate and compare the independent hemisphere activities improves the discrimination between normal variants and pathological responses. The effect of a cortical lesion on the VER appears to depend exclusively on the presence of damage to the primary projection pathways or visual cortical generators. The resulting asymmetries parallel the type and extent of the visual field defect. The effects on amplitude and latency appear to be dissociated and few pathological responses have prolonged component latencies. The major effect appears to be attenuation of responses from the abnormal fields. The pattern VER appears to be indifferent to cortical lesions which spare the specific visual pathways. The method is limited by the high variance associated with subdivisions of the visual half-field but represents a significant advance over the flash technique.

Doc. Ophthal. Proc. Series, Vol. 27, ed. by H. Spekreijse & P.A. Apkarian   347
© 1981 Dr W. Junk Publishers, The Hague/Boston/London

INTRODUCTION

The relationship between the scalp recorded visual evoked response (VER) and abnormalities of the human cerebral cortex has generated much conflicting and controversial data. This is not surprising considering the inaccessible and complex structure of the visual cortex and the widely varied stimulation and recording techniques that have been used by many investigators. Most workers in this field are conversant with the divergent results of studies into the effects of cerebral lesions on the flash evoked potentials which were carried out in the 1960s (see Halliday 1975 for a review of this topic). This is perhaps best summed up by the pessimistic but considered view of Öosterhuis, Ponsen, Jonkman and Magnus (1969) who, after a careful study of patients and controls, concluded that it was rarely possible to identify responses as definitely abnormal even in the presence of severe hemisphere lesions.

The present paper will be restricted to a discussion of our as yet limited experience of the effect of hemisphere lesions on the responses evoked by structured stimuli. The most widely applied clinical technique has been that of checkerboard pattern reversal, the exquisite sensitivity of which for the detection of optic nerve (Halliday, McDonald & Mushin 1972; 1973) and chiasmal lesions (Halliday, Halliday, Kriss, McDonald & Mushin 1976) has now been well established. However, its application to the objective study of cortical lesions has, with few exceptions (Holder 1980; Howe & Mitchell 1980), been limited to anecdotal reports of single cases (Chain, Lesèvre, Leblanc, Rémond and Lhermitte 1972; Bodis-Wollner, Atkin, Raab & Wolkstein 1977; Ashworth, Maloney & Townsend 1978) or to small series of patients where the cortical lesions were not accurately localised (Regan & Heron 1970; Wildberger, Van Lith, Wijngaarde & Mak 1976; Celesia & Daly 1977).

As pattern reversal was more widely applied in clinical neurophysiology in the 1970s it became increasingly important to clarify the effects of post-chiasmal lesions on the VER to avoid misinterpreting results. This was also the decade where it became possible to accurately define the localisation and extent of lesions of the cerebral hemispheres by computerised axial scanning (CAT scan). It is important to know whether the pattern VER is capable of objective confirmation of a post-chiasmal lesion in a useful proportion of patients. Limitations and pitfalls of the technique need defining. Do 'silent' areas within the hemisphere exist and do different pathologies in the posterior visual pathways have specific effects on the VER? Has this laboratory technique anything to offer the clinician in this context or is it merely a sophisticated research tool?

In this paper we would like to present and discuss some of the results obtained in a study of a group of patients with a variety of well-demarcated lesions of the cerebral hemispheres.

METHODS

The stimulation and averaging techniques used in this study are unchanged from those previously reported for both healthy subjects and patients (for details see Blumhardt & Halliday 1979).

The *standard montage* consisted of a transverse chain of five occipital electrodes placed 5 cm above the inion and 5 cm apart so that two electrodes were situated 5 and 10 cm to either side of the midline electrode. Extra electrodes to a total of 16 were symmetrically disposed in subsidiary chains above and below this level. All electrodes were referred to a common mid-frontal reference placed 12 cm above the nasion in the midline. Subjects or patients requiring refraction wore their glasses during the recording. The radius of the full- and half-field stimulus screens subtended 16 degrees and the subtense of the black and white checks was 50 minutes.

Analysis of results and parameters studied

The results to be discussed here are limited to the potentials recorded at the standard transverse occipital chain of five electrodes. The components obtained on full- and half-field stimulation were defined in a multichannel study of 50 healthy subjects, the detailed analysis of which has been published elsewhere (Blumhardt & Halliday 1979). Peak latencies were estimated at all electrode sites and normal limits (2.5 SD) established for all components at the electrodes which gave the least variable results. For the major full-field positivity this gave upper limits for latency of 115.2 msec and 117.5 msec, for the left and right eye respectively, at the midline electrode. The variance increased dramatically over the lateral scalp so that the upper limit increased to 131.8 msec. The half-field $\overline{P100}$ latency limits (2.5 SD) were estimated in the ipsilateral channel 5 cm from the midline and varied slightly with the eye/field combination to a maximum of 117.9 msec (for further details see Blumhardt & Halliday 1979).

Component amplitudes were determined peak-to-peak from the preceding wave of opposite polarity. Asymmetries of the full-field response were analysed by comparing the amplitudes of the major positivities on the two sides in the channels 5 cm lateral to the midline. An upper limit for this data was set at a ratio of 1:3 (Table 1). Asymmetries of ratio between nasal and temporal half-field responses within each eye were similarly determined using the amplitude of the $\overline{P100}$ components at the 5 cm electrodes ipsilateral to the half-field stimulated (Blumhardt & Halliday 1979). This data allowed an upper limit for the amplitude asymmetries between the half-field responses to be set at 1:2 (Table 1).

Table 1. Normal limits of the $\overline{P100}$ amplitude asymmetry[a] (n = 50)

	Eye	Ratio	2.5 SD
Full-field major	left	1.58 ± 0.559	2.98
positive wave	right	1.60 ± 0.553	2.93
Half-field[b]	left	1.36 ± 0.331	2.19
$\overline{P100}$	right	1.34 ± 0.296	2.08

[a]Ratio of larger/smaller wave at electrodes 5 cm from midline.
[b]Heteronymous field comparisons.

Clinical material

Thirty-two patients with well-demarcated lesions determined by CAT scans, angiography and clinical data, were studied. They included ten patients recorded after the surgical excision of various tumours, arteriovenous malformations or cerebral abscesses, four with in situ space-occupying lesions, sixteen following old vascular infarctions or haemorrhages and two with acute post-chiasmal plaques of demyelination. Four patients had bilateral occipital pathology. Twenty-seven of these patients had visual field defects while five had no clinically detectable defect of their visual fields despite severe cerebral pathology.

Most of the patients were recorded at a time remote from the pathological event thus minimising the possible non-specific effects of the acute lesion, for example, by pressure, displacement or oedema.

RESULTS

The interpretation of pathological full-field responses in patients with homonymous visual field defects is complicated by the asymmetries that occur in the responses of healthy subjects (Blumhardt, Barrett, Halliday & Kriss 1978; Blumhardt & Halliday 1979). These are common and invariably homonymous. They reduce the accuracy with which one can distinguish normal from pathological evoked potentials. Asymmetries come about by the cancellation of the ipsilateral and contralateral components of the half-field responses which are recorded at electrodes over the lateral scalp. The degree of asymmetry depends on the relative amplitudes of the components of opposite polarity at the same latency which arise from each hemisphere. These variations in amplitude and topography which can be attributed to the underlying anatomy of the cortical generator area, place severe restraints on the usefulness of the full-field response in detecting unilateral lesions of the cerebral hemispheres. The amplitude ratio at the 5 cm electrodes must exceed at least 3:1 before a pathological asymmetry may be detected.

The major effect of a cortical lesion which is associated with an homonymous hemianopic field defect is an 'uncrossed' or homonymous asymmetry (Fig. 1) in which the distribution of the potentials is the same for each monocular response. In cases where the homonymous hemianopia is complete this asymmetry of distribution is entirely attributable to the activity evoked from the *intact* half-field (or hemisphere). The latter potentials will also dominate over the residual activity from the affected half-field in patients where homonymous defects are incomplete. Thus in all patients, typical ipsilateral activity (negative-positive-negative or NPN complex) is recorded from the scalp ipsilateral to the intact half-field while variable results are obtained from the contralateral electrodes in parallel with the findings on half-field stimulation in healthy subjects. On full field stimulation some hemianopic patients will show phase reversed components (a positive-negative-positive or PNP complex) contralateral to the intact field (e.g. in the most lateral channel on the right in Fig. 1). The late and

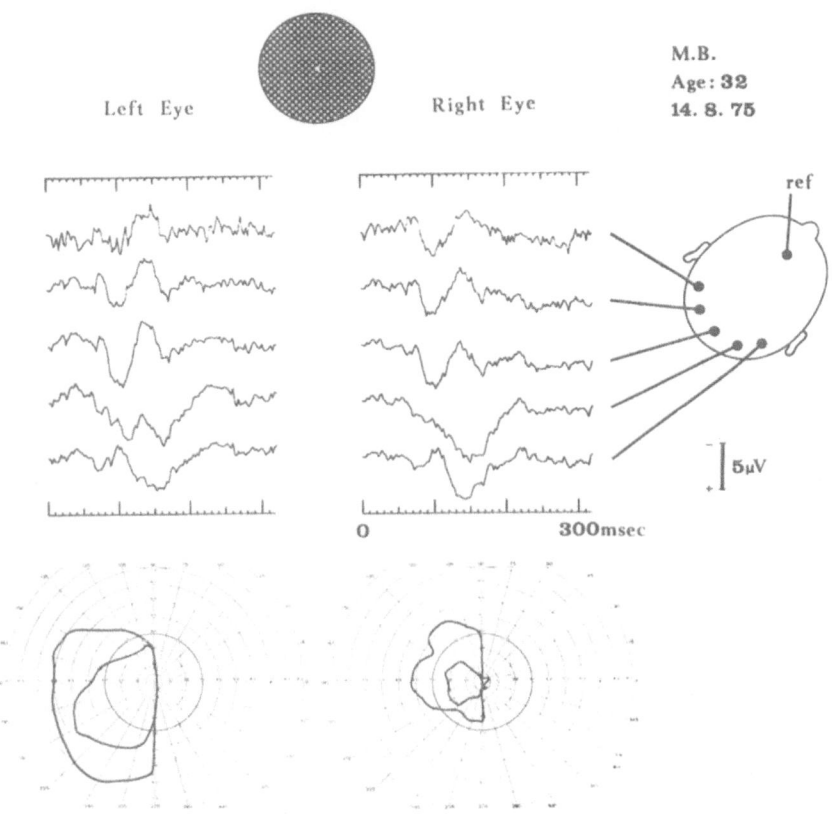

Left Eye   Right Eye

M.B.
Age: 32
14. 8. 75

ref

5µV

0   300msec

Fig. 1. Typical 'uncrossed' asymmetry in patient with right homonymous hemianopia. Note similar asymmetrical distribution of monocular full-field responses from each eye. P100 and accompanying negativities are distributed widely over scalp ipsilateral to intact half-fields while 'phase-reversed' contralateral components are seen at the most lateral channel on the right side of the scalp. The responsible lesion is a post-chiasmal plaque of demyelination on the left side but the P100 is undelayed because the response is generated by the right hemisphere from stimulation of the preserved areas of the left half-field. (From Halliday 1978).

often dominant positivity ipsilateral to the defective field should not be confused with a delayed P100. It can be shown to be due to the contralateral component P135, which is at normal latency in such responses. Half-field stimulation is essential to check the origin of such components. The results from the *intact* half-fields of all subjects with unilateral hemisphere lesions were indistinguishable, on the grounds of amplitude, latency and distribution criteria, from the asymmetrical responses of healthy subjects (e.g. Fig. 2). Further confirmation that stimulation of the intact half-field in patients with hemisphere lesions gave indistiguishable results from those in healthy subjects came from patients following surgical ablations which involved

351

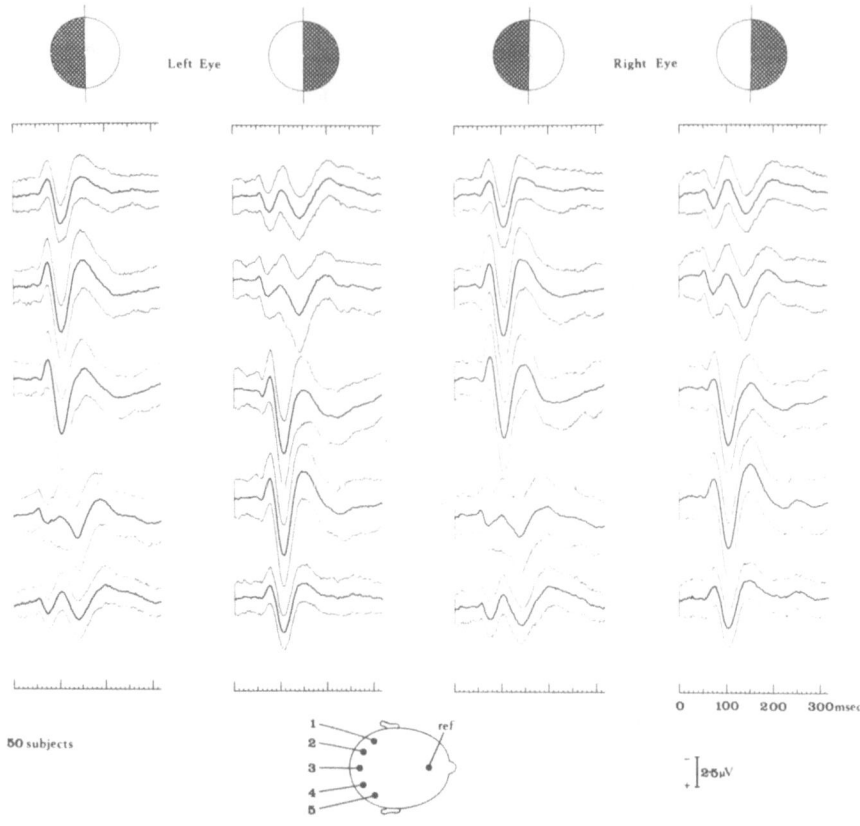

Fig. 2. Mean waveform and standard deviation for half-field responses of 50 healthy subjects. The ipsilateral (NPN), contralateral (PNP) and 'transitional' waveforms are clearly defined. (From Blumhardt & Halliday 1979).

the visual cortex or the whole hemisphere. No evidence was obtained that any of the major half-field potentials had a significant contribution from trans-callosally conducted signals (Fig. 3).

Surgical resections of a more limited nature which involved restricted areas of the visual cortex gave similar results to those obtained in patients after total hemispherectomy. Allowing for some run-to-run variability the similarity of the full- and half-field responses confirmed the absence of any detectable contribution to the half-field response from the largely intact ipsilateral hemisphere in these cases. Where hemianopic field defects were incomplete due to small areas of focal cortical destruction the results were consistent with those obtained in major resections provided the stimulus on that side was limited to the affected area of the field (Fig. 4). This patient illustrates one of the difficulties created by the variable topography of normal half-field potentials. If stimulation is limited to the use of a symmetrical full-field stimulus some severe hemianopic defects will be hidden

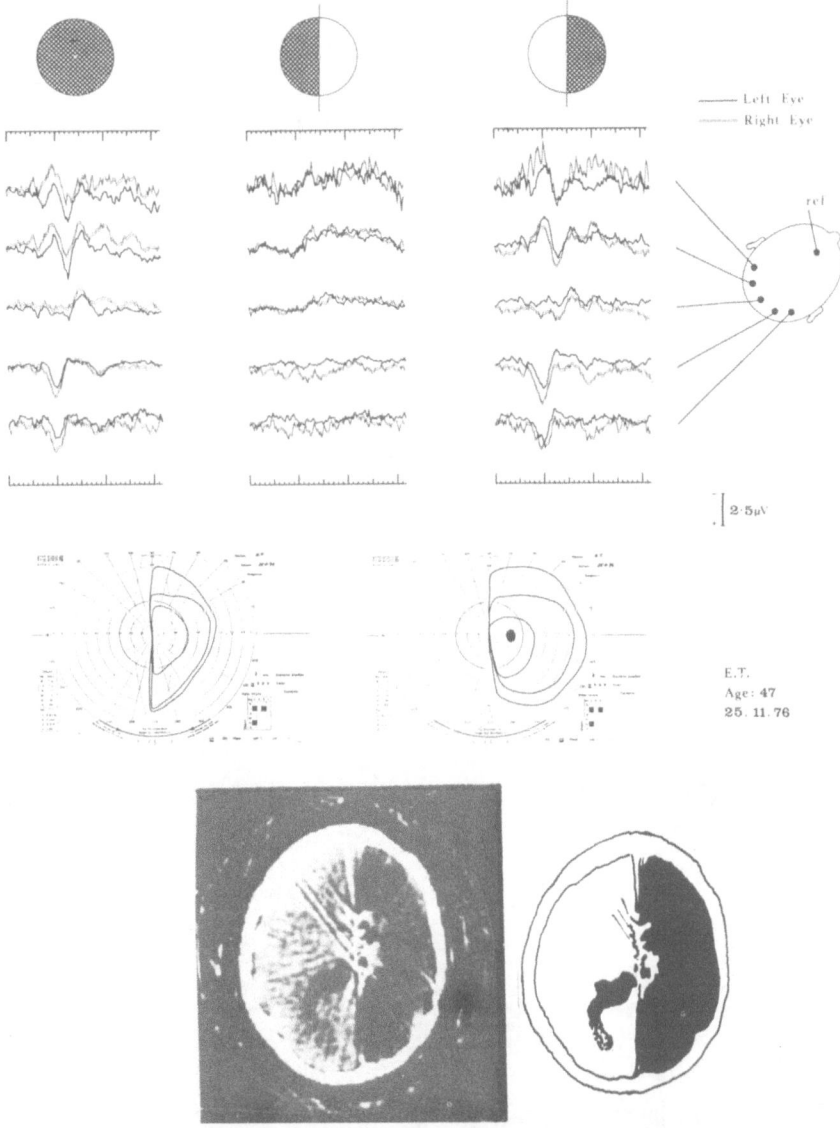

Fig. 3. Full- and half-field responses after 'total' right hemispherectomy. Perimetry shows macular-splitting left homonymous hemianopia. CAT scan shows that the occipital pole of the left hemisphere is in the normal position. No clearly recognisable components are detected above the background noise on stimulation of the left half-fields. This is confirmed by the virtually identical full- and right half-field responses. Note that the right half-field response has a 'transitional' midline waveform due to dominant contralateral components as found in 16% of healthy half-field responses. Note that the ipsilateral complex (NPN) is recorded from the scalp overlying the excised hemisphere and that all components are at normal latency.

353

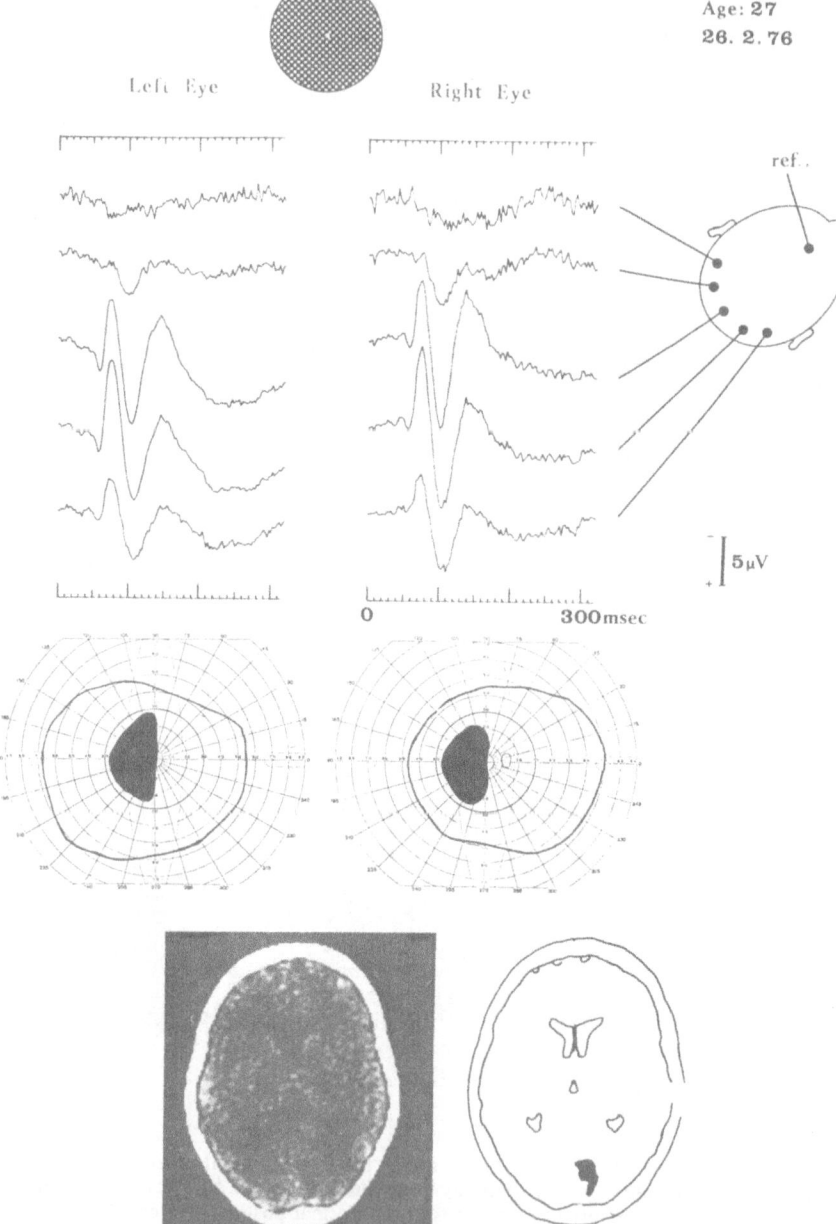

Left Eye   Right Eye

ref.

5μV

0   300msec

354

by the spread of the ipsilateral half-field complex (NPN) across the midline of the scalp. Such a wide-spreading half-field response may mimic a healthy but asymmetric full-field response. Such cases are clearly separated from physiological asymmetries by comparison of the ipsilateral potentials from each half-field (Fig. 5). The poorly lateralized ipsilateral complex in some healthy hemispheres appears to be predominantly due to activity arising from the foveal representation near the pole of the occipital lobe. If this area extends round the tip of the lobe so that its generator neurones are on the lateral surface of the hemisphere, the ipsilateral NPN complex may spread to a variable degree across the midline. This proposition is supported by the clearer lateralisation of the NPN complex in some patients when the foveal $0-2°$ is excluded by eccentric fixation. The variable foveal response is particularly likely to create difficulties for workers who persist in using the 10–20 electrode placements 0_1 and 0_2 which are too close to the midline to allow clear separation of ipsilateral and contralateral activities. Provided half-field stimulation was carried out, all severe hemianopic field defects resulted in amplitude asymmetries which were clearly beyond the upper limit of normal variability.

With less severe lesions of the posterior visual pathways the abnormality of the VER depended on the extent and location of the visual field defect and the pre-existing anatomical asymmetry. Residual potentials arising from preserved areas of the visual fields, particularly from the macula and areas adjacent to the vertical meridian will reduce the response asymmetry (Fig. 6). Patients with large areas of macular sparing or with small ratios of abnormal to normal half-field responses did not exceed the limits of the amplitude asymmetry criteria.

Similar problems were posed by homonymous quadrantic field defects as the potentials produced by quadrantic stimulation in healthy individuals are highly variable (Blumhardt & Halliday 1979). In some normal subjects one entire half-field response may arise exclusively from the lower quadrant while the upper quadrant of the opposite half-field gives rise to readily detectable ipsilateral and contralateral components. Thus while some quadrantic hemianopias are clearly revealed by analysis of the half-field response amplitudes (Fig. 7), others will go undetected (Fig. 8). Of eight patients with homonymous quadrantanopias (four upper and four lower field defects), five had abnormal amplitude asymmetries (two with upper and three with lower field defects). By extension of the principle of the generation of the full-field response by half-field summation, an increased sensitivity would be expected by comparing the separated quadrant

Fig. 4. Monocular full-field responses after excision of right occipital cystic arteriovenous malformation. Pre-operative CAT scan shows the position of the small lesion on the medial aspect of the right occipital lobe. Following excision of a small block of tissue measuring 2.5 cm × 1 cm × 1 cm a dense homonymous macular-splitting scotoma extending to about 25° radius ensued. Potentials are asymmetrically distributed, being maximally recorded from the right scalp overlying the damaged hemisphere. Note that the spread of potentials across the midline tends to partially reduce the marked asymmetry which is clearly revealed by half-field stimulation in Fig. 5. Note the radius of stimulating field is only 16°, well within the scotomatous area on the left.

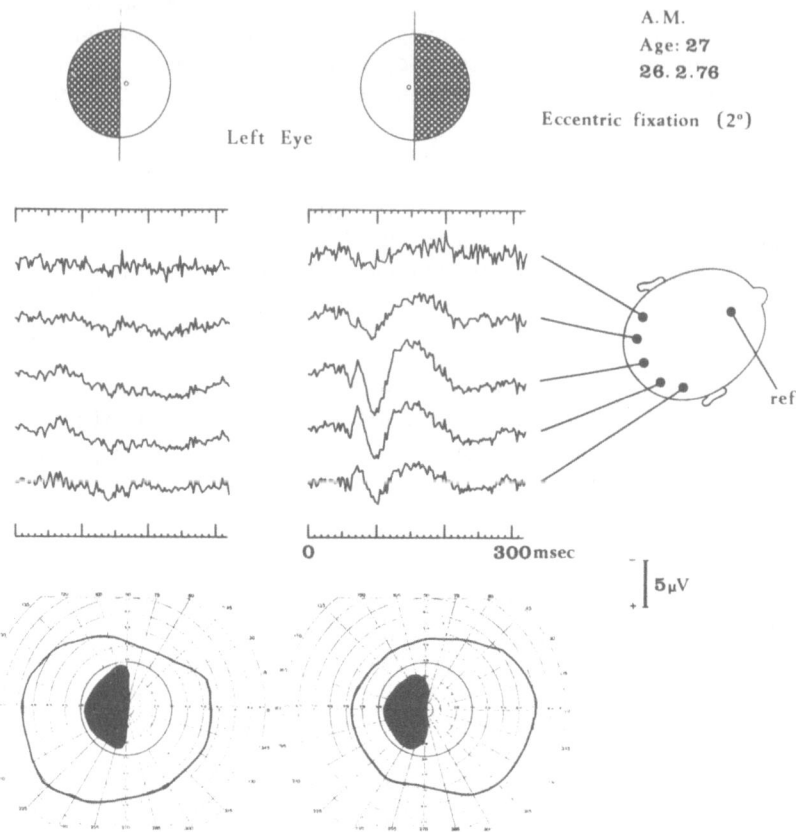

A.M.
Age: 27
26.2.76

Eccentric fixation (2°)

Left Eye

ref.

0   300 msec

5 μV

Fig. 5. Half-field responses from the patient whose full-field responses are shown in Fig. 4. With eccentric fixation the response amplitude is reduced due to loss of activity from the foveal 2° strip. Left half-field stimulation is within the scotomatous field defect and there is no detectable response above noise level (left hand record). Stimulation within preserved right half-fields produces small but typical ipsilateral (NPN) complex from scalp overlying hemisphere with surgical defect. Electrodes over *intact hemisphere* recorded little activity. (from Blumhardt, Barrett & Halliday 1977).

responses. It was found, however, that the great variability, particularly of the upper field activity, in healthy subjects limited the usefulness of such comparisons.

Several patients were recorded with bilateral hemisphere damage. In each case the distribution of the potentials reflected the visual field defect rather than the extent of the pathological hemisphere lesion. In one case with bilateral, gross, symmetrical occipital lesions the VERs paralleled the more marked involvement of striate cortex in the right hemisphere, as reflected in the more severe involvement of the left half-fields, and appeared normal when the other hemisphere was stimulated, despite an otherwise comparable lesion on that side. In another patient in whom perimetry showed grossly

356

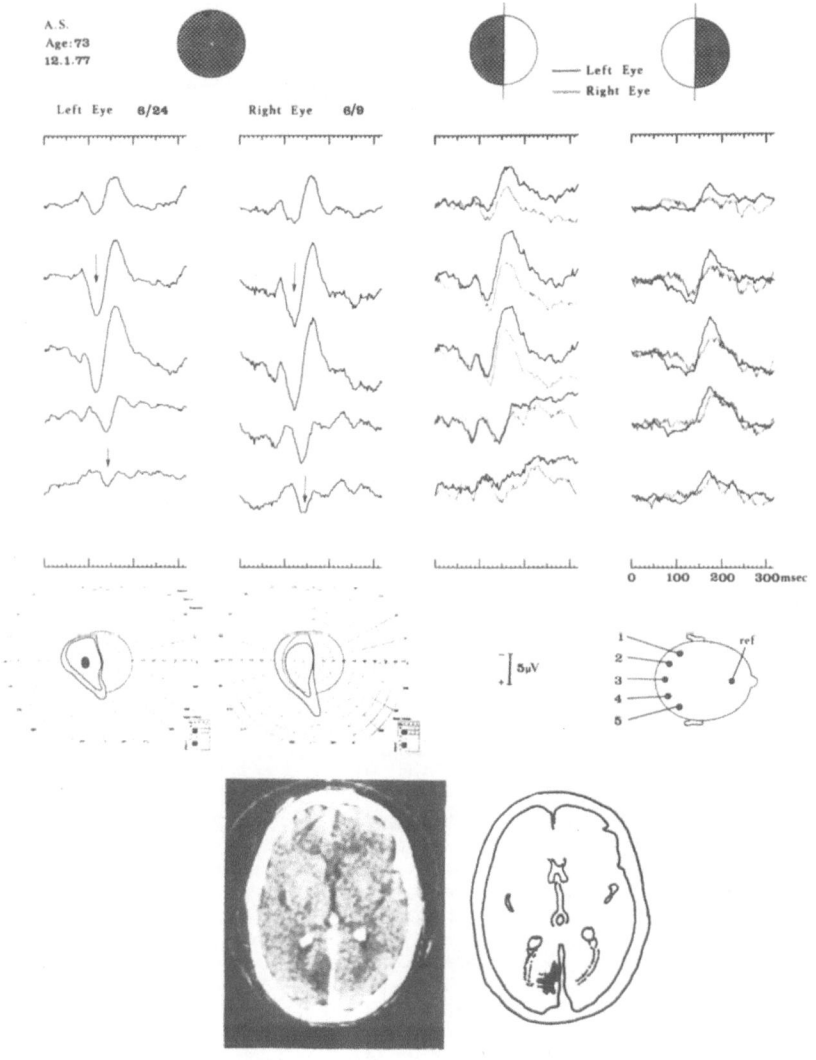

Fig. 6. Uncrossed asymmetry with residual activity from hemianopic visual field. CAT scan shows irregular infarction in the calcarine cortex anterior to the left occipital pole. There is a slight degree of macular sparing on perimetry. As would be expected from the field defect most activity arises from intact left half-fields, the responses from which closely resemble full-field activity. Apparent 'delay' of the positive wave in right-sided channels is shown to be a contralateral $\overline{P135}$ wave at normal latency (Column 3). Although considerable residual activity (particularly a late surface negative wave) arises from the affected half-fields the $\overline{P100}$ in ipsilateral channels is completely attenuated.

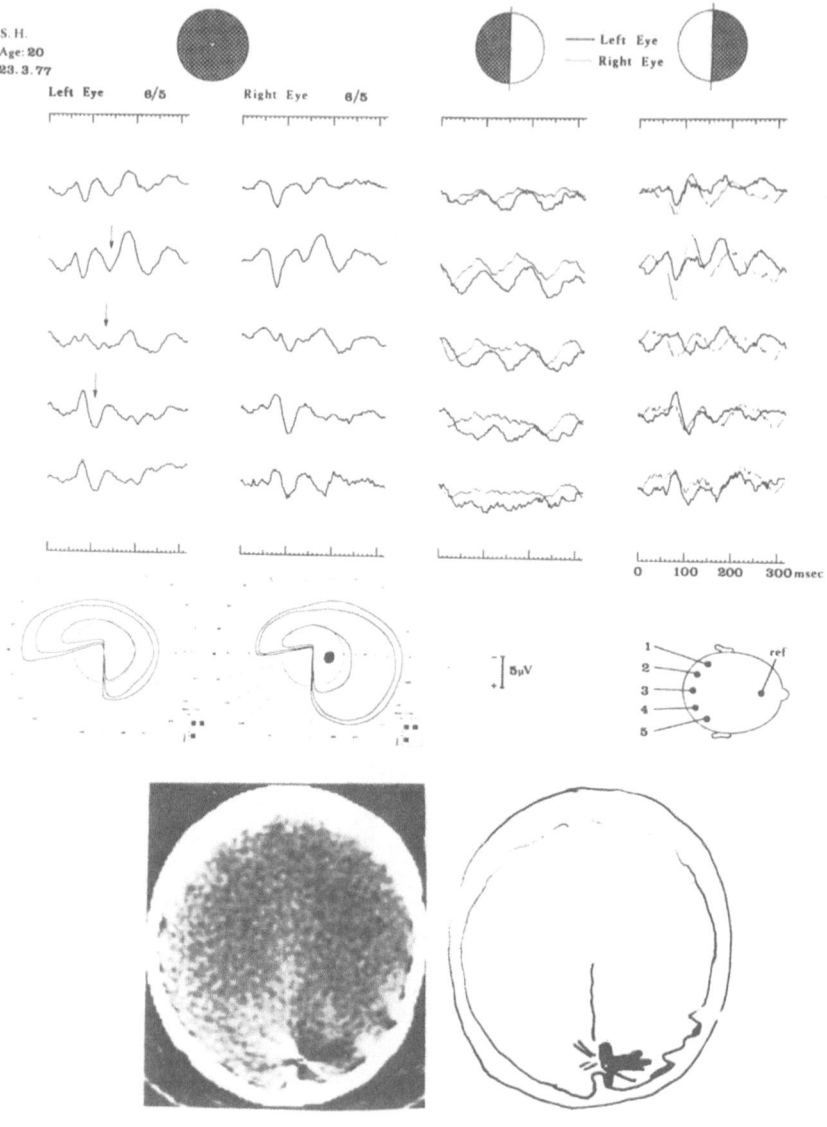

Fig. 7. Uncrossed asymmetry in lower quadrantanopia. CAT scan shows post-surgical defect high in right occipital lobe following surgical drainage of a cerebral abscess. Full-field responses show an uncrossed asymmetry with clearly defined ipsilateral (NPN) and contralateral (PNP) right half-field complexes (Channels 2 and 4 in column 1). Note midline responses are transitional in waveform (Arrow, channel 3, column 1). Stimulation of the affected left half-field shows only an asymmetric time-locked alpha rhythm, while the right half-field responses closely parallel the waveform on full-field stimulation, with some incongruencies in the responses from the left and right eye.

358

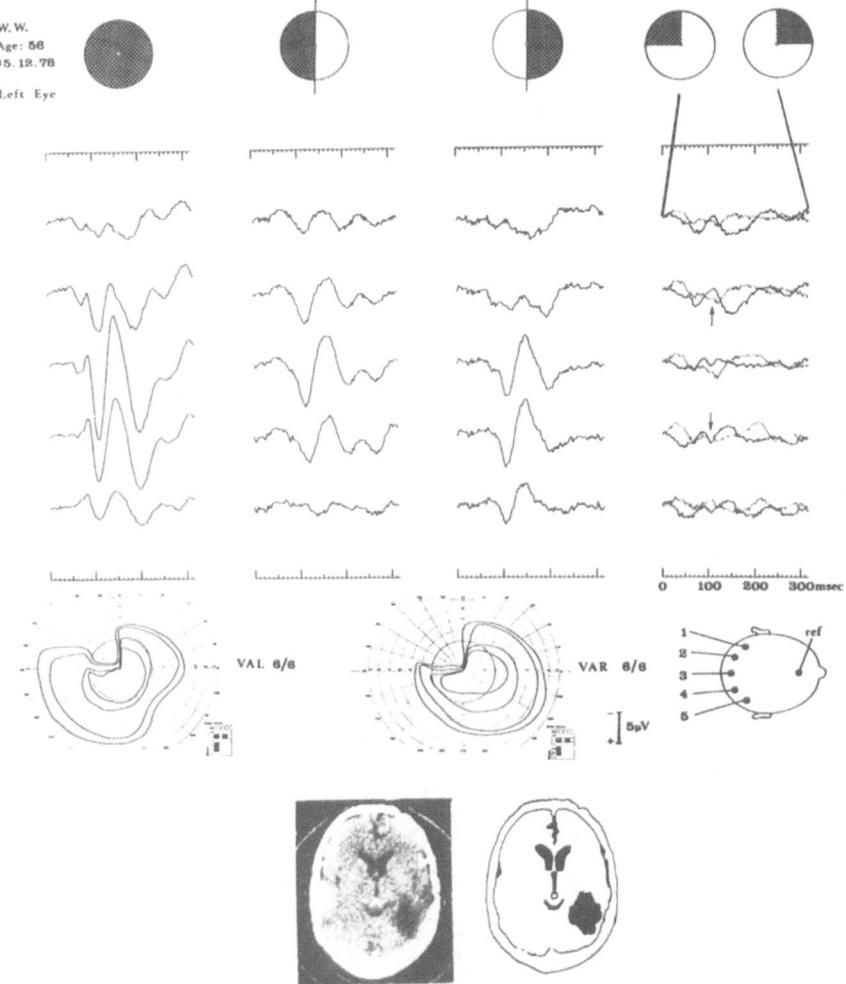

Fig. 8. Symmetrical responses in upper quadrantanopia. CAT scan shows right parieto-occipital infarction. Full- and half-field responses are within normal limits for amplitude ratio asymmetries and latencies. Quadrantic stimulation shows differences between upper field responses in direction predicted from field defects; ipsilateral and contra-lateral waves are only obtained from right upper field, (arrows, dark trace).

constricted but asymmetric fields, the evoked potentials, though small, showed an uncrossed asymmetry consistent with the perimetry (Fig. 9).

Gross hemisphere destruction from such lesions as massive infarction of middle cerebral artery territory, space-occupying lesions such as temporal lobe gliomas and extensive parietal and frontal arteriovenous malformations or thalamic haemorrhages had no detectable effect on the distribution or amplitude of the responses provided that no clinical defect of the visual

359

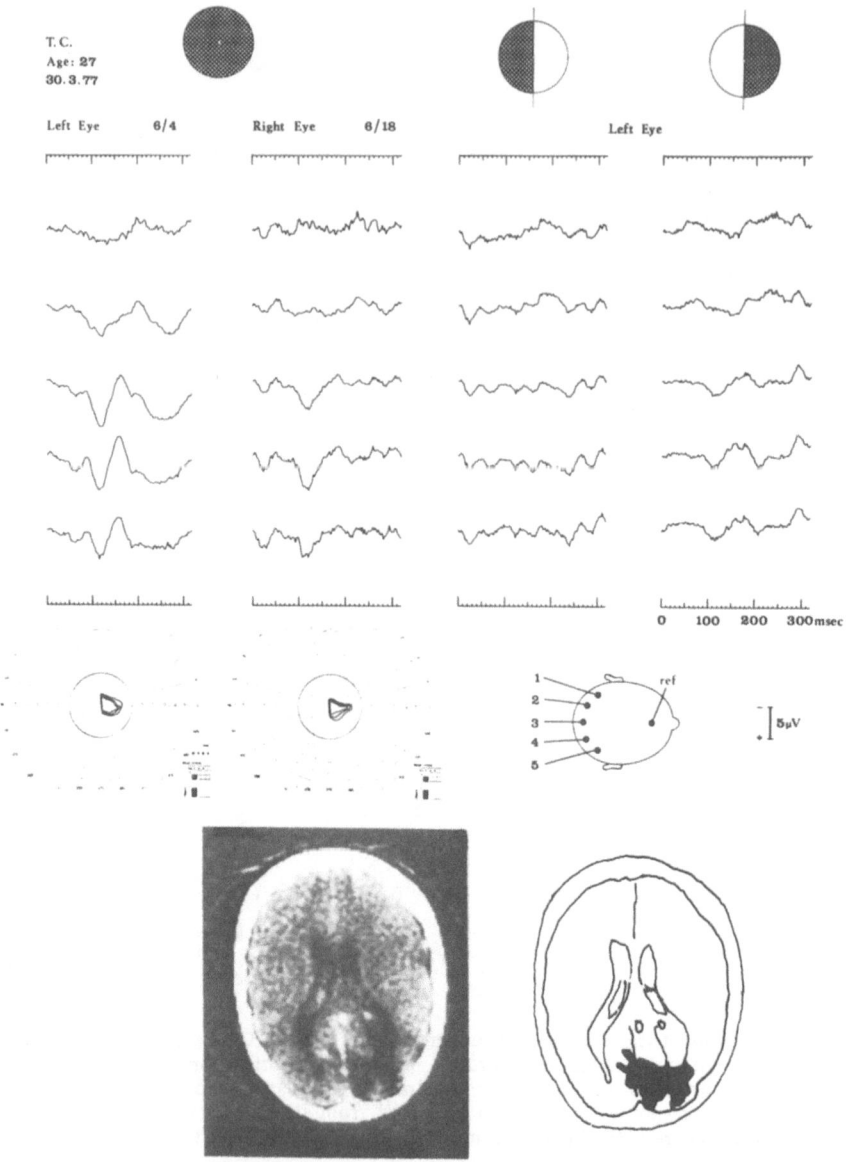

Fig. 9. Evoked potentials in bilateral occipital lobe damage due to open head injury. The CAT scan shows an extensive low density lesion in the right occiptal lobe and a small lesion in the anterior aspect of the left striate cortex. Visual fields are consistent with these lesions and show a total left homonymous hemianopia and peripheral constriction of the right half-fields. Despite the very small fields and rather variable responses a clear uncrossed asymmetry is confirmed by half-field stimulation with a P100 at normal latency recorded from the scalp overlying the most extensively damaged hemisphere.

fields was present. One case with a right thalamic haemorrhage but no field defect had a slightly delayed response.

In summary, the full-field responses revealed pathological amplitude asymmetries from each eye in only 14 of 26 patients (54%) with homonymous visual field defects. If monocular asymmetries were included this increased to 16 of 26 (62%). Using half-field criteria this hit rate was increased to 84% (Table 2). The patients whose responses remained within

Table 2. Number of abnormalities of amplitude ratio according to extent of visual field defect.

	Complete homonymous Hemianopia (n = 16)		Incomplete homonymous field defect (n = 10)[a]		All field defects (n = 26)	
Full field response	11(1)[b]	69%	5(1)	50%	16(2)	62%
Half-field response	15(1)	100%[c]	6(2)	60%	21(3)	84%

[a]Includes 8 with quadrantanopic defects and two with subtle homonymous scotomata.
[b]Figures in brackets represent number of those included in total who exceeded ratio limits for one eye only.
[c]One case did not have half-field recordings.

normal limits had cortical abnormalities which were associated either with normal visual fields or peripheral or quadrantic field defects. By contrast the majority of patients had undelayed responses (Table 3). In the 26 half-field responses in which there were consistent component peaks on stimulation of the affected half-fields, there were no delays. From the 50 half-field responses obtained from the unaffected hemispheres in these cases there were seven slight delays (14%) which were of the order of 2–3 msec. Even in patients where one would expect a delayed conduction velocity on the basis of the underlying pathology, the responses were not invariably delayed. For example, in one patient with a post-chiasmal plaque of demyelination, all components of the response in which a marked amplitude asymmetry parallelled the visual field defect, were at normal latency (e.g. Fig. 1).

DISCUSSION

This limited study has provided some insight into the value and limitations of the pattern reversal technique as applied to hemisphere lesions. It is clear from the multi-channel recordings that the gross alteration of waveform which occurs with hemianopic field defects can cause major problems in interpretation and wide divergence of conclusions, especially where recordings are made from single electrodes positioned either at or near the midline. Many previous results of studies on the VER of patients with hemisphere lesions have suffered from an over-simplified concept of the relationship between the anatomy of the visual pathways and the scalp distribution of the VEP. Thus it has been widely assumed that all or most of the electrical activity evoked from one visual half-field should be recorded

361

Table 3. Number of patients with delayed major positive-wave or $\overline{\text{P100}}$ in cortical lesions

	Patients with homonymous visual field defects (n = 26)		Patients with clinically intact visual fields (n = 5)	
Full-field response (midline electrode)	6/52	12%	2/10	20%
Response from abnormal $\frac{1}{2}$ fields	0/27*	0%	1/10	10%
Response from intact $\frac{1}{2}$ fields	7/50	14%	1/10	10%

*The remainder had absent responses from the affected fields.

from the scalp which overlies the contralateral hemisphere. This idea assumes that the distribution of evoked potentials is solely determined by the crossed arrangement of the geniculo-cortical projection *pathways* and ignores the importance of the position and orientation of generator neurones in the visual cortex. Studies using common reference recordings have clearly demonstrated that activity from each visual half-field is *invariably* recorded on *both* sides of the scalp, whether to flash stimulation (Biersdorf & Nakamura 1971) or to pattern (Michael & Halliday 1971; Jeffreys & Axford 1972; Barrett, Blumhardt, Halliday, Halliday & Kriss 1976; Shagass, Amadeo & Roemer 1976). Another widely-held view is that the largest waves will be lateralised over the hemisphere contralateral to the stimulated field. This however, does not apply to the pattern reversal potentials. Lateralisation of maximal amplitudes on the scalp have no constant relationship to the hemisphere of origin. For example, while the ipsilateral $\overline{\text{P100}}$ or $\overline{\text{N145}}$ potentials are the largest waves recorded in the majority of half-field responses, up to 16% of such recordings may have a dominant contralateral component. When stimulus conditions are held constant it is the *form* and *polarity* of the recorded complexes on the scalp which have consistent relationships to the stimulated hemisphere (Blumhardt, Barrett, Halliday & Kriss 1978). An understanding of the variation of the healthy hemisphere responses is important for the interpretation of the effects of cortical lesions on the VER.

Hemisphere lesions which affect the visual pathways appear to result primarily in asymmetries of distribution of scalp recorded activity principally because of an effect on the amplitude of potentials. In contrast with previous reports on the flash evoked potential these appear to be largely dissociated from any effect on component peak latencies. The latter is a very unreliable indicator of posterior visual pathway lesions (cf Kooi, Güevener & Bagchi 1965).

Investigators who use only full-field stimuli will have difficulty separating almost half their patients with homonymous field defects from normals. This problem can be entirely attributed to the variability of the healthy full-field responses together with a tendency for half-field potentials to spread across the midline in some subjects. Direct comparison of the hemisphere potentials evoked by independent half-field stimulation allows a better separation of normals and hemianopic patients. The hit rate in dense hemianopics approaches 100% but falls off according to the incompleteness of the field defect. The usefulness of the half-field technique is limited by the increasing variance as the half-field is fractionated so that the detection rate for quadrantic defects falls off again to about 50%. The intersubject and interhemisphere variation becomes so great for smaller segments of the visual field that quantitative analysis, even with multichannel recordings, seems unlikely to detect smaller than quadrantic defects reliably (cf Regan & Milner 1978).

A striking feature of the pattern reversal technique appears to be its insensitivity to even widespread cortical destruction provided that the geniculocortical pathways and occipital generator areas in the cortex are intact. Abnormalities of the VER in patients with dense homonymous hemianopic field defects are broadly similar whether they are caused by discrete, multifocal or widespread hemisphere damage. The end result is the loss of all recordable activity arising from the affected hemisphere over *both* sides of the scalp. The requirement for abnormality to be registered by the pattern evoked potential appears to be a field defect and its type and extent determines the degree of response asymmetry. The pattern VER appears to provide no information on the extent and the localisation of lesions outside the specific visual pathways. This conclusion contrasts with the reports of abnormalities of the flash evoked potential in cases with hemisphere lesions but no visual field defects (eg. Ebe, Mikami, Ito, Aki & Miyazaki 1963; Vaughan & Katzman 1963; Kooi, Güevener and Bagchi 1965; Creutzfeldt, Kugler, Morocutti & Sommer-Smith 1966; Richey, Kooi & Tourtellotte 1971). Whether this represents a fundamental difference between the flash and pattern potentials or the failure accurately to identify and compare analogous components in the abnormal flash waveform, remains to be clarified.

This study has shown that common reference recording of half-field responses from a simple transverse chain of occipital electrodes can provide objective confirmation of most, if not all, severe lesions associated with hemianopia, together with a useful proportion of lesser field defects. Although this method is unlikely to have a wide clinical application we have found it useful in small groups of patients suspected of psychiatric or mixed organic/psychiatric disease to confirm or exclude a subjectively-determined visual field defect. It is also of considerable importance to recognise the abnormal waveforms caused by lesions of the posterior visual pathways in order to avoid erroneous pathophysiological conclusions. The pattern reversal technique provides a simple and reasonably sensitive method for the functional examination of the primary visual projection pathway and the cortical generators of the VER. Whether a further development of the technique or the discovery of an appropriate visual stimulus will allow the detection of lesions beyond the primary visual projection pathway remains a challenge for future investigation.

REFERENCES

Ashworth, B., Maloney, A.F.J. & Townsend, H.R.A. Delayed visual evoked potentials with bilateral disease of the posterior visual pathway. J. Neurol. Neurosurg. Psychiat. 41: 449–451 (1978).

Barrett, G., Blumhardt, L.D., Halliday, A.M., Halliday, E. & Kriss, A. A paradox in the lateralisation of the visual evoked response. Nature 261: 253–255 (1976).

Biersdorf, W.R. & Nakamura, Z. Electroencephalogram potentials evoked by hemi-retinal stimulation. Experientia 27: 402–403 (1971).

Blumhardt, L.D. & Halliday, A.M. Hemisphere contributions to the composition of the pattern evoked potential waveform. Exp. Brain Res. 36: 53–69 (1979).

Blumhardt, L.D., Barrett, G. & Halliday, A.M. The asymmetrical visual evoked potential to pattern reversal in one half-field and its significance for the analysis of visual field defects. Br. J. Ophthal. 61: 454–461 (1977).

Blumhardt, L.D., Barrett, G., Halliday, A.M. & Kriss, A. The effect of experimental 'scotomata' on the ipsilateral and contralateral responses to pattern reversal in one half-field. Electroenceph. clin. Neurophysiol. 45: 376–392 (1978).

Bodis-Wollner, I., Atkin, A., Raab, E. & Wolkstein, M. Visual association cortex and vision in man: pattern evoked occipital potentials in a blind boy. Science 198: 629–630 (1977).

Celesia, G.G. & Daly, R. Visual electroencephalographic computer analysis (VECA). Neurology 27: 637–641 (1977).

Chain, F., Lesèvre, N., Leblanc, M., Rémond, A. & Lhermitte, F. Etude topographique des réponses évoquées visuelles dans un cas de lobectomie occipitale. Rev. Neurol. 126: 372–378 (1972).

Creutzfeldt, O., Kugler, J., Morocutti, C. & Sommer-Smith, J.A. Visual evoked potentials in normal human subjects and neurological patients. Electroenceph. clin. Neurophysiol. 20: 99P (1966).

Ebe, M., Mikami, T., Ito, H., Aki, M. & Miyazaki, M. Photically evoked potentials (PEP'S) in brain disorders. Tohoku J. Exp. Med. 80: 323–372 (1963).

Halliday, A.M. The effect of lesions of the visual pathway and cerebrum on the visual evoked response. In: Evoked potentials. Handbook of electroencephalography and clinical neurophysiology. (Ed. W.S. Van Leeuwen, F.H. Lopes da Silva & A. Kamp) Amsterdam Elsevier 8A: 119–129 (1975).

Halliday, A.M. Commentary: evoked potentials in neurological diagnosis. In: Event-related brain potentials in man (Ed. E. Callaway, S.H. Koslow, & P. Tueting.) Academic Press, New York. 197–213 (1978).

Halliday, A.M., Halliday, E., Kriss, A., McDonald, W.I. & Mushin, J. The pattern evoked potential in compression of the anterior visual pathways. Brain 99: 357–374 (1976).

Halliday, A.M., McDonald, W.I. & Mushin, J. Delayed visual evoked responses in optic neuritis. Lancet, 1: 982–985 (1972).

Halliday, A.M., McDonald, W.I. & Mushin, J. The visual evoked response in the diagnosis of multiple sclerosis. Br. Med. J., 4: 661–664 (1973).

Holder, G.E. Abnormalities of the pattern visual evoked potential in patients with homonymous visual field defects. In: Evoked potentials (Ed. C. Barber) MTP Press, Lancaster. 285–291 (1980).

Howe, J.W. & Mitchell, K.W. Visual evoked potentials from quadrantic field stimulation in the investigation of homonymous field defects. In: Evoked potentials, (Ed. C. Barber) MTP Press, Lancaster. 279–283 (1980).

Jeffreys, D.A. & Axford, J.G. Source location of pattern specific components of human visual evoked potentials. I: Component of striate cortical origin. Exp. Brain Res. 16: 1–21 (1972).

Kooi, K.A., Güvener, A.M. & Bagchi, B.K. Visual evoked responses in lesions of the higher optic pathways. Neurology 15: 841–854 (1965).

Michael, W.F. & Halliday, A.M. Differences between the occipital distribution of upper and lower field pattern evoked responses in man. Brain Res., 32: 311–324 (1971).

Oosterhuis, H.J.G.H., Ponsen, L., Jonkman, E.J. & Magnus, O. The average visual response in patients with cerebrovascular disease. Electroenceph. clin. Neurophysiol. 27: 23–34 (1969).

Regan, D. & Heron, J.R. Simultaneous recording of visual evoked potentials from the left and right hemispheres in migraine. In: Background to Migraine. Heinemann. London 66–77 (1970).

Regan, D. & Milner, B.A. Objective perimetry by evoked potential recording: limitations. Electroenceph. clin. Neurophysiol. 44: 393–397 (1978).

Richey, E.T., Kooi, K.A. & Tourtellotte, W.W. Visual evoked responses in multiple sclerosis. J. Neurol. Neurosurg. and Psychiat. 34: 275–280 (1971).

Shagass, C., Amadeo, M. & Roemer, R.A. Spatial distribution of potentials evoked by half-field pattern reversal and pattern onset stimuli. Electroenceph. clin. Neurophysiol. 41: 609–622 (1976).

Vaughan, H.G. & Katzman, R. Pathology of the visual evoked potential in man. Electroenceph. clin. Neurophysiol. 15: 146 (1963).

Wildberger, H.G.H., Van Lith, G.H.M., Wijngaarde, R. & Mak, G.T.M. Visual evoked cortical potentials in the evaluation of homonymous and bitemporal visual field defects. Br. J. Ophthal. 60: 273–278 (1976).

Authors' address:
Medical Research Council,
National Hospital,
Queen Square,
London WC1N 3BG, U.K.

THE EFFECTS OF TEMPORAL FREQUENCY CHANGES ON HUMAN PATTERN VECPs IN RESPONSE TO UPPER AND LOWER HALF FIELD STIMULATION

E. ADACHI-USAMI, J. CHIBA & K. YANASHIMA

(Bad Nauheim, F.R.G./Hamamatsu, Japan)

ABSTRACT

Visually evoked cortical potentials (VECPs) were studied in response to checkerboard pattern reversal stimuli of upper and lower visual fields for different temporal frequencies. It was found that the amplitude vs. temporal frequency curves for the upper and lower half field were similar, although VECP amplitude attenuation was significant in the upper field. The amplitude was highest at around 5–6 Hz with a sharper decrease of amplitude at higher frequencies. It was also found that a positive wave showing a peak latency of 130 ms with stimulation of the lower half field was delayed by 10–30 ms in the upper half field. The origination of upper and lower half field responses was discussed.

INTRODUCTION

Polarity reversal of VECP components has been observed with stimulation of the upper and lower visual fields both with flash and pattern stimuli (Schreinemachers & Henkes 1968; Jeffreys 1971; Michael & Halliday 1971; Chiba, Chiba, Kuroda & Adachi-Usami 1979; Chiba & Adachi-Usami 1979). Jeffreys (1971) and Michael & Halliday (1971) suggested the polarity inversion arises from two sets of generators positioned as geometrically opposed dipoles (spatial domain) while Lehmann et al. (1977) suggested latency changes of components with constant polarity and similar surface distributions (time domain). The phenomenon is rather complicated and previous studies (Chiba & Adachi-Usami 1979; Jeffreys & Smith 1979; Lesèvre & Joseph 1979) have led to equivocal conclusions. The fact that experimental conditions among these investigations considerably differ also makes the problem more confusing.

The present study attempts to locate the positions of the presumed generators for the upper and lower half field responses by studying temporal factors in the VECP.

METHODS

A TV display system (Medelec, England) was used to produce checkerboard pattern stimuli. A semi-circular pattern was presented to either the upper or lower half of the visual field and viewed binocularly from a distance of 127 cm or 270 cm. At these distances the angular subtense of the diameter of the semi-circular field was 15 or 7 degrees, respectively. Check size was generally 14 minutes. Mean luminance was kept at 68.3 cd/m². Patterns were reversed independently from the display frame rate in a square wave mode. Contrast in per cent was calculated as

$$\frac{Lmax - Lmin}{Lmax + Lmin} \times 100$$

by measuring the maximum and minimum luminance with an SEI photometer. Contrast was 23 per cent unless stated otherwise. Temporal frequencies examined were from 1.6 Hz to 14 Hz. It should be noted that the temporal frequency indicated in the present study is the sweep frequency which is half of the pattern reversal frequency.

VECPs were recorded monopolarly from each of four midline electrodes placed at the inion, Oz, Pz and Cz with either a right earlobe reference or a midfrontal reference electrode positioned 30 per cent above the nasion on the midline. Potentials were led into a pre-amplifier (Tektronix AM 502) with a band pass filter of 1–100 Hz and then averaged (n = 128) by an averager (Nicolet, Model 1072). Upward deflection in the records indicates positivity of the scalp electrode with respect to the reference electrode. Mydriaticum Roche was used to control the size of the pupil and changes of accommodation. An artificial pupil of 4 mm also was used. The subject investigated gazed at a small fixation point in the middle of the chord. Six well trained normal observers served as subjects.

RESULTS

Fig. 1 shows a representative set of the responses to increasing temporal frequencies of the stimuli for upper (left) and lower (right) half fields at four different electrode positions. The upper half of the figure represents the data obtained with the right earlobe reference electrode, and the lower half the data obtained with the midfrontal reference electrode. For the same recording condition it was found that the responses to lower half field stimulation were generally greater than responses to upper field stimulation in the posterior electrode position (inion and Oz), while the responses to upper half field stimulation were generally greater in the anterior position (Pz and Cz).

For all electrode positions examined, the VECP amplitude was highest at around 5–6 Hz with a more pronounced decrease of amplitudes at higher frequencies. No measurable VECPs were obtained at frequencies higher than 14 Hz.

The effect of position of the reference electrode most clearly could be seen in the records obtained at the inion and Cz. The amplitudes obtained at the inion were smaller in the lower frequency range with the earlobe reference electrode than those with the midfrontal one.

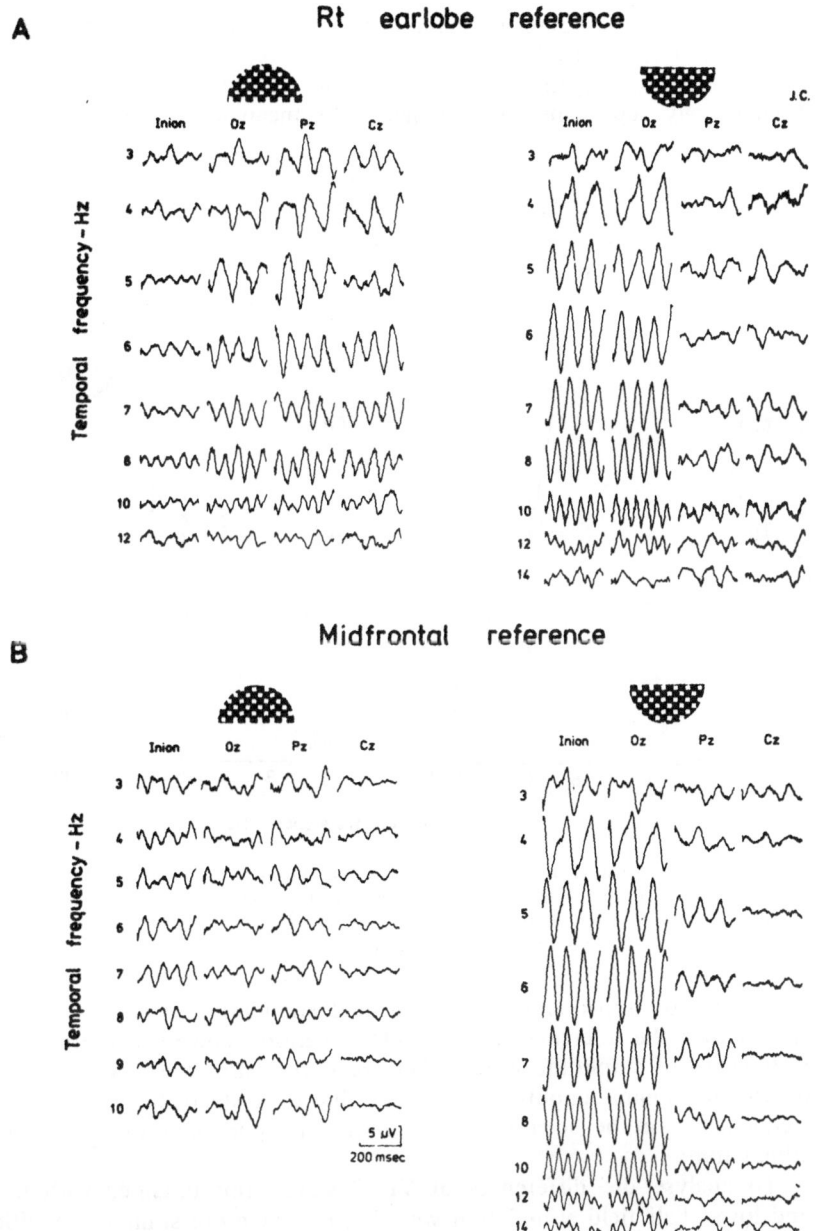

Fig. 1. VECPs to upper and lower half field stimuli of different temporal frequencies. Recordings were made from 4 midline electrodes with reference to the right earlobe (A) and midfrontal position (B). Positivity of active electrode upwards. Stimulus field 7° in diameter, check size 14', contrast 23 per cent. Binocular viewing from a distance of 270 cm.

Similarly, the responses obtained at Cz were much smaller with the mid-frontal reference electrode than with the earlobe reference.

The results of experiments performed on six subjects were similar. Fig. 2 graphically represents for 6 subjects the mean amplitude vs. temporal

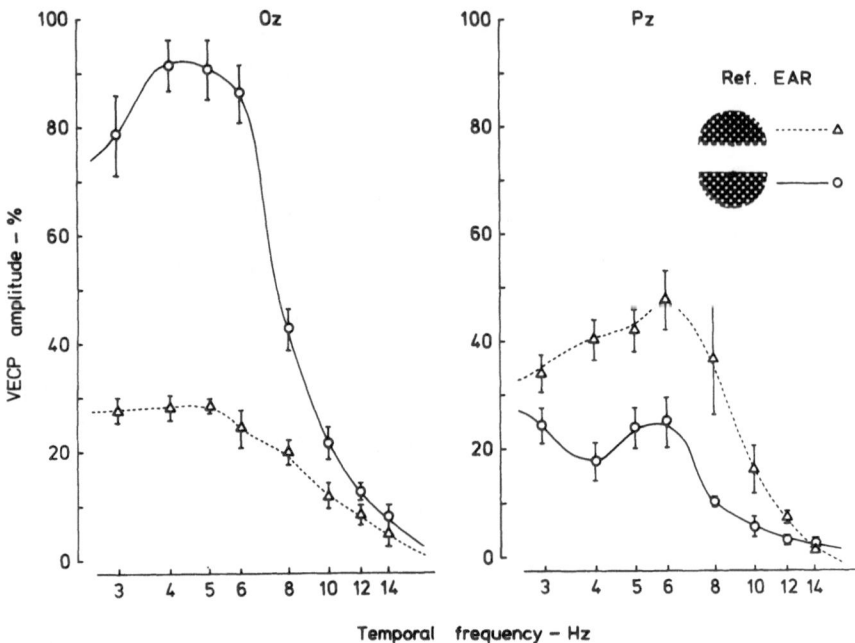

Fig. 2. VECP amplitudes in per cent of the maximum against various temporal frequencies for 6 subjects with upper and lower half field stimulation. Bars indicate standard errors. Monopolar recording from Oz and Pz with reference electrode at the right earlobe. Stimulus conditions same as in Fig. 1.

frequency for upper and lower half field stimulation at Oz (left) and Pz (right) with the reference electrode at the earlobe. Since the interindividual differences of amplitude were rather great, they are expressed in per cent of the maximum amplitude in each subject. A steep decrease at higher frequencies can be seen to occur both for upper and lower half field stimulation.

To analyse the differences of VECP wave-forms obtained with upper and lower half field stimulation we tried to match our stimulus conditions as closely as possible to those of Lehmann et al. (1977), who used a mirror galvanometer for the pattern stimuli instead. In order to achieve comparable conditions we used a patterned field subtending 15°, monocular viewing at a distance of 127 cm, check sizes of 56', temporal frequencies of 1.6 and 3.2 Hz a contrast level of 86 per cent and a mean luminance of 68.3 cd/m². Stimuli of a smaller check size (14') and a lower contrast (23 per cent) also were presented to assess the effects of a smaller check size and a lower contrast on the results. In addition, steady-state VECPs with 6 Hz stimulus were used.

Fig. 3 shows representative responses from subject, S.H. investigated under the above conditions. It was seen that instead of a polarity inversion there was a clear latency difference for the upper and lower half responses. At low frequencies of stimulation (1.6 and 3.2 Hz) a surface positive wave was prominent with a peak latency of about 110–140 ms (indicated by arrows in the uppermost records of A and B) which varied with the conditions of the stimulus. The latency of this component was markedly shorter in the response to the lower half field than to the upper field as observed in the responses recorded from Oz where amplitudes were big enough to be estimated. In the steady-state responses to 6 Hz stimulation it was seen that the sinusoidal responses to stimulation of the lower half field were generally shifted in the direction of shorter latencies. Therefore, it is more acceptable to presume that the difference in waveform with stimulation of upper and lower field are merely due to a shortening of latency of the responses showing the same polarity as the upper field responses.

Clearly the peak latency difference between the upper and lower field responses became greater as the temporal frequency increased. The corresponding values were 10–14, 18–26 and 26–30 ms for 1.6, 3.2 and 6 Hz stimulation, respectively. This was due to the fact that on increasing the stimulus frequency the peak latency in the upper field response became longer, while that in the lower field response shortened. No essential difference was evident between our initial stimulus conditions (smaller check size, lower contrast) and those of Lehmann (larger checks, higher contrast). In fact, the data with the larger check size and higher contrast showed shorter peak latencies than those with the smaller check size and lower contrast.

DISCUSSION

In a previous study Adachi-Usami & Morita (1979) determined the VECP pattern reversal contrast sensitivity vs. temporal frequency for full field stimulation, showing a steep attenuation of sensitivity in the frequency range of 6–12 Hz. No signal could be detected with simulus frequencies exceeding 12 Hz, whereas a certain amount of attenuation was observed at low frequencies (cf. Sternheim & Cavonius 1972). A comparison of these VECP data with psychophysical De Lange curves has been made elsewhere (Adachi-Usami & Morita 1979).

Since a contrast level of around 20 per cent was suggested to be physiological (Spekreijse 1966; Adachi-Usami 1979), the present study also determined the VECP amplitude for various temporal frequencies at a constant contrast of 23 per cent. The resulting curve for lower half field stimulation showed a low frequency attenuation similar to results reported previously (Adachi-Usami & Morita 1979). No low frequency attenuation, however, was found for upper half field stimulation. Such temporal frequency properties of responses recorded at different electrode positions over the

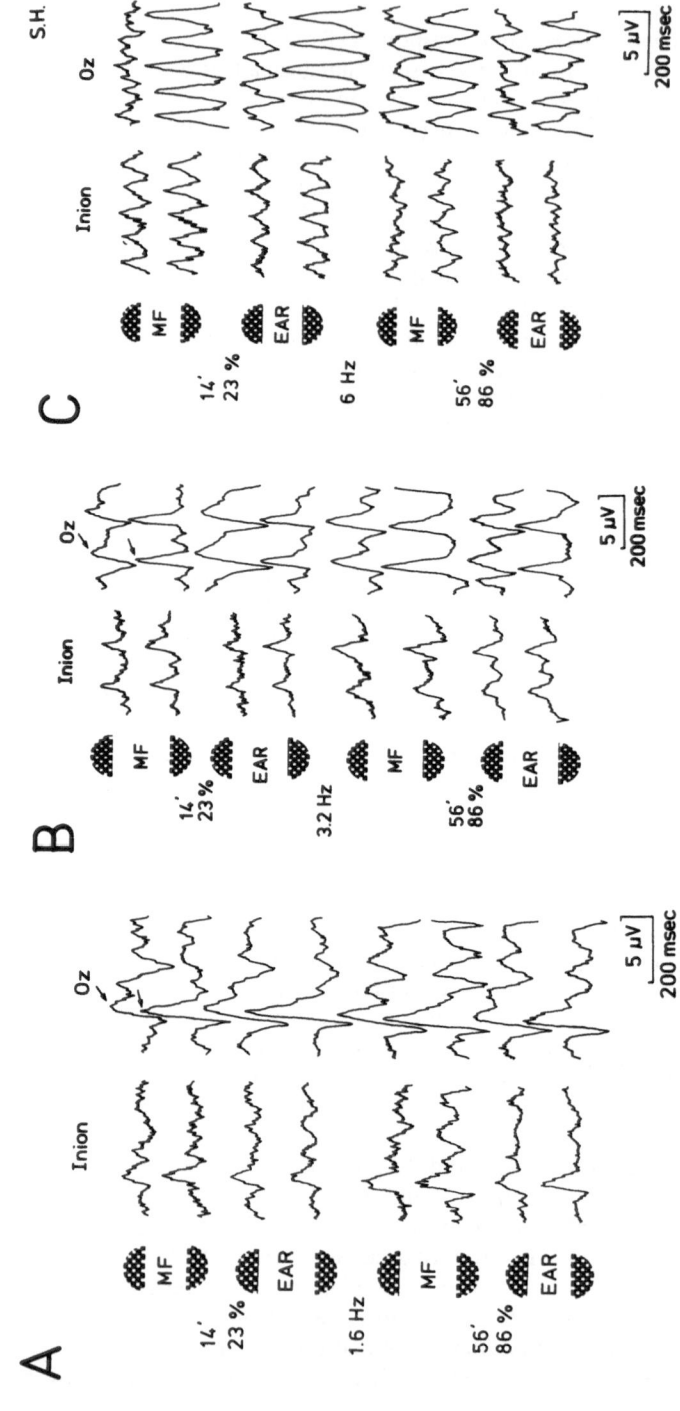

Fig. 3. VECPs to upper and lower half field pattern reversal stimuli of different temporal frequencies of 1.6 Hz (A), 3.2 Hz (B) and 6 Hz (C). Comparison of the responses to stimuli of small check size (14′) and low contrast (23%) with those of large check size (56′) and high contrast (86%). Monopolar recording from 2 different active electrode positions, reference electrode at the right earlobe (EAR) or at midfrontal position (MF). Stimulus field 15° in diameter, monocularly viewed from a distance of 127 cm.

midline of the scalp were found to be similar. It is, therefore, suggested that neurons responding to half field stimulation of frequencies greater than 4 Hz are similar in their temporal frequency behaviour, as far as pattern responses are concerned. It should be noted, however, that sensitivity differences at the same electrode position were clearly seen for responses to upper and lower half visual fields. This finding agrees with previous observations that the scalp distribution of responses to stimuli of the lower half field is highest at the posterior portion of the scalp, while the responses to the upper field are higher at the anterior portion (Jeffreys & Axford 1972; Michael & Halliday 1971; Lehmann & Skrandies 1979; Chiba & Adachi-Usami 1979).

This finding has been discussed by several authors using component analysis of pattern VECPs. For transient responses Halliday & Michael (1970) suggested reversal of polarity for a component wave with a peak latency of 100 ms for upper and lower half field stimulation which probably resulted from activation of two sets of neuronal elements in the extra-striate cortex. For pattern onset responses Jeffreys & Axford (1972) identified two distinct components of different peak latencies at 80 ms (CI) and 110 ms (CII) which were concluded to originate from the striate cortex and the extra-striate cortex, respectively.

The similarity of temporal frequency properties and the sensitivity differences between the upper and lower half field responses found in frequency ranges between 4 and 14 Hz suggests that the upper and lower field VECPs originate from neurons of similar temporal behaviour, situated in a different cortical area. It is most likely that the upper field responses originate from the extra-striate cortex and the lower field responses from neurons in the striate cortex. This speculation has an anatomical basis. The extra-striate cortex, particularly, the para-striate cortex where the lower retina (upper visual field) projects, locates anteriorly and deeply from the occipital pole, while the central half of the upper retina (lower visual field) projects to the striate cortex and to the part of the para-striate cortex which is closely located posteriorly and at the occipital pole. The finding of overall amplitude attenuation of responses to stimulation of the upper field indicates a more distant and deeper origin and a smaller number of neurons than for the responses of the lower half field.

Using the stimulus conditions of Lehmann et al. (1.6 Hz) (1977) the wave of peak latency 130 ms in response to lower field stimuli was delayed by 10–30 ms in the response to stimuli of the upper field, depending on the temporal frequency used. With higher temporal frequencies (3.2 Hz) the peak latency of response to the upper field became longer while that of the lower field became shorter. This is in contrast to Lehmann & Skrandies (1979) showing latency changes restricted to the responses of the upper field. Moreover, different phase characteristics in the two half fields for 6 Hz stimulation were shown in the present investigation. This allows the presumption that the origin of responses to stimuli of the upper and lower field are spatially different.

With regard to the suggestion of inverted polarity the present data support the description of Lehmann et al. (1977) of latency differences of components with constant polarity. However, we are still left with many questions with respect to waveform and site of origin of the upper and lower field responses.

REFERENCES

Adachi-Usami, E. Comparison of contrast thresholds of large bars and checks measured by VECPs and psychophysically as a function of defocusing. Albrecht v. Graefes Arch. klin. exp. Ophthal. 212: 1–9 (1979).

Adachi-Usami, E. & Morita, Y. Temporal contrast sensitivity characteristics of human vision as obtained by VECPs to checkerboard stimuli. In: 16th ISCEV Symposium (Ed. Tazawa) Jap. J. Ophthal. 249–257 (1979).

Chiba, J. & Adachi-Usami, E. Pattern reversal VECPs to stimulation of the upper and lower half field. Acta. Soc. Ophthal. Jap. 83: 2215–2224 (1979).

Chiba, Y., Chiba, J., Kuroda, N. & Adachi-Usami, E. Checkerboard pattern reversal VECP in humans hemispheric asymmetry, electrode position and half field stimulation. Folia. Ophthal. Jpn. 30: 669–673 (1979).

Halliday, A.M. & Michael, W.F. Pattern-evoked responses in man associated with the vertical and horizontal meridians of the visual field. J. Physiol. 208: 499–513 (1970).

Jeffreys, D.A. Cortical source locations of pattern-related visual evoked potentials recorded from the human scalp. Nature, 229: 502–504 (1971).

Jeffreys, D.A. & Axford, J.G. Source locations of pattern specific components of human visual evoked potentials. II. Component of extrastriate cortical origin. Exp. Brain Res. 16: 22–40 (1972).

Jeffreys, D.A. & Smith, A.T. The polarity inversion of scalp potentials evoked by upper and lower half field stimulus patterns: latency or surface distribution differences? Electroencephal. clin. Neurophysiol. 46: 409–415 (1979).

Lehmann, D., Meles, H.P. & Mir, Z. Average multichannel EEG potential fields evoked from upper and lower hemiretina: latency differences. Electroencephal. clin. Neurophysiol. 43: 725–731 (1977).

Lehmann, D. & Skrandies, W. Multichannel evoked potential field show different properties of human upper and lower hemiretina systems. Exp. Brain Res. 35: 151–159 (1979).

Lesèvre, N. & Joseph, J.P. Modifications of the pattern-evoked potential (PEP) in relation to the stimulated part of the visual field (clues for the most probable origin of each component) Electroencephal. clin. Neurophysiol., 47: 183–203 (1979).

Michael, W.F. & Halliday, A.M. Differences between the occipital distribution of upper and lower field pattern evoked responses in man. Brain Res. 32: 311–324 (1971).

Schreinemachers, H.P. & Henkes, H.E. Relation between located stimuli and the visual evoked response in man. Ophthalmologica 155: 17–27 (1968).

Spekreijse, H. Analysis of e. e. g. responses in man, evoked by sine wave modulated light. Junk, The Hague (1966).

Sternheim, C.E. & Cavonius, C.R. Sensitivity of the human ERG and VECPs to sinusoidally modulated light. Vis. Res. 12: 1685–1695 (1972).

Author's address:
Department of Ophthalmology
Chiba University School of Medicine
Inohana 1-8-1
280 Chiba
Japan

VISUALLY EVOKED CORTICAL POTENTIALS TO HALF-FIELD STIMULATION IN NORMALS AND AMBLYOPES

K. YANASHIMA & B. DEGERING

(Frankfurt/M. and Bad Nauheim, F.R.G.)

ABSTRACT

In order to localize defects in the human visual system by evoked cortical potentials half-field patterned stimuli were applied to compare the projection of the macula in normals and amblyopes by latency measurement. Steady-state conditions were chosen for stimulation of the temporal and nasal half-fields with and without occluding a 3° central retinal field. With *retino-temporal* half-field stimulation the EP amplitude recorded from the *contralateral* visual cortex was larger and the latency was shorter than at the ipsilateral visual cortex. With *retino-nasal* half-field stimulation the EP amplitude recorded from the *ipsilateral* visual cortex was larger and the latency was shorter than at the contralateral visual cortex. In all normal subjects investigated stimulation of the retino-temporal half-field led to larger cortical responses at both hemispheres than stimulation of the retino-nasal half-fields.

INTRODUCTION

The cortical projection of both hemi-retinas and the bilateral representation of the macula region has previously been investigated by recording visually evoked cortical potentials (VECP) from different positions of the human scalp. Authors generally agree that pattern reversal stimulation permits separation of the responses from both hemispheres (Cobb & Morton 1970). Blumhardt et al. (1977) and other investigators tried to apply this observation to the evaluation of visual field defects (Wildberger, Van Lith, Wijngaarde & Mak 1976; Blumhardt, Barrett & Halliday 1977). However, in order to achieve the biggest advantage for diagnosis, we feel that statistical evaluation of VECP parameters is needed and is more promising than case reports. To do this more than 60 responses were evaluated by means of Fast Fourier Transform (F.F.T., Cooly & Tukey 1965) and by latency as well as amplitude histograms. The procedure led us to results of small redundancy, i.e., big reliability.

Doc. Ophthal. Proc. Series, Vol. 27, ed. by H. Spekreijse & P.A. Apkarian   375

© 1981 Dr W. Junk Publishers, The Hague/Boston/London

After stimulation of the temporal hemi-retina the VECP amplitude was previously shown to be bigger on the contralateral occipital lobe and smaller on the ipsilateral lobe, whereas after stimulation of the nasal hemi-retina the VECP amplitude was bigger on the ipsilateral hemisphere. This discrepancy between the anatomical projection of visual nerve fibers and electrophysiological findings has been called lateralization of the VECP but is typically reported mainly in terms of VECP amplitude and not latency.

The following report should be regarded as an attempt to explore, in normals and amblyopes, the projection from the retina to brain by measurement of the changes in latency after stimulating the nasal and temporal half retina.

METHODS

Visually evoked cortical responses were recorded and averaged (n = 48) from 10 healthy individuals (age 20 to 34 years) and 5 strabismic amblyopes (age 18 to 27 years). Three of the amblyopes were exotropic, two were esotropic. Visual acuity ranged from 0.3 to 0.6 with fully corrected glasses; the angle of deviation ranged from $3°$ to $10°$.

The electrodes were placed on O_1, O_2 and referred to F_P, according to the international 10–20 electrode convention. The right ear lobe was connected to the ground. A black and white checkerboard pattern, presented on a TV-screen, was masked to produce a full $(12°)$ or half-field with or without occluding a center field of $3°$. The subject was seated at a fixed distance (1 m) in front of the TV; vision was optically corrected by glasses. The rate of reversal of the pattern presented was 12 Hz, the contrast ratio of the brighter and darker checks was 32 per cent. Each square of the checkerboard subtended an angle of 34 min of arc. The mean luminance of the TV-screen was 0.86 log ft. Lambert. Recording and evaluation was done by means of a PDP 11/40 computer. A sweep time of 5120 ms was employed to calculate the F.F.T. and the autopower-spectrum. The power spectrum was smoothed by the use of the Hanning window function. The latency was calculated by using the following formula: latency (ms) = one trigger interval (ms) + duration from trigger to peak (ms).

RESULTS

The plots shown in Fig. 1 illustrate the VECP findings in normals and amblyopes, exposing the nasal and temporal hemi-retina to checkerboard stimulation. The findings are in general agreement with the observation of Barret et al. (1976) and Beauchamps et al. (1976) and support the notation of a paradoxical lateralization of the VECP, i.e., the amplitude of the evoked cortical potential upon stimulation of one half of the retina is bigger on that lobe of brain where fibers do not project anatomically. In amblyopes (open circles in Fig. 1) this phenomenon is even more striking. In respect to the latencies measured, the present results indicate a more frequent occurrance

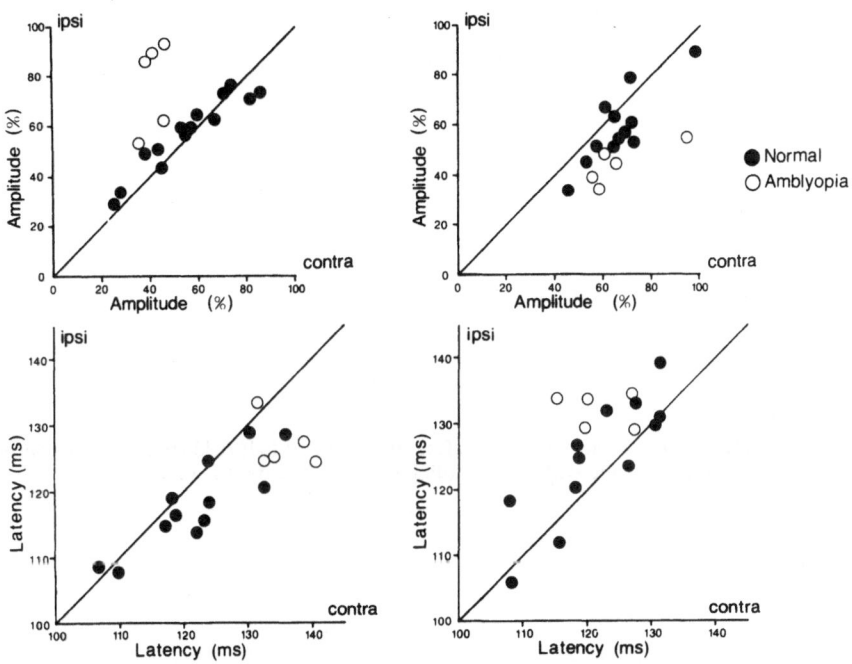

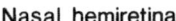

Fig. 1. Relative amplitudes (above) and absolute latencies of VECPs (below) recorded on ipsi- and contralateral hemispheres after retinal half-field stimulation in normals and amblyopes. Amplitudes (in per cent) were calculated as the amplitude of half-field stimulation/the amplitude of full-field stimulation.

of earlier responses on that lobe of the visual brain where bigger amplitudes were recorded.

Fig. 2 demonstrates more in detail the relation between the absolute latencies of the VECP in normals and amblyopes after full-field and half-field stimulation. It shows that the paradoxical lateralization of the VECP is present not only in amplitude but also in latency. Fig. 2 also shows that with occluding the center (dashed columns) all latencies became longer, without affecting the phenomenon of lateralization. Fig. 3 shows the different contribution of the nasal and temporal retina to the VECP amplitude. In all normal subjects investigated the VECP amplitude was bigger after stimulation of the temporal half-field of the retina than of the nasal hemi-retina.

DISCUSSION

Comparing the VECP in response to retinal half-field stimulation longer latencies were observed after occluding the center. This may be caused by

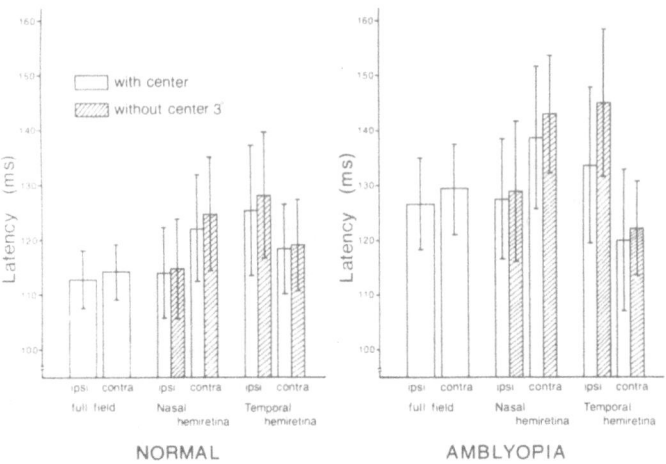

Fig. 2. Measured latencies of VECPs after full-field and half-field stimulation in normals and amblyopes with and without occluding the retinal center (3° in diameter).

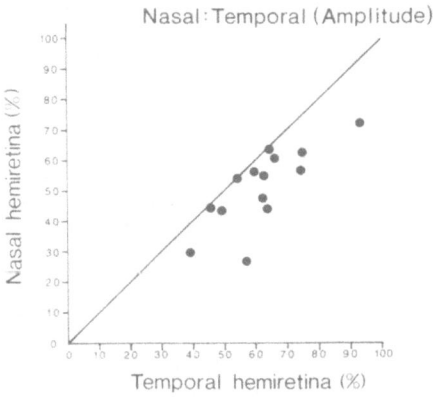

Fig. 3. Comparison of VECP amplitudes evoked by nasal and temporal retinal half-field stimulation in normals.

the omission of the faster conducting macula fibers of the visual pathway. In amblyopes the latencies in response to half-field stimulation were even longer than in normals which points to the functional failure of the central retinal area in amblyopes. With retino-temporal half-field stimulation the latency of response as measured at the contralateral lobe of the visual brain is shorter than at the ipsilateral lobe which indicates that the retinal fiber connections of the peripheral field may suppress the visual brain cells connected to nerve fibers of the retinal center. In amblyopes this suppression may be even stronger than in normals.

Retino-nasal half-field stimulation leads to shorter latencies of VECP than retino-temporal stimulation which may be attributed to the longer interocular distance of unmedullated nerve fibers serving the temporal retina.

From the differences in VECP amplitude and latency after stimulating the nasal and temporal retinal half-field we conclude the presence of two separate nerve fibers systems converging to the visual brain. Such a suggestion is also supported by cybernetics. According to Braitenberg (1965) the projection of the temporal hemi-retina to the occipital lobe is younger in evolution than the projection of crossed fibers from the nasal hemiretina. Following Braitenberg the advantage of the new uncrossed nerve fiber projection from the temporal hemi-retina would be a more flexible reaction to visual stimuli of the outside world.

In order to extract more detailed information out of the VECP records appropriate stimulus conditions like half-field stimulation are advantageous, and evaluation procedures by using computers should be improved. We feel that the frequency analysis methods used in this study for data evaluation permit extraction of more information out of the VECP especially for the clinical Ophthalmologist.

REFERENCES

Barret, G., Blumhardt, L., Halliday, A.M. Halliday, E. & Kriss, A. A paradox in the lateralization of the visual evoked response. Nature 261: 253–255 (1976).

Blumhardt, L.D., Barret, G. & Halliday, A.M. The asymmetrical visual evoked potential to pattern reversal in one half field and its significance for the analysis of visual field defects. Br. J. Ophthal. 61: 454–461 (1977).

Braitenberg, V. Taxis, Kinesis and Decussation. Progr. Brain Res. 17: 210–222 (1965).

Bunt, A.H., Minckler, D.S. & Johanson, G.W. Demonstration of bilateral projection of the central retina of the monkey with horseradish peroxidase neurography. J. Comp. Neurol. 171: 619–630 (1977).

Cobb, W.A. & Morton, H.B. Evoked potentials from the human scalp to visual half-field stimulation. J. Physiol. 208: p 39–40 (1970).

Cooly, J.W. & Tukey, J.W. An algorithm for the machine calculation of complex Fourier series. Math. Comp. 19: 297–301 (1965).

Wildberger, H.G.H., Van Lith, G.H.M., Wijngaarde, R. & Mak, G.T.M. Visually evoked cortical potentials in the evaluation of homonymous and bitemporal visual field defects. Br. J. Ophthal. 60: 273 (1976).

Authors' address:
Dr. K. Yanashima
MPI für Physiol. und Klin. Forschung
W.G. Kerckhoff – Institut
Parkstr. 1
D-6350 Bad Nauheim, F.R.G.

B. Degering
Augenklinik
Zentralkrankenhaus
St. Jürgenstrasse
D-2800 Bremen, F.R.G.

379

PROPERTIES OF FOVEAL PATTERN STIMULI WHICH DETERMINE THE MORPHOLOGY AND SCALP DISTRIBUTION OF VISUAL EVOKED POTENTIALS

N. DRASDO

(Birmingham, England)

ABSTRACT

A foveal stimulus field with an adapting surround is used to present luminance compensated pattern stimuli. The signals derived from electrodes placed to sample schematic striate and pre-striate foveal projections show noticeable differences in morphology with expected inter-individual variations (Drasdo 1980), but the consistency of form of the signal elicited by any specified pattern for one individual is remarkable. A series of effective patterns which have been selected by empirical observation have been examined to demonstrate their main spatial frequency components. Other patterns generated to include known spatial frequencies in one or many meridians have been compared in an attempt to identify the most effective stimuli for clinical purposes and to relate the observed phenomena to hypothetical mechanisms in the generation of the visual evoked potential.

INTRODUCTION

Cortical potentials evoked by pattern presentation, in the absence of mean luminance fluctuations, are dependent on many stimulus variables. Authorative reports have been given by Spekreijse, Estévez & Reits (1977), Spekreijse (1980), Jeffreys (1977; 1980) and Kulikowski (1977). The nomenclature proposed by Jeffreys for pattern onset components has won wide acceptance, but some doubts have been expressed on the suggestion that CI, the first major positive component, originates necessarily in the striate cortex (Leserve & Joseph 1980; Drasdo 1980).

Assembled and experimental evidence was presented by Drasdo (1980) to support the view that a lateral line of electrodes 5% above the inion and at 10% intervals could directly sample the average projections of a foveal stimulus in the striate and circumstriate areas. (These are percentages of vertical and horizontal inion-nasion distances). The relatively uniform properties of foveal vision were considered advantageous for analytical studies and produced highly defined signals, but considerable individual

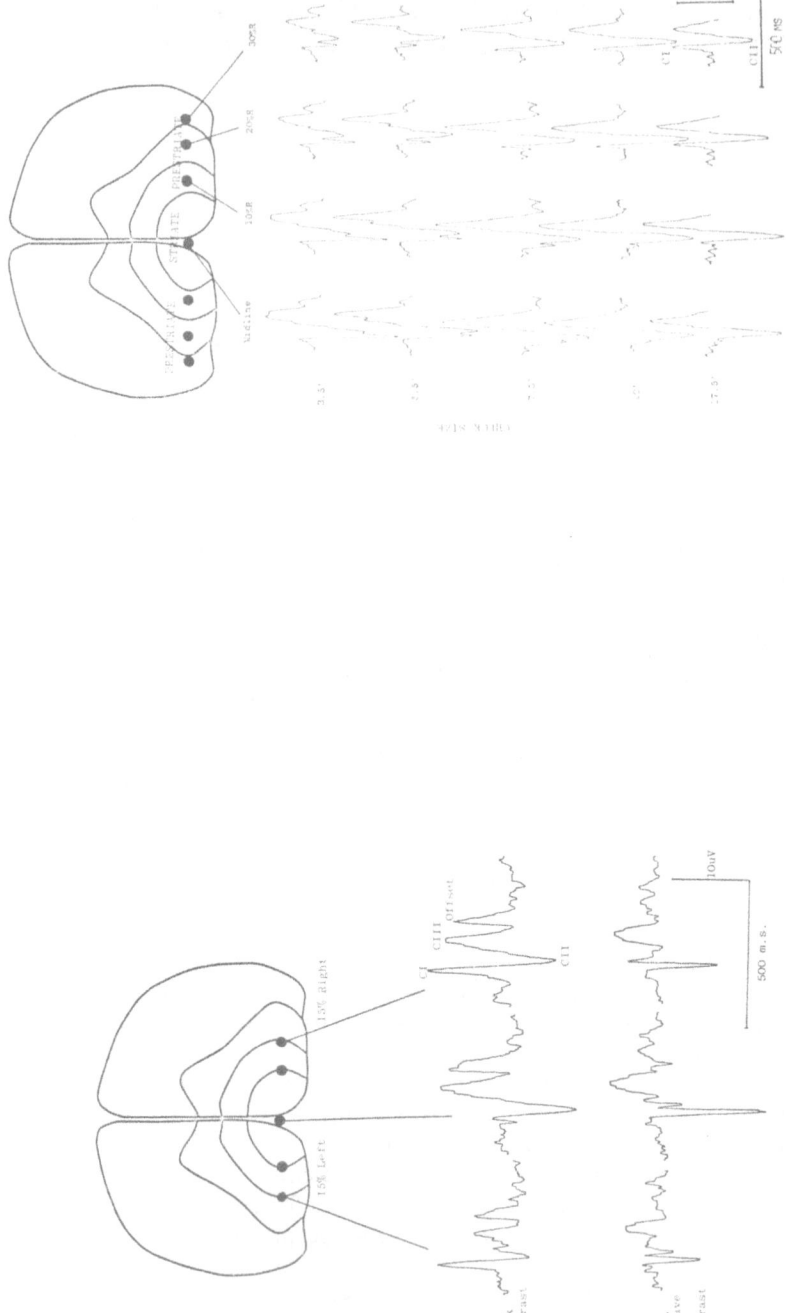

Fig. 1. a) The CI component elicited by a 14 minute checkerboard is maximal on electrodes corresponding to the pre-striate areas, whereas the steep negative transient elicited in many subjects by a 14 cycle per degree square wave grating is maximal on the mid-line electrode corresponding to the striate area. This negative transient appears to be the leading edge of the CII component, often concealed by an overlapping CI as shown in b) in which the relative positions of CI and CII are changed by the electrode position and the check size of the stimulus. CI, CII and CIII are in the conventional positions with large checks and laterally placed electrodes (lower right).

variation occurred, perhaps reflecting underlying striate and prestriate projections. CII, the major negative component, was usually found to be maximal on the mid-line electrode and CI was more predominant on the electrodes corresponding to the average positions of areas 18 and 19 (Fig. 1a, b). It was also shown that CI appeared to move independently across CII when changing the dimensions of the stimulus details or when recording from different electrodes (Fig. 1b).

Jeffreys has reported less temporal overlap between CI and CII but emphasised that the components must be separated for analytical study (Jeffreys 1980). Spekreijse and Jeffreys have shown that whereas CI responds primarily to luminance, CII is primarily responsive to pattern. However, the variable of pattern structure produces innumerable possibilities so that empirical exploration is unattractive. It seems appropriate to reconsider in principle what the nature of the ideal pattern stimuli might be.

Many neurones in the visual cortex respond maximally to a pattern stimulus with a specific orientation and spatial frequency. DeValois (1977) characterised these responses in a polar-plot resembling a 2-dimensional Fourier transform (Fig. 2a).

We could imagine that if the receptive fields of all the foveally projected neurones in a human were plotted on such a diagram, the majority would probably be concentrated between about 3 and 20 cycles per degree. These arbitrary estimates receive some support from the fact that such responses have been recorded in primates (Poggio, Doty & Talbot 1977), and contrast sensitivity at the fovea in humans peaks at about 8 to 12 cycles per degree (Koenderink, Bouman, Bueno de Mesquita & Slappendel 1978; Sjostrand 1978).

This distribution of neurons would correspond to an annular region on the polar plot, but the existence of the oblique effect renders high spatial frequencies ineffective at oblique angles (Campbell, Kulikowski & Levinson 1966) so the polar plot would be deficient in neurones in the outer regions along oblique axes. The neurones which correspond to low spatial frequencies would be more centrally located and would have lower contrast thresholds (Fig. 2b). It seems clear that this hypothetical plot of cortical neurone receptive field properties approximately determines the 2-dimensional Fourier transform of the optimal pattern stimulus, which would excite the maximum number of neurones. Evidently, therefore, we should examine the Fourier components of various patterns in conjunction with the evoked potentials which they produce.

Optical Fourier transforms of patterns can be obtained by Fraunhoffer diffraction (Lipson 1972) or non-coherent optics (Rogers 1979). The procedure is, however, fairly time consuming and after studying the latter method it seemed that use might be made of superimposed optical zone plates for rapid detection of the components of many patterns by visual inspection.

The moire fringes instantly identified the orientations and spatial frequencies. The phase and amplitude of the components could be roughly assessed. The spatial frequency is linearly arranged, so the moire pattern nodes directly represented the Fourier transforms. (Fig. 3).

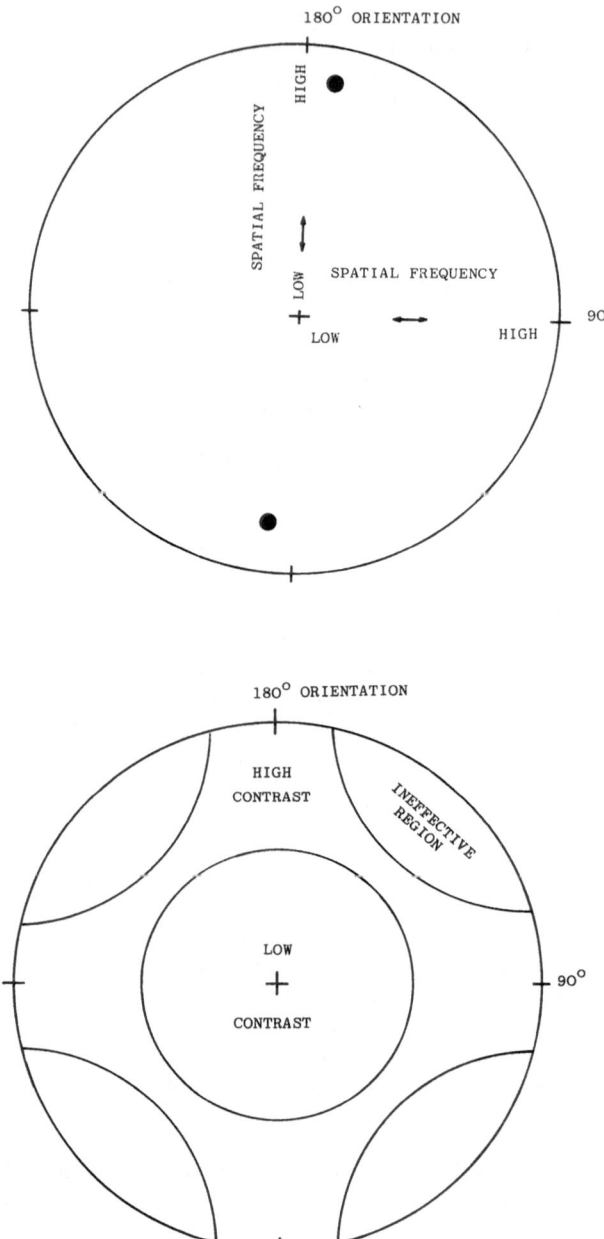

Fig. 2. a) Hypothetical plot of spatial frequency and orientation characteristics of neurones (after DeValois). the discs represent the orientation (170°) and spatial frequency (high) of a neurone.
b) Scheme for Fourier transforms of optimal visual stimulus, outlines the frequency space which would excite the maximum number of spatially tuned neurones.

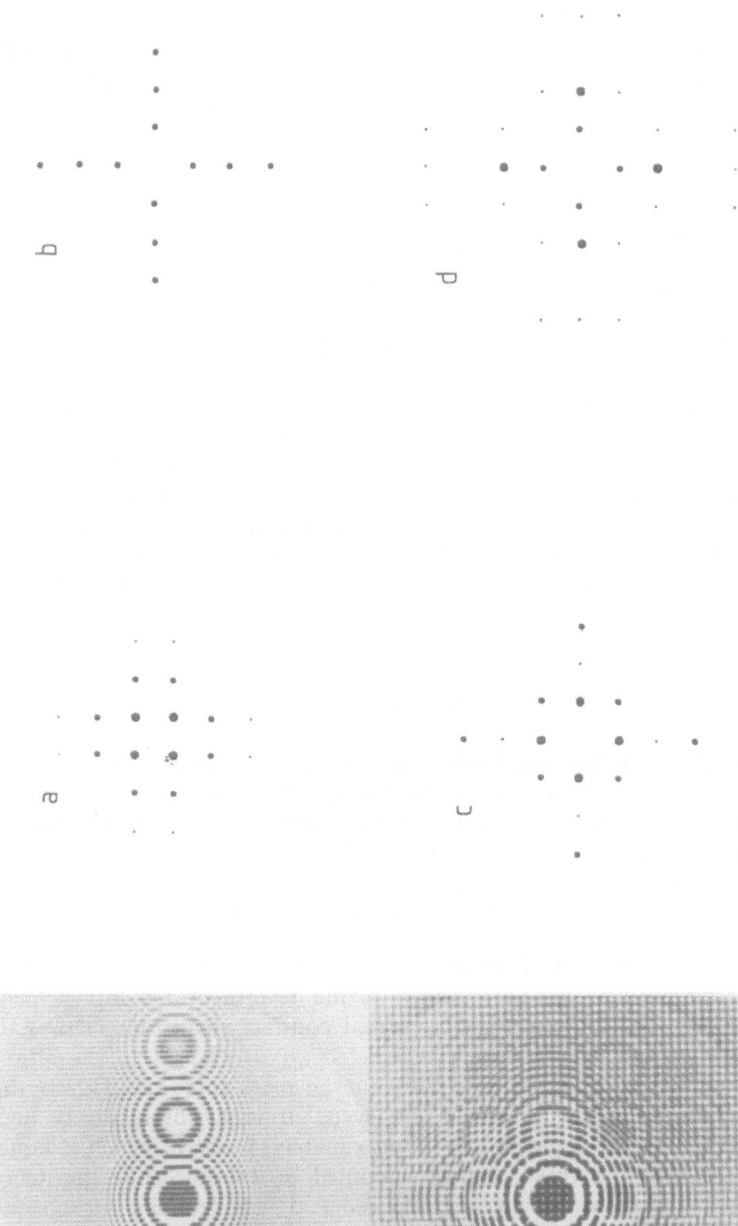

Fig. 3. Fourier transforms produced by optical zone plate. The Moiré patterns show that that the asymmetric rectangular wave (upper left) has a high amplitude second harmonic, and the complicated transform of a polka dot pattern is revealed (lower left). The schematic examples roughly portray the transforms of the patterns discussed: a) checkerboard; b) grid; c) isolated squares; d) outlines. The dot size represents the subjectively judged magnitude of the most significant components.

Another method of identifying the spatial frequencies of a pattern is to synthesize it from known components by photographic summation or spatial filtering. Only the first method has so far been used in this study. Photographic emulsion gives a non-linear response and an elaborate technique was required to produce sine waves of high contrast and fidelity.

METHODS AND MATERIALS

Selected patterns were presented by means of a projector with a diffusing shutter which provided luminance compensated stimuli (Drasdo 1976). The duration of exposure was normally retained at 150 milliseconds to separate the 'on' and 'off' components. All recordings were made with mid-frontal reference, right ear and active electrodes designed to sample the striate and circumstriate projections of a $3°$ foveal stimulus fixated at $0.5°$ above the centre (Drasdo 1980). The mean luminance of the stimulus was $600 \, cd/m^2$; the surround luminance was $50 \, cd/m^2$. The stimulus was presented 64 times at an average interval of 550 milliseconds. The results were recorded positive upwards using a time constant of 0.3 seconds and a 50 Hz filter with a 4 channel averager. A pre-stimulus delay of 25 ms. was used.

RESULTS

The Fourier transforms and evoked potentials from many pattern stimuli have been inspected. Using sine wave gratings the VEP recorded from the midline electrode usually has a prominent negative feature which changes latency according to spatial frequency and contrast (Kulikowski 1977). Adding the same spatial frequency in several meridians produced only slight differences (Fig. 4a & b) and single square waves and sine waves produced similar results. The checkerboard has a complicated transform which could be related to the larger VEP signal which it produces. The high frequencies have low amplitudes, however, which is the reverse of the arrangement shown in Fig. 2b, and the high integrated contrast change emphasises CI which detracts from a clearly defined CII.

Asymmetric rectangular waves (with uneven mark space ratios) have the advantage of producing both odd and even harmonics of relatively high amplitude. These are separated by approximately 1 octave which is equal to the bandwidth of a visual channel (Campbell & Robson 1968). Inevitably the integrated contrast change is also reduced, which would favour the isolation of CII. The Fourier components of a rectangular grid can be deduced from this and these are seen to approximate those of the hypothetical model (Fig. 2 & 3) having high energy, high frequency components along the vertical and horizontal meridians. Such patterns have previously been shown to be related to the CII component of the VEP (Jeffreys 1977; Spekreijse 1980), and have been found to be the most effective pattern for augmenting a flash stimulus in photosensitive epilepsy (Jeavons, Harding,

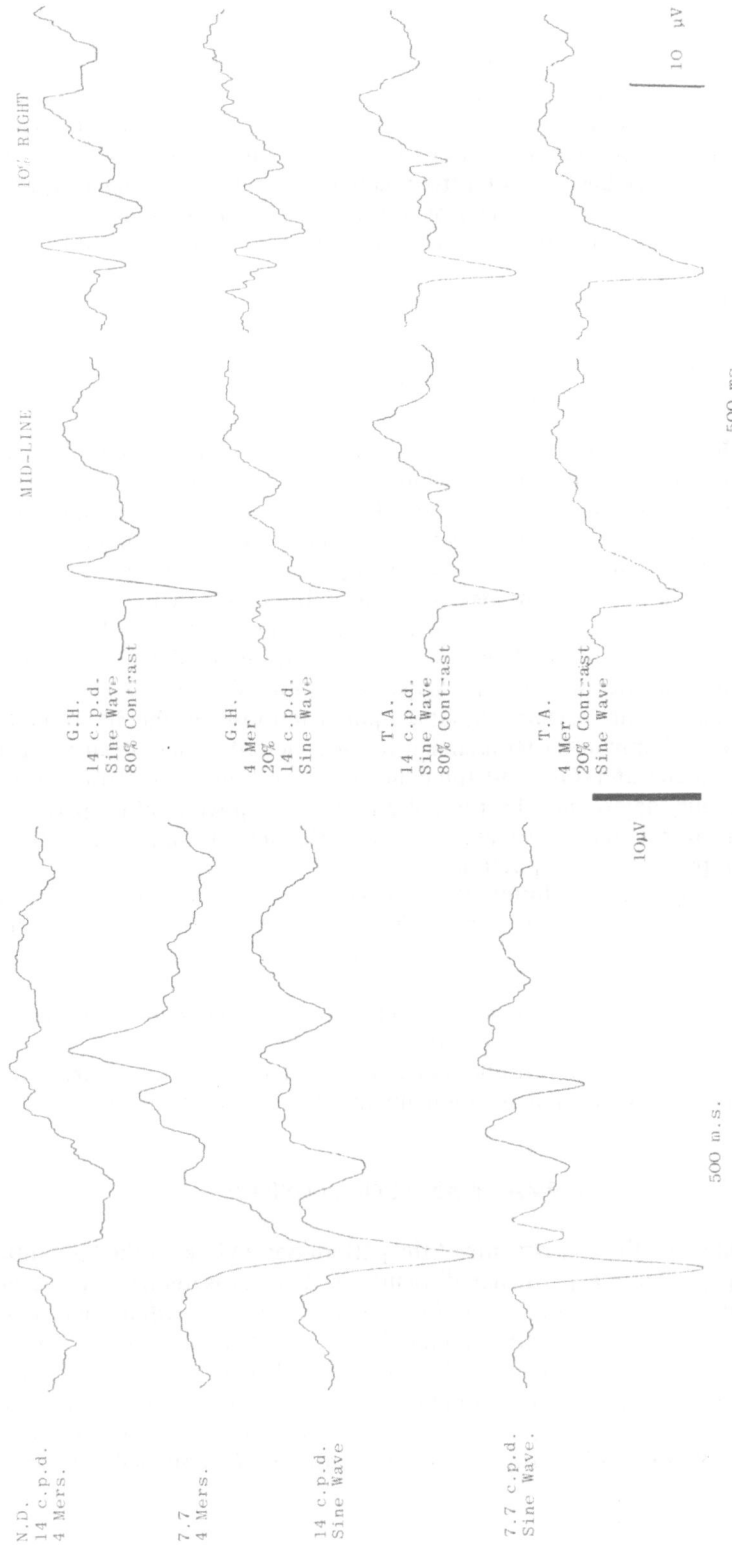

387

Fig. 4. a, b. Sinusoidal gratings with four combined orientations (4 mers) tend to produce a broader CII than single vertical gratings. This may be difficult to demonstrate with higher spatial frequencies due to the lower amplitude in the combined gratings (Fig. 4a. Subject ND 14 cycles per degree). Note: Subject TA has the maximal CII displaced from the mid-line which is slightly atypical.

Panayiotopoulos & Drasdo 1972). The grid with a 10:1 ratio gives a clear CII (Fig. 5), but the pattern has few components in oblique directions. To introduce these the lines can be widened. The result is similar to the isolated square pattern reported by Jeffreys (1977) to elicit large VEPs, but this produces considerable CI and off-set activity due to its higher integrated contrast change. However, the isolated square outline pattern devised by Jeffreys to adapt contour detectors seems to approach the desired arrangement of spatial frequencies without undue contrast effects, so that the CII component is more effectively isolated.

DISCUSSION

Due to the large number of variables in pattern stimuli, and the character of the responses, studies of individuals are a justifiable method, though care must obviously be taken in relating these to others. With the appropriate modes of stimulation it seems possible that the individual differences in the occipital region can be related more directly to variations in the underlying projections. The transient inputs coinciding with the expected position of the prestriate areas are also of particular interest. With subjects who show a clear CII component on the midline electrode, an obvious tendency is observed for CII to become broader and larger and more defined as the Fourier components of the pattern stimulus approach those of the hypothetical model Fig. 5. Stimulus patterns similar to those described have been reported elsewhere in the literature, but the concept of the Fourier transform of the ideal stimulus, determined by the polar plot of receptive field properties of cortical neurones seems valuable for the selection of new experimental stimuli for pattern evoked potentials.

The fact that the amplitude of the signal does not increase in proportion to the number of wave components in the pattern is not surprising, since these would vary in latency according to the spatial frequency and there might be electrical and neurological reasons why they should not summate directly. On the other hand some increase in amplitude and a considerable extension of the negativity of CII seems to be associated with patterns satisfying these complex criteria and it is hoped that the ideas mentioned in this paper can be pursued in a more quantitative way in the future.

SUMMARY AND CONCLUSIONS

The tendency of the components of the pattern onset visual evoked potential to overlap produces a particular difficulty in their measurement. It appears that the relationship changes with different stimuli and recording conditions. The structure of the pattern stimulus is an important determinant of the morphology of the CII component. It is proposed that the two-dimensional Fourier transform of the ideal stimulus for CII may be deduced from neurophysiological and psychophysical data. When this has been approximately identified, Fourier transforms of various patterns are obtained by use of

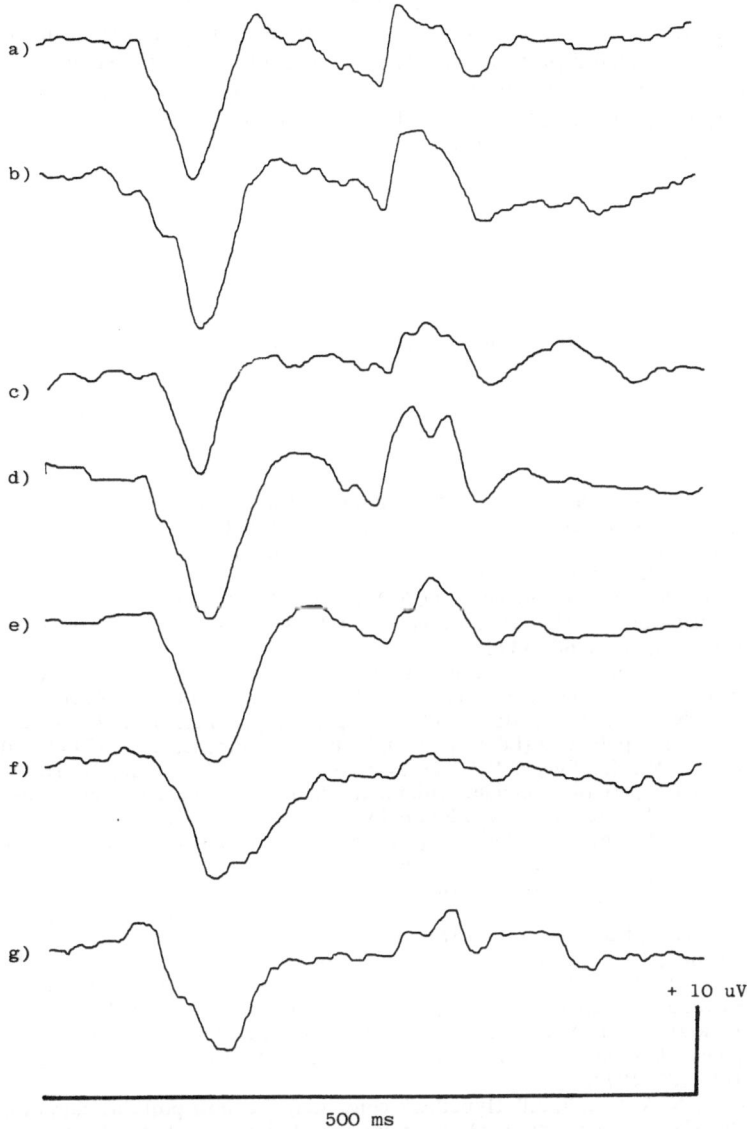

Fig. 5. Potentials evoked by patterns with complicated Fourier transforms (mid-line electrodes 90% contrast).
a) Rectangular Grid, 1′ white line, 12′ black squares.
b) 2 grids as in a) combined 45°.
c) Negative of a).
d) Isolated squares, 10′ white square, 10′ black space.
e) 1′ outline of 10′ square with 10′ space.
f) Negative of above.
g) Polka-dot rectangular matrix 2′ white dot, 10′ intercentre separation.

optical zone plates. Pattern onset VEPs to a 3° field have been recorded with electrodes situated over the average positions of foveal cortical projections. Using the selected patterns the clarity and amplitude of the signals, and other corresponding results in the literature appear to support the value of the hypothesis, and it seems likely that new and more effective pattern stimuli may be identified by use of these methods.

ACKNOWLEDGEMENTS

The author is indebted to Professor G.L. Rogers of the Physics Department, University of Aston for the loan of a zone plate and for useful discussion.

REFERENCES

Campbell, F.W., Kulikowski, J.J. & Levinson, J. The effect of orientation of the visual resolution of gratings. J. Physiol. 187: 427–436 (1966).

Campbell, F.W. & Robson, J.G. Application of fourier analysis to the visibility of gratings. J. Phyisol. 197: 551–556 (1968).

DeValois, R.L. Spatial tuning of LGN and cortical cells in monkey visual system. In: Spatial Contrast (Ed. H. Spedreijse & L.H. Van der Tweel). North Holland Pub. Co., Amsterdam. 60–63 (1977).

Drasdo, N. A method of eliciting pattern specific responses and other electrophysiological signlas in human subjects. Br. J. Physiol. Opt. 31: 14–22 (1976).

Drasdo, N. Cortical potentials evoked by pattern presentation in the foveal region. In: Evoked potentials (Ed. C. Barber). MTP Press, Lancaster. 167–174 (1980).

Jeavons, P.M., Harding, G.F.A., Panayiotopoulos, C.P. & Drasdo, N. The effect of geometric patterns combined with intermittent photic stimulation on photo-sensitive epilepsy. Electroenceph. clin. Neurophysiol. 33: 221–224 (1972).

Jeffreys, D.A. The physiological significance of pattern visual evoked potentials. In: Visual evoked potential in man: new developments. (Ed. J.E. Desmedt). Clarendon Press, Oxford. 134–167 (1977).

Jeffreys, D.A. The nature of pattern VEPs. In: Evoked potentials (Ed. C. Barber). MTP Press, Lancaster. 149–157 (1980).

Koenderink, J.J., Bouman, M.A., Bueno de Mesquita, A.E. & Slappendel, S. Perimetry contrast detection thresholds of moving spatial sine wave patterns. III. The target extent as a sensitivity controlling parameter. J. Opt. Soc. Am. 68: 854–860 (1978).

Kulikowski, J. Visual evoked potentials as a measure of visibility. In: Visual evoked potentials in man: new developments (Ed. J.E. Desmedt) Clarendon Press, Oxford. 168–183 (1977).

LeServe, N. & Joseph, J.P. Hypothesis concerning the most probable sites of origin of the various components of the pattern evoked potential. In: Evoked potentials (Ed. C. Barber). MTP Press, Lancaster. 159–166 (1980).

Lipson, H. Optical Transforms. Academic Press, London (1972).

Poggio, G.F. Doty, R.W. Jr. & Talbot, W.H. Foveal striate cortex of behaving monkeys, single neurone responses to square wave gratings during fixation of gaze. J. Neurophysiol. 40: 1369–1391 (1977).

Rogers, G.L. Non-coherent optical processing. Wiley, New York. (1977).

Sjöstrand, M.D. Contrast sensitivity in amblyopia; A preliminary report. Met. Ophthal. 2: 135–137 (1978).

Spekreijse, H., Estevez, O. & Reits, D. Visual evoked potentials and the physiological analysis of visual processes in man. In: Visual evoked potentials in man: new developments (Ed. J.E. Desmedt). Clarendon Press, Oxford. 16–89 (1977).

Spekreijse, H. Pattern evoked potentials: principles methodology and phenomenology. In: Evoked potentials (Ed. C. Barber). MTP Press, Lancaster. 55–74 (1980).

Authors' address:
Clinical Neurophysiology Unit,
Department of Ophthalmic Optics
University of Aston in Birmingham,
Birmingham, England.

THE CONTRAST ORIGIN OF PATTERN EPs
IN AWAKE RHESUS MONKEYS

H. VAN DER MAREL, G. DAGNELIE & H. SPEKREIJSE

(*Amsterdam, The Netherlands*)

ABSTRACT

Considering the close correspondence to man in cortical architecture rhesus monkeys seem to be a good experimental model for localizing the sources of the various components in the contrast EP. Previous studies have shown, however, that contrast specific EPs cannot be recorded in the monkey under conditions of nembutal anaesthesia. To record under awake conditions, therefore, four rhesus monkeys were trained to fixate a TV-screen on which checkerboard patterns of various sizes and contrasts could be presented. Simultaneous half-field stimulation was employed to establish the quality of fixation and the topological representation of the responses. Pattern evoked potentials which could be distinguished from those evoked by luminance variations were obtained. In the monkey, these contrast-specific responses proved to have an outspoken contralateral representation.

INTRODUCTION

In man checkerboard patterns elicit a visually evoked cortical potential essentially different from that to stimulation with homogenous illuminated fields (Spehlman 1965; Spekreijse 1966). the difference can be deduced from the fact that the appearance and disappearance of a pattern generate differently shaped evoked potentials (EPs), although from a luminance point of view the onset of the pattern cannot be distinguished from the pattern offset. Thus, if luminance is the prime parameter, identical responses would be expected to both pattern on- and offset (Spekreijse & Estévez 1972). Of the two response types, the pattern onset response has been studied more extensively. In the positive-negative-positive (PNP) complex of this response, three components can be distinguished on the basis of topological representation. The first positive component (denoted CI) is generally accepted to have a striate origin, whereas the two other components (the negative CII and the positive CIII) are assumed to be of extrastriate origin (Jeffreys & Axford 1972a, b). Thus far the neuronal bases of these components have not been established. Such a search has to be carried out with invasive recording techniques. The rhesus monkey (*Macaca mulatta*) seems to be a suitable animal for these experiments because of its highly developed visual system and the resemblance with the human visual cortex. In a previous study (Padmos, Haaijman & Spekreijse 1973) an attempt was made to determine with conventional scalp recordings whether the rhesus monkey has contrast and luminance responses as found in man. The study was undertaken in animals anaesthetized with nembutal. Under these conditions no genuine contrast evoked potentials could be detected. The responses to both pattern on- and offset had the same shape. Furthermore, they could not be distinguished from the responses evoked by pure luminance stimulation. From these findings it was concluded that no contrast EPs could be recorded in anaesthetized monkeys.

Additional reports about contrast responses in awake monkeys (Doddington 1972; Lieb & Karmel 1974; Perryman & Lindsley 1977; Short, Lieb & Wilson 1977) are ambiguous as the contrast stimuli used were presented under stimulus flash conditions. Spekreijse et al. (1973) demonstrated that in man a flashed-on pattern does not generate a contrast EP but rather an enhanced luminance EP. Thus, the presence of an EP to a patterned flash may not be conclusive about the luminance or contrast origin of the response.

We therefore decided in our search for contrast EPs in the monkey to use a) awake animals that were trained to fixate and accommodate at the screen on which the patterns were presented and b) pattern presentations without overall changes in mean luminance level.

METHODS AND MATERIALS

Stimulus

Both the pattern and luminance stimuli were generated on a TV-screen subtending 9° by 12° of visual angle with a mean luminance of $63 \, cd/m^2$. In the middle of the screen was positioned a red light emitting diode (LED) subtending 6 min of arc which the monkey was required to fixate. The monkeys were seated at a distance of 1.7 m from the screen. Pattern stimulation consisted of abruptly appearing and disappearing checkerboard and bar patterns at a constant mean luminance level. Luminance stimulation consisted of a stepwise increase and decrease of the whole field luminance, having the same time profile as the pattern on- and offset stimuli. The pattern onset-offset rate was low to avoid contamination of the appearance responses by the disappearance responses. Simultaneous left and right half field pattern stimulation was employed to check for fixation quality and to study topological representation.

Animal training

The training of the monkeys (3–5.5 kg *Macaca mulatta* with normal visual acuity) starts with the presentation of a 350 Hz tone for half a second. This tone is followed after 1–8 sec at random by a 2 second-brightness increase of a red LED subtending 6 min of arc. As long as the LED is on, the monkey, seated in a primate chair, can depress a handle bar and each time it does so, 0.25 cc of apple juice is delivered through a tube located in the proximity of its mouth. After a random period of 5 to 10 sec this sequence is repeated. If, however, the response key is depressed when the LED is not on, it takes longer for the next sequence to start again. The monkeys were regarded suitably trained for the experimental sessions when an 85% correct response level was obtained.

Recording

The EPs were recorded with tinned/copper cup electrodes of 3.5 or 5 mm diameter attached to the scalp with collodion. The electrode placements are indicated in the figures; the reference electrode was always placed on the vertex. The bandwidth of the EEG amplifiers was 1.6 Hz to 35 Hz. The high cut-off frequency was set by a fourth-order Butterworth filter, which introduces an increase of the peak latency in the recording of 14 msec. The filtered signals were averaged with an HP 2100 computer and displayed in real time. Usually 64 to 128 averages were sufficient to obtain a clear response. The criterion for this was set by the experimenter's judgement. Positivity of the response is depicted upwards in the figures. The human EPs presented for comparison are derived from a female subject, 25 years old, in good health and with normal visual acuity.

RESULTS AND DISCUSSION

Fig. 1 shows for comparison the evoked potentials derived in monkey (left) and man (right) upon the appearance and disappearance of either checker-board (upper records) or horizontal bar (lower records) patterns. We believe that these responses are conclusively of contrast origin. As indicated in the traces at the bottom of Fig. 1, the onset and offset of the pattern were not accompanied by an overall change in mean luminance. If local luminance changes would have generated the EPs depicted, then a symmetrical response would have been obtained. The EPs to the onset of the patterns clearly differ, however, in shape from those to the offset of the patterns. Further-more, larger responses are generated by the presentation of small checks (12 min of arc, top curves) than by the onset of large checks (48 min of arc, bottom curves). If these EPs were generated by local luminance variations, then according to a simple receptive field model a greater response amplitude might be expected for larger check sizes (Spekreijse 1966); the data suggest otherwise. On the basis of these two arguments, in awake monkeys as in man, EPs to pattern presentation can be derived that have contrast origin. There are, however, differences in the dependence on stimulus parameters. For example, in monkey narrow bars generate EPs with about the same amplitude as checkerboards. In man, however, bar patterns are generally a much less effective stimulus.

The data in Fig. 2 derived from a previous study (Padmos, Haaijman & Spekreijse 1973) show that in the anaesthetized monkey the contrast specific

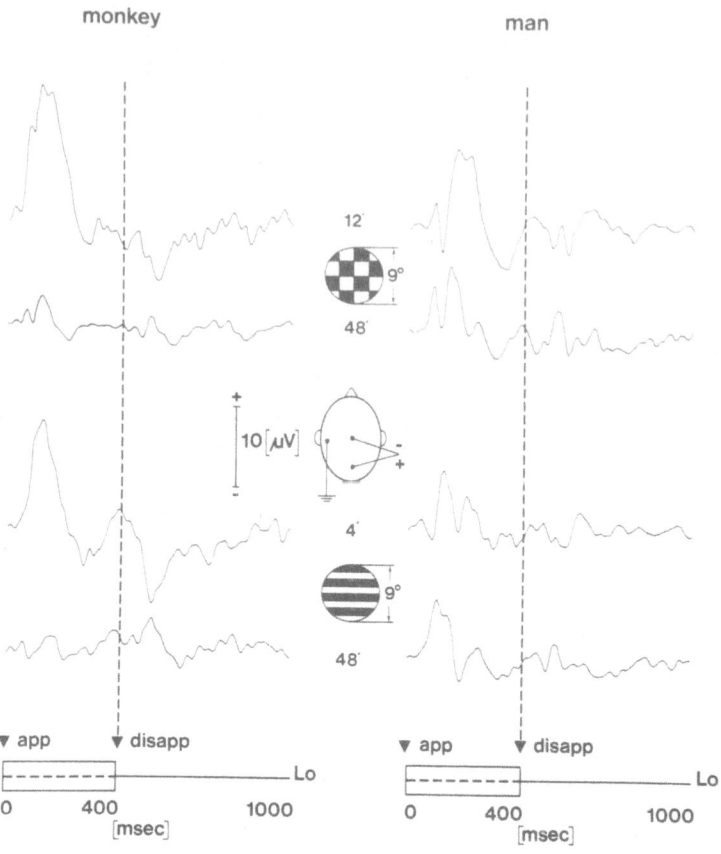

Fig. 1. Checkerboard and bar pattern evoked potentials derived from monkey and man, with surface electrodes on the occiput as indicated. The top half of the figure gives the responses to small (12 min of arc) and large (48 min of arc) checks. The bottom half displays the responses to narrow (bar width 4 min of arc) and wide (48 min of arc) horizontal bars. The contrast in all patterns is close to 100%, field size 9° × 12°. App refers to the appearance of the pattern; disapp refers to the disappearance of the pattern. The luminances of the two sets of checks return to the same value of $L_0 = 63$ cd/m^2. The patterns were presented for 400 msec once per 1000 msec.

component in the response to pattern stimulation is lost. Under nembutal anaesthesia the responses to both pattern appearance and pattern disappearance are the same (Fig. 2, upper left half). They are also rather similar in shape to the responses from luminance on- and offset (Fig. 2, bottom half). Since the luminance contribution in the EP to contrast presentation cannot be estimated without knowledge about the spatial organization of the visual system in the monkey, the luminance EP depicted was selected from a series of recordings obtained at different contrast modulation depths. A modulation depth of 50% generated the EPs presented in the bottom traces. The right-hand traces are the contrast and luminance responses obtained in the awake

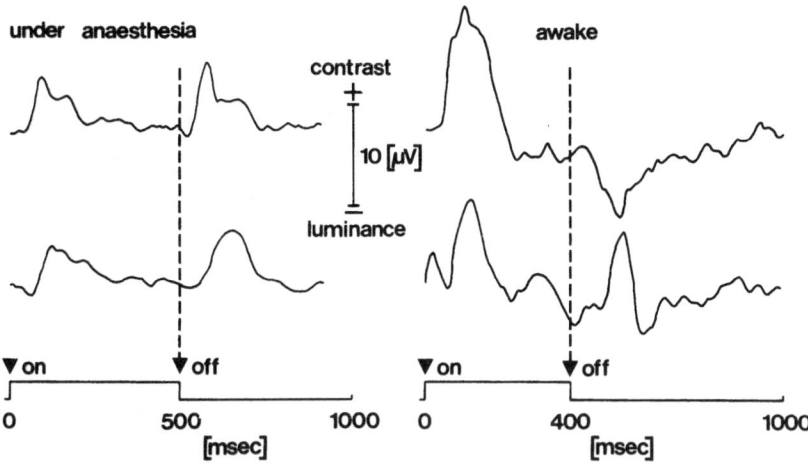

Fig. 2. Contrast (top half) and luminance (bottom half) evoked potentials from anaesthetized (left half) and awake (right half) monkeys. The evoked potentials recorded
under nembutal anaesthesia are from a previous study (Padmos, Haaijman & Spekreijse
1973). The contrast responses (upper traces) were obtained to stimulation with checkerboard patterns. A 12° field consisting of 24' checks of 50% contrast and a mean
luminance of 20 cd/m² was used in the anaesthetized condition: a 9° field with 12'
checks of nearly 100% contrast and mean luminance of 63 cd/m² was used in the awake
situation. The luminance EPs were generated by a 50% square wave modulated
homogeneous field of the same size, time profile and mean luminance as the
corresponding patterned stimuli. On and off refer to pattern onset and offset or to the
stepwise increase and decrease of the luminance stimulus. The left hand EPs were derived
with a surface electrode over the foveal projection (position T6 see Fig. 3), the right
hand EPs with an inion electrode (position I).

condition. The first interesting point is the larger response amplitude in the
awake situation. The second and more important point is the difference in
shape between the EPs to luminance and contrast presentation. From these
data it can be concluded that a) nembutal anaesthesia severely affects the
amplitude and frequency contents of the visual evoked potentials and b)
under nembutal anaesthesia the contrast component in the EPs to pattern
presentation is lost.

To investigate the topological representation of the contrast EP
simultaneous responses from 12 electrodes were measured. Fig. 3 gives an
example of the responses to simultaneous right and left half field stimulation.
From each electrode two responses could be derived simultaneously since the
presentation onsets of each half field (Fig. 3, top) had no fixed time relation.
Thus, two averaging procedures could be carried out simultaneously, one
locked to the onset of the pattern in the left half field (Fig. 3, dashed line)
and the other to the pattern in the right half field (Fig. 3, solid line). This
form of stimulation is a sensitive method for fixation control because only
when the fixation is correct at the middle of the screen, may a contralateral
representation be expected. Since such a representation can clearly be seen in
Fig. 3, it can be concluded that the monkeys had good fixation. Furthermore,

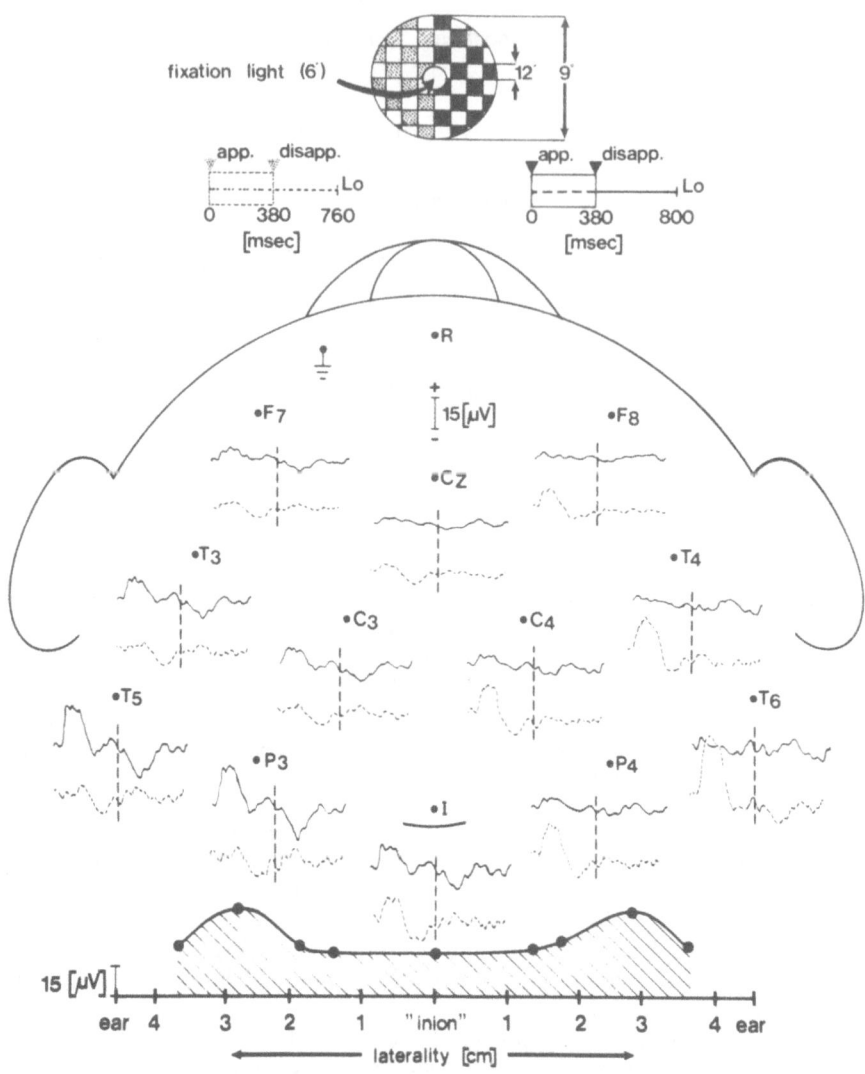

Fig. 3. Responses to simultaneous left and right half field stimulation. Both right (solid) and left (dashed) half visual fields were stimulated with an appearing and disappearing checkerboard pattern (check size 12 min of arc). The presentation times of the two patterns were chosen in such a way that the onset-offset instants of the two patterns had no fixed time relation (top Fig.). In this way from each of the 12 electrodes the responses to simultaneous right and left half field stimulation could be averaged separately. The right temporal electrodes yield greater amplitude responses from left half field (dotted lines), the left temporal electrodes from right half field stimulation (solid lines). At midline electrodes (see e.g. position I) the responses to both half fields are approximately equal. For illustrative purposes lateral electrode positions are displayed obliquely; during recording they were positioned in horizontal rows.

the responses at electrode positions T5 and T6 have a greater amplitude than the responses at the 'inion' electrode. This is in accordance with the anatomical finding that foveal projection areas in the monkey have a parieto-temporal location (Daniel & Whitteridge 1961). In the bottom graph of Fig. 3 the amplitude of the appearance response to full field stimulation is plotted as a function of laterality. This graph shows that the largest responses can be recorded at about 2.8 cm to the left and the right of the inion, most likely just over the foveal projection areas in the monkey studied. Since in monkey, foveal projection varies with body weight, the largest responses are obtained between 2.5 and 3.0 cm lateral from the midline which is in the proximity of electrode positions T5 and T6. Similar findings have been reported recently by Coppola & Nakamura (1979).

CONCLUSIONS

(a)   In awake rhesus monkeys genuine contrast responses, as found in man, can be obtained.

(b)   The response to pattern appearance can be distinguished clearly from that to pattern disappearance.

(c)   The contrast EP amplitude varies with the size of the elements in the pattern.

(d)   That Padmos et al. (1973) could not detect contrast EPs in their study can be attributed to the use of nembutal anaesthesia.

(e)   The largest contrast EPs in monkey can be recorded from parieto-temporal electrodes overlying the foveal projection regions.

ACKNOWLEDGEMENTS

We are grateful to Hans Meester and Peter Brassinga for technical support and to Jos Verkerk for assisting in animal caretaking.

REFERENCES

Coppola, R. & Nakamura, R.K. Electrocortical responses to visual spatial frequency in behaving monkeys. Society for Neuroscience Abstracts 5: 780 (1979).

Daniel, P.M. & Whitteridge, D. The representation of the visual field on the cerebral cortex in monkeys. J. Physiol. 159: 203–221 (1961).

Doddington, H.W. Activity evoked in the visual system of human, rhesus monkey and cat by spatially patterned and non-patterned visual stimuli. Dissertation. University of Florida (1972).

At the bottom the amplitude of the appearance response to full field stimulation is plotted as a function of laterality; the inion electrode (position I) is 5 mm above the anatomical inion. This graph is based on data obtained at different electrode positions from the same monkey during several sessions. Note that normalisation of response amplitude across sessions was not necessary.

Jeffreys, D.A. & Axford, J.G. Source location of pattern-specific components of human visual evoked potentials. I. Components of striate cortical origin. Exp. Brain Res. 16: 1–21 (1972a).

Jeffreys, D.A. & Axford, J.G. Source location of pattern-specific components of human visual evoked potentials. II. Components of extrastriate cortical origin. Exp. Brain Res. 16: 22–40 (1972b).

Lieb, J.P. & Karmel, B.A. The processing of edge information in visual areas of the cortex as evidenced by evoked potentials. Brain Res. 76: 503–519 (1974).

Padmos, P., Haaijman, J.J. & Spekreijse, H. Visually evoked cortical potentials to patterned stimuli in monkey and man. Electroenceph. clin. Neurophysiol. 35: 153–163 (1973).

Perryman, K.M. & Lindlsey, D.B. Visual responses in geniculo-striate and pulvino-extra-striate systems to patterned and unpatterned stimuli in squirrel monkeys. Electroenceph. clin. Neurophysiol. 42: 157–177 (1977).

Short, R.A., Lieb, J.P. & Wilson, W.A. Effects of light intensity and edge density on visually evoked potentials in rhesus monkeys. Psychophysiol. 14(6): 531–536 (1977).

Spehlman, R. The averaged electrical response to diffuse and to patterned light in the human. Electroenceph. clin. Neurophysiol. 19: 559–560 (1965).

Spekreijse, H. Analysis of EEG responses in man. Junk. The Hague (1966).

Spekreijse, H. & Estévez, O. The pattern appearance-disappearance response. Trace 6: 13–19 (1972).

Spekreijse, H., van der Tweel, L.H. & Zuidema, T.H. Contrast evoked responses in man. Vis. Res. 13: 1577–1601 (1973).

Authors' address:
The Netherlands Ophthalmic Research Institute
Department of Visual System Analysis
P.O. Box 6411
1005 EK Amsterdam, The Netherlands

CHANGES IN THE VISUAL EVOKED RESPONSE DURING NITROUS OXIDE INHALATION

J.W. HOWE, K.W. MITCHELL & M.J.M. ENGLISH

(*Newcastle upon Tyne, England*)

ABSTRACT

In a group of normal, healthy volunteers the effects of inhalation of nitrous oxide on the VER have been studied. The subjects inhaled N_2O at concentrations of 10%, 20% and 40%. Prior to recording the subjects were allowed to stabilize for 10 minutes. At each level the VERs to flash and pattern-reversal were recorded. Even at 40% concentration of N_2O the subjects remained fully conscious and co-operative, and were able to fixate the stimulus adequately. Each subject was examined on at least two separate occasions in order to assess the consistency of the results.

The major consistent change in the flash VER was an enhancement of later components VI–VII. The major consistent change in the pattern VER was a gradual reduction in amplitude, particularly noticeable in the P100 component. Latency changes were primarily noticeable in the N130 component. The results obtained using each stimulus mode are presented and the findings relating to varying pattern and field sizes discussed.

INTRODUCTION

The purpose of this study was to assess the effects of inhalation of various concentrations of nitrous oxide (N_2O) on the visual evoked response (VER). It is part of a wider investigation being performed to ascertain whether visual evoked cortical potentials can be regarded as an electrophysiological index of sedation caused by various drugs. This is, therefore, an interim report on our findings thus far.

Only a few workers have investigated the effect of inhalation of N_2O on the VER. Domino et al. (1963), in a basically qualitative study, reported that N_2O at deep anaesthetic levels had little or no effect on the VER elicited by stroboscopic flash stimuli. Kulikowski & Leisman (1973) investigating the effects of N_2O inhalation at 50% concentration also reported little change on the contrast thresholds to grating onset-offset stimuli. Quantitative studies concerning the effect of various concentrations of N_2O on evoked responses

Doc. Ophthal. Proc. Series, Vol. 27, ed. by H. Spekreijse & P.A. Apkarian   401

© *1981 Dr W. Junk Publishers, The Hague/Boston/London*

were reported by Lader & Norris (1969) and Jarvis & Lader (1971). They measured audiometric evoked responses (AER) and observed significant reductions in the amplitude of A.E.R. components at various concentrations up to 30%.

To our knowledge, our study is the first to examine the quantitative changes in the cortical responses evoked by checkerboard pattern reversal and stroboscopic flash at levels of N_2O inhalation up to 40%.

MATERIALS AND METHOD

Five healthy members of staff were used in the present investigation, their ages ranging from 23 to 35 years. Each had a sound knowledge of the purpose of the study and the methods to be employed. Visual acuities in all were 6/6 or better in each eye and the fields of vision were full.

Silver/silver chloride disc electrodes were attached to the scalp with collodion in the following positions (Jasper 1958): active — Oz, reference — Cz, earth — Fpz.

A Medelec electrophysiological unit was used to amplify, store and average the signals. The amplifier bandwidth was 0.8 Hz–80 Hz and 128 (1000 sample points) epochs of 400 msec. length were averaged. The responses were recorded on an X-Y plotter.

Both flash and pattern reversal stimuli were used. The flash stimulus was provided by a stroboscope lamp with an energy of 0.2 Joules. The light was diffused by an opalescent cover. The lamp was placed 0.35 metres in front of the subject and subtended an angle of $22°$ in the visual field. The flash rate was set at 2 per second. As the lamp emitted an audible click at each flash presentation, 'ear-muffs' were used in order to obviate the possibility of contaminating the VER with the auditory evoked responses.

A video pattern generator produced a checkerboard stimulus which was displayed on a high quality TV monitor. The reversal rate was 2 per second, each change being locked to the 50 Hz monitor frame rate. The space average luminance of the blank screen was $42 \, cd/m^2$ and the relative contrast of the checkerboard, about this mean value, was fixed at 90%. The subject was seated 1.7 metres from the monitor at which distance the TV screen subtended an angle of $17° \times 13°$. Investigations were performed with (a) $50'$ checks and large field ($17° \times 13°$) stimulation and (b) $25'$ checks and small field ($5°$) stimulation.

A small marker was attached to the centre of the screen and the subject instructed to fixate, binocularly, at all times during the recording of the responses. After the electrodes had been attached to the subject pre-adaptation to the luminance of the blank screen was performed for about 10 minutes (mins). A series of initial responses were then recorded with the subject breathing air. Following this, a 10% N_2O–90% O_2 mixture was administered using a non-return system and for a period of 10 mins. the subject was allowed to equilibrate. The evoked responses were once again recorded. This procedure was repeated at 20% and 40% concentrations of N_2O. Throughout the investigation the subject was reminded of the

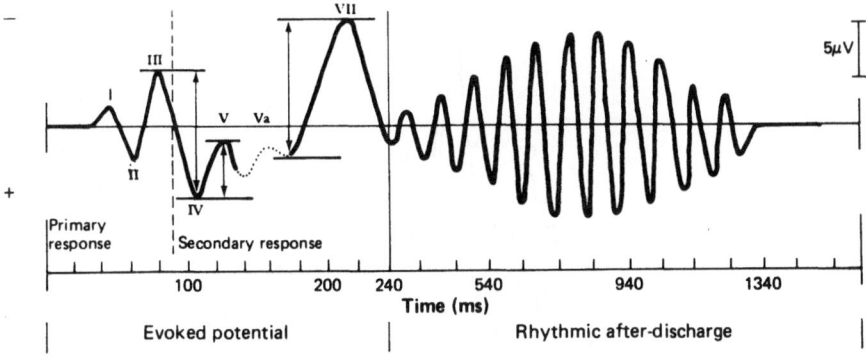

Fig. 1. Schematic representation of human flash VER showing the main primary and secondary components (modified after Cigánek).

importance of maintaining accurate fixation during recording. In addition to this an independent observer monitored fixation, and averages were excluded where fixation wandered significantly.

At the end of the investigations, when the subject was returned to air inhalation, responses were recorded to compare with the initial values, as a control. Two independent investigations were performed on each subject and the quantitative results reported herein, were obtained from the average of the two runs.

RESULTS

Flash evoked responses

The responses we obtained showed some variation regarding the occurrence of the very early components (I and II) described by Cigánek (1961), but we were usually able to identify those occurring later (III–VII).

These components, which were consistently present in the evoked responses of all the subjects, were chosen for measurement of peak to peak amplitude and latency. In analysing the results we have paid particular attention to the amplitude measurements of components III–IV, IV–V and VI–VII (Fig. 1).

In Fig. 2 the evoked responses of one of our subjects and the effects of N_2O inhalation are shown.

Fig. 3 shows the range of the absolute values of the amplitude of component III–IV plotted against N_2O concentration for the five subjects, and the amplitude values normalised at 0% N_2O concentration. It can be seen that three of the subjects showed considerable enhancement of this component and two subjects a reduction, with increased concentrations of N_2O. Component III–IV was observed to show a similar variability.

In Fig. 4 the data for component VI–VII are illustrated. This was the

403

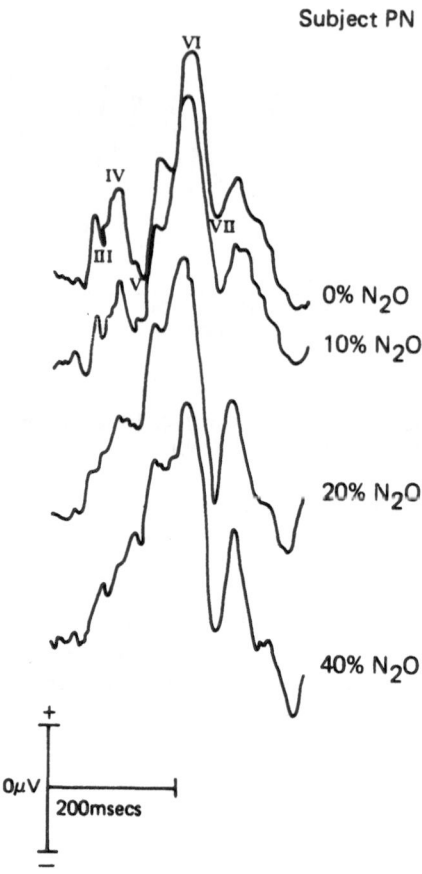

Subject PN

0% N$_2$O

10% N$_2$O

20% N$_2$O

40% N$_2$O

10μV

200msecs

Fig. 2. Flash VER at varying N$_2$O concentrations, showing reduction in components III–IV and IV–V, but enhancement of VI–VII.

largest and the most easily identifiable component in the evoked responses of this group of subjects. All subjects demonstrated an enhancement of this component and the shape of the curves would tend to suggest a saturation effect in the amplitude – dose characteristic at about the 20% level. The graph of the mean values of the normalised amplitudes against N$_2$O concentration helps to visualize this, even though the standard deviations are rather large.

Measurements of latency of these flash components was attempted but no consistent changes with increased concentrations of N$_2$O were observed outside the normal variability of latencies in an individual.

Pattern reversal response

In the results from checkerboard pattern reversal stimulation the amplitude measure chosen was that between components P100 and N130. In Fig. 5

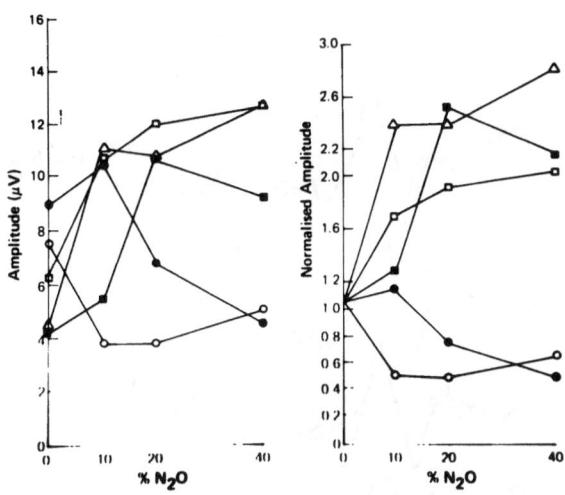

Fig. 3. Absolute and normalised amplitudes of component III–IV plotted against N_2O concentration. Latency 70–120 msec.

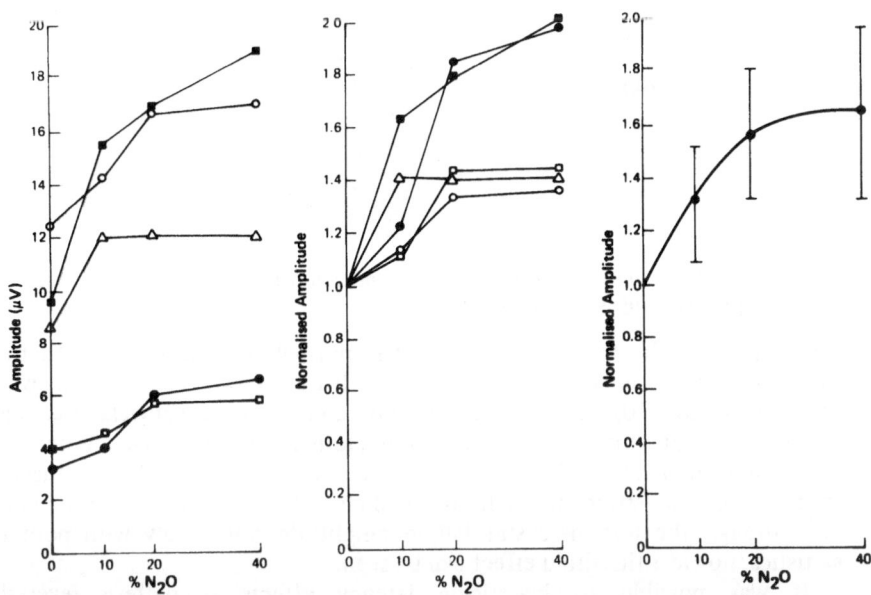

Fig. 4. Absolute and normalised amplitudes of component VI–VII plotted against N_2O concentration. Latency 200–250 msec.

the pattern reversal evoked responses are shown at different concentrations of N_2O inhalation for one subject using 50′ checks and $17° \times 13°$ field. The effects upon amplitude can be clearly seen. The results for all our subjects are shown in Fig. 6, the three graphs and their constituent parameters being

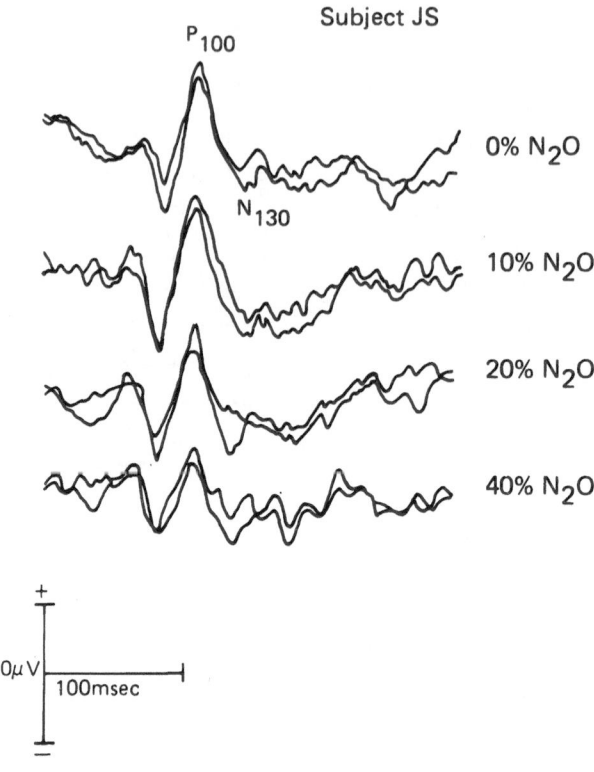

Fig. 5. VER's from one patient during one examination showing amplitude reduction of N_2O with increasing N_2O concentration.

the same as in the flash experiments. The normalised data illustrate that a threshold effect seems to occur, in that little change in amplitude was observed below 10% N_2O concentration, and in some subjects even an enhancement at this value (though not statistically significant) before a common proportional fall off in amplitude with increasing N_2O concentration. Fig. 7 illustrates the data for small check/small field stimulation, and even though the responses still fall in amplitude, admittedly with poorer statistics, no clear threshold effect can be seen.

It was possible to investigate latency effects as pattern reversal components are much more consistent and reproducible than flash evoked components. Latency measures of components P100 and N130 are shown for large check/large stimulation in Fig. 8. They illustrate that no change could be seen in the peak latency of P100, but show that reduction in N130 latency with increasing N_2O concentration was observed. Similar effects were observed for small check/small field stimulation.

The observed changes in evoked potential amplitude due to inhalation

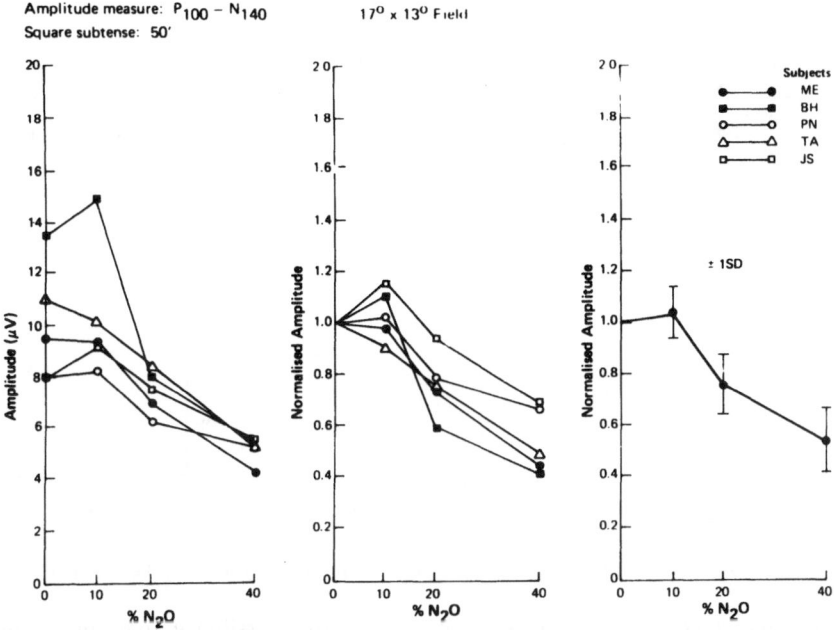

Fig. 6. Absolute and normalised amplitudes of P100 plotted against N_2O concentration. Large field/large check stimulation.

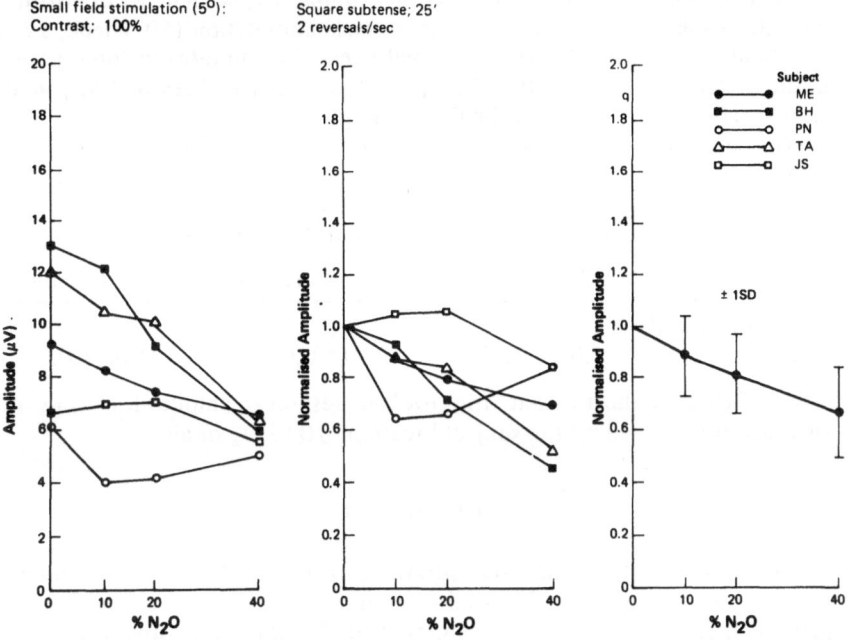

Fig. 7. Absolute and normalised amplitudes of P100 plotted against N_2O concentration. Small field/small check stimulation.

407

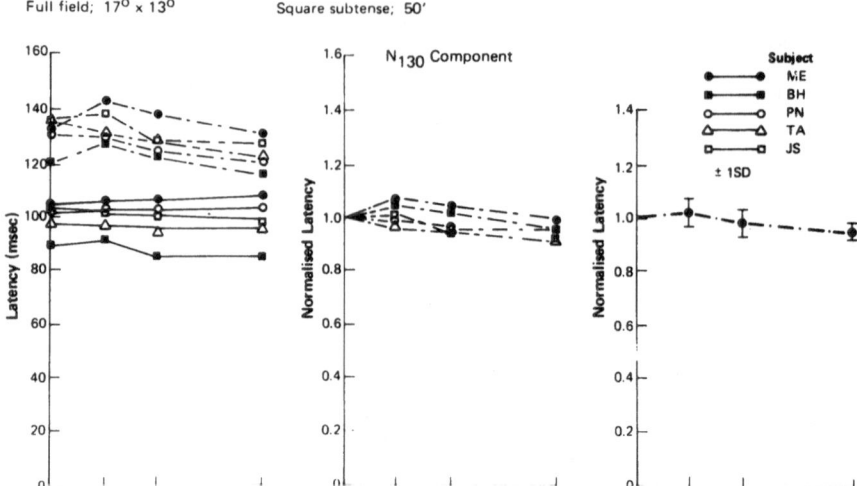

Full field; 17° x 13°   Square subtense; 50'

Fig. 8. Absolute and normalised latencies of N130 plotted against N_2O concentration.

of the $N_2O–O_2$ mixture, do not exclude the possibility that the changes are influenced by the increased oxygen concentration i.e. from 100% air to 90% O_2, 80% O_2 and 60% O_2.

To investigate the effect of oxygen a simple experiment was performed whereby evoked responses to pattern reversal stimulation (50' check, 17° x 13° field, 90% contrast) were obtained every five minutes in three periods lasting 20 mins. each. In the first period the subject breathed air, in the second, 100% oxygen, and in the third, air again.

The amplitudes of the evoked potentials were normalised to the initial value obtained on air inhalation and the mean and standard deviations of the values recorded in each 20 min. period were calculated. The results from tests performed on three subjects are shown in the table below:

	Air (20 mins.)	Oxygen (20 mins.)	Air (20 mins.)
Mean normalised amplitudes	1.04 ± 0.08	1.00 ± 0.06	1.02 ± 0.07

These figures indicate that the evoked response amplitudes were not significantly changed by the subject breathing 100% O_2 or air.

DISCUSSION

In our initial investigations, concentrations of up to 50% N_2O were administered to two subjects. At this level we found, as did Kulikowski and Leisman (1973), that problems were encountered. Both subjects became drowsy and reported great difficulty in concentrating on the fixation target. Subsequent

408

studies were therefore limited to a maximum concentration of 40% N_2O at which levels accurate fixation was still possible.

The flash evoked potentials which we have obtained show significant differences in amplitude with increasing concentrations of N_2O. Analysis of the early components (III–IV) and (IV–V) showed some interindividual variation. There was an enhancement of the responses in three patients, but a reduction in the other two. The later components (VI–VII) were much more consistent in that all subjects showed an enhancement, and in fact appear to demonstrate a saturation effect at 20% N_2O concentration. These results would appear to be at variance with those reported by Domino et al. (1963), but it must be borne in mind that their studies were carried out at much higher concentrations of N_2O (80%) than we have employed.

The pattern reversal studies show that the responses elicited by foveal stimulation appear to fall in a roughly linearly related amplitude–dose relationship. This effect was also noted by Lader & Norris (1969) and by Jarvis & Lader (1971) in their audiometric evoked response work. For larger field stimulation, however, the relationship is certainly not linear at low N_2O concentrations, exhibiting a threshold effect at 10% (even a possible enhancement in some subjects), before we see a proportional fall off in amplitude occurring with greater concentrations of N_2O.

The latency measurements suggest that the P100 component is unaffected, but that the latency of the N130 component is somewhat reduced, inferring a shorter conduction time along the visual pathways for this component.

REFERENCES

Cigánek, L. Die elektroencephalographische lichtreizantwort der menschlichen Hirnrinde. Slovenskej Adademie Vied, Bratislava. (1961).

Domino, E.F., Corssen, G. & Sweet, R.S. Effects of various general anaesthetics on the visually evoked responses in man. Anaesthesia and Analgesia. 42: 735–747 (1963).

Jarvis, M.J. & Lader, M.H. The effects of nitrous oxide and the auditory evoked response in a reaction time task. Psychopharmacol. (Berl.) 20: 201–212 (1971).

Jasper, H.H. Report of the committee on methods of clinical examination in electro-encephalography. Electroenceph. clin. Neurophysiol. 10: 370 (1958).

Kulikowski, J.J. & Leisman, G. The effect of nitrous oxide on the relation between the evoked potential and contrast threshold. Vis. Res. 12: 2079–2086 (1973).

Lader, M. & Norris, H. The effects of nitrous oxide on the human auditory evoked response. Psychopharmacol. (Berl.) 16: 115–127 (1969).

Authors' address:
University of Newcastle upon Tyne
Royal Victoria Infirmary
Queen Victoria Road
Newcastle upon Tyne, NE1 4LP, U.K.

VISUALLY EVOKED AND SPONTANEOUS POTENTIALS
OF THE HUMAN CORTEX

R.P. STODTMEISTER, I. WILMANNS & M.P. BAUR

(*Bonn-Venusberg, F.R.G.*)

ABSTRACT

The spontaneous brain potentials can be influenced by light stimuli (Adrian & Matthews 1934). By inspection of VECP recordings possible changes of the spontaneous brain activity can usually not be recognized. These changes, however, may influence the responses from the visual pathways (Bishop 1933). To evaluate the interaction between EEG and VECP, visually evoked potentials were recorded with periodic and non-periodic stimulation at different stimulus repetition frequencies in 30 human volunteers. The results of these experiments are demonstrated and the possibility of interaction between the EEG and VECPs as suggested by Trimble & Potts (1975) is discussed.

INTRODUCTION

In 1934 Adrian and Matthews had shown that the spontaneous brain potentials can be influenced by periodic light stimuli. When visually evoked potentials are recorded, however, it is widely assumed that the spontaneous brain potentials are not influenced by the periodic light stimuli necessary to evoke potentials from the visual system. The influence of spontaneous brain potentials on the visually evoked cortical potential (VECP) cannot always be recognized by inspection of response curves. The experiments presented here were made to examine a possible interaction between spontaneous brain potentials and evoked potentials. Preliminary experiments have shown that there may be a clear interaction in the initial part of the response; the study, therefore, was designed to confirm the above mentioned results.

METHODS AND MATERIALS

The experiments were carried out in 30 human volunteers. The stimuli were binocular Ganzfeld discharge flashes with a luminance integral of 0.4 cdsec/m^2. The pupils were maximum dilated. For periodic stimulation, the stimulus repetition frequency was 1 Hz, 2 Hz, 3.2 Hz and 4 Hz. Non-periodic stimulation was achieved by the following method (Wilmanns, 1979). After each stimulus there was an interval during which the next stimulus could not occur. It did occur during a second interval which we name the random interval. The time of occurrence during this interval was determined by a random interval generator. By this method each stimulus interval consisted of a fixed interval and a variable interval, the longest duration of which was set in our experiments to 100 msec. The variable intervals had an even distribution. The fixed interval was set to appropriate values to obtain mean stimulus repetition frequencies of 1 Hz, 2 Hz, 3.2 Hz and 4 Hz.

The VECP was recorded with a needle electrode 15% above the inion and a silver-clip electrode on the left earlobe. The bandpass of the amplifier and display system was 0.3–300 Hz (−3 dB). The responses were manually digitized with intervals of 13.65 msec during the first 259 msec after the stimulus onset. Quantitative measures of the bioelectrical activity were obtained from the absolute value of the area between the response curve and the baseline drawn through the point of the curve at stimulus onset to the first 68 msec after stimulus onset.

RESULTS

Original recordings of VECPs with periodic and non-periodic stimulation are shown in Fig. 1. With periodic stimulation there are voltage changes

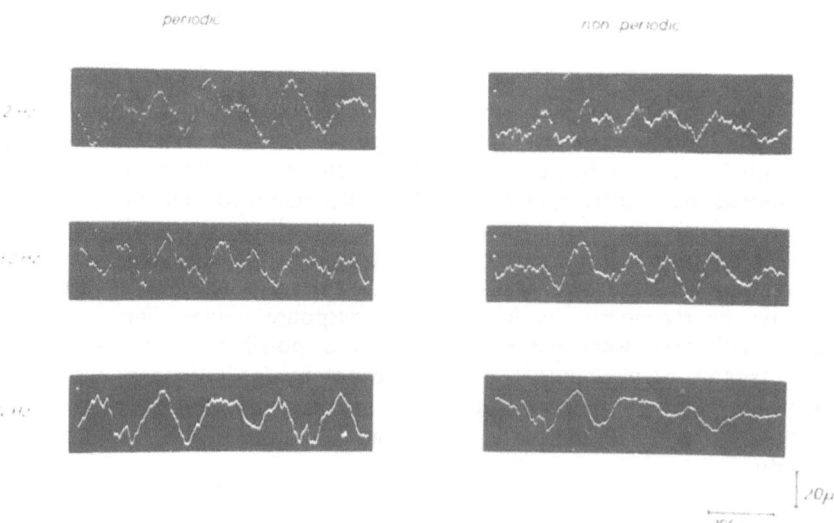

Fig. 1. VECP responses with periodic and non-periodic stimulation. Stimulus repetition frequency and mean stimulus repetition frequency is given to the left of the recordings. The stimulus flash occured at the start of the trace. Each curve is the average of 64 single responses.

without latency. With non-periodic stimulation the baseline changes of the initial part of the curves are within the range of the biological noise.

The arithmetic mean curves shown in Fig. 2, each calculated from 30 response curves, show practically no difference with periodic and non-periodic stimulation. The standard deviations for the initial values, however,

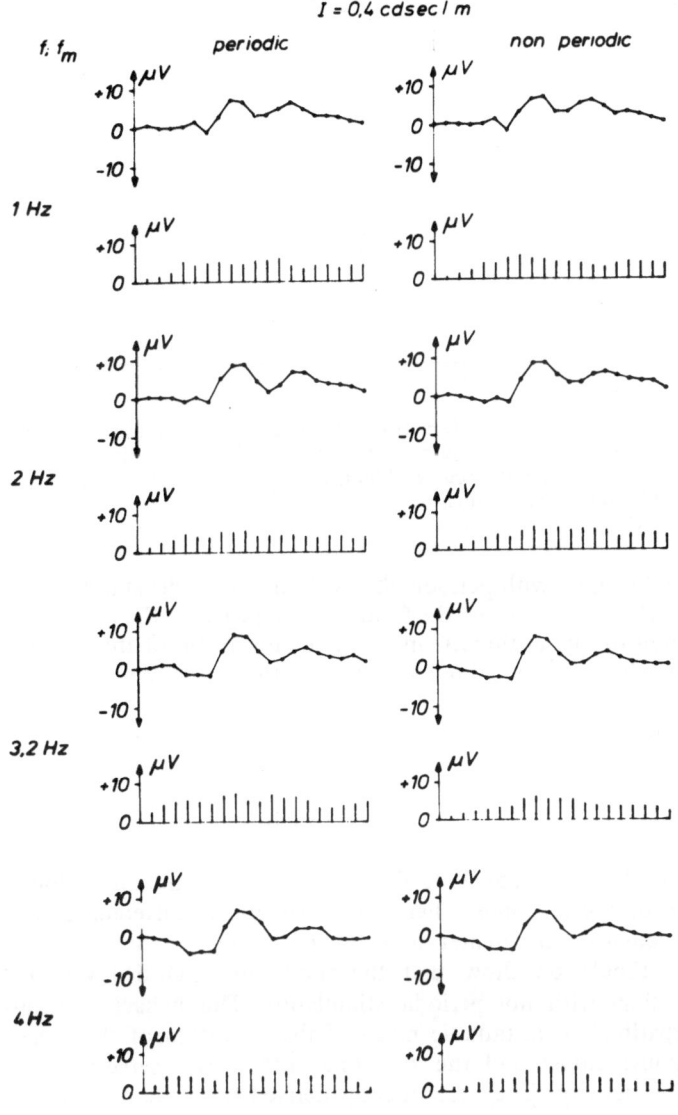

Fig. 2. Mean curves and standard deviations from 30 subjects. f = stimulus repetition frequency, f_m = mean stimulus repetition frequency. The stimulus flash occured at the start of the traces.

413

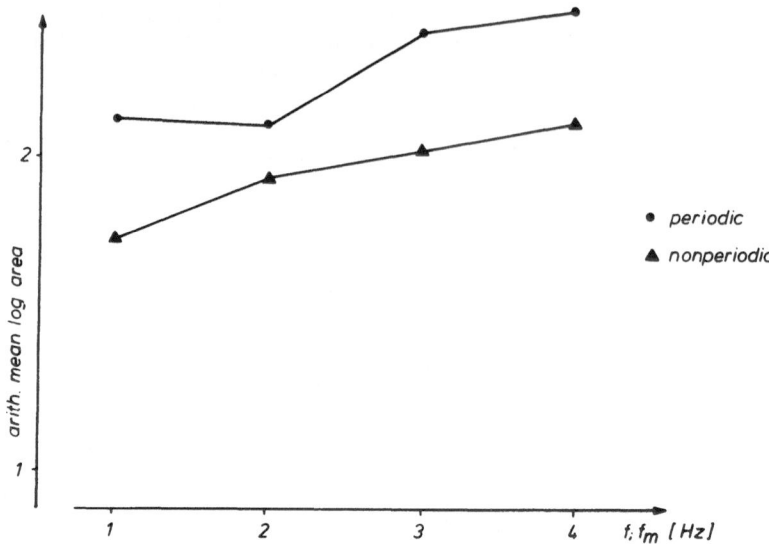

Fig. 3. Ordinate: Arithmetic mean from 30 subjects of the logarithm of the absolute values of the areas between the response curves and the zero line drawn through the initial point of the response curve. Abscissa: f = stimulus repetition frequency, f_m = mean stimulus repetition frequency.

are generally larger with periodic than with non-periodic stimulation.

Fig. 3 shows that across the frequency range tested the bioelectric activity represented by the arithmetic mean of the logarithm of the mentioned areas is higher with periodic stimulation than with non-periodic stimulation. This difference is significant at the 5% level as calculated by analysis of variance (Kirk 1968).

DISCUSSION

From Fig. 2 we can conclude that non-periodic stimulation does not alter the form of the response. There are no significant differences in amplitude or peak latency. The greater standard deviations for the initial values with periodic stimulation show that the amplitudes recorded vary more with periodic than with non-periodic stimulation. This behaviour is also shown by comparing the arithmetic mean of the logarithm of the areas between the response curves and the zero line. These areas serve as a measure of bioelectric activity. They are directly derived from the response curves and they can be subjected to analysis of variance as done in this study. According to the presumption generally accepted, the spontaneous EEG potentials are not related to the stimulus repetition frequency of periodic stimulation, i.e. the voltage deviations caused by spontaneous activity vary at random. In our experiments we superimposed on this supposed random process a second known random process. The superimposition of a random process to a random process results in a random process. Theoretically the result should not be changed by the addition of this random process. If however an altered response occurs by addition of a known random process to a supposed random process it must be assumed that the supposed random process does not fulfill the requirements of randomness.

If we apply these theoretical considerations to our experiments we see that the addition of a known random process (the non-periodicity of the stimuli) to a supposed random process (the spontaneous brain activity with respect to the periodic stimuli) induces a change in the results. Therefore we may conclude that there is an interaction between the periodic stimuli and the spontaneous brain activity.

Thus our experiments demonstrate that one important pre-requisite for averaging evoked responses (i.e. independence between the EEG and VECPs) cannot always taken for granted. From inspection of VECPs it cannot easily be concluded whether the response is contaminated by the influence of spontaneous brain activity. Ruchkin (1965) has shown in a theoretical analysis that non-periodic stimuli may improve the recording of evoked potentials. Our study experimentally confirms the considerations of this author.

Our study also confirms the conclusions of Trimble and Potts (1975) who stated that alpha activity influences the initial part of the VECP. In analyzing VECPs this possibility should always be considered.

REFERENCES

Adrian, E.D. & Matthews, B.H.C. The Berger rhythm: potential changes from the occipital lobes in man. Brain 57: 355–384 (1934).
Bishop, P.O. Cyclic change in the excitability of the optic pathway of the rabbit. Amer. J. Physiol. 103: 211 (1933).
Kirk, R.E. Experimental design. Brooks/Cole, Belmont. 237 (1968).
Ruchkin, D.S. An analysis of average response computations based upon aperiodic stimuli. IEEE Trans. Bio. Med. Engin. 12: 87–94 (1965).
Trimble, J.L. & Potts, A.M. Ongoing occipital rhythms and the VER. I. Stimulation at peaks of the alpha-rhythm. Invest. Ophthalmol. Vis. Sci. 14: 537–546 (1975).
Wilmanns, I. Pseudorandom stimulation. Ophthal. Res. 11: 154–158 (1979).

Authors' address:
I. Wilmanns & M.P. Baur
Universitäts-Augenklinik
Klinisches Institut für experimentelle Ophthalmologie
Institut für medizinische Statistik Dokumentation und Datenverarbeitung
Bonn-Venusberg, F.R.G.

Prof. Dr. R. Stodtmeister
Univ. Augenklinik
Prittwitzstr. 43
D-7900 Ulm, F.R.G.

EVALUATION OF PLASTICITY IN HUMAN BRAINS

VECP changes by training in normal subjects

B. DEGERING & K. YANASHIMA

(*Frankfurt/Bad Nauheim, F.R.G.*)

ABSTRACT

In 15 healthy subjects cortical potentials evoked by patterned stimuli were recorded from both hemispheres of the visual cortex. Each subject was exposed for five hours, once a week, to the same stimulus (reversing checks of 19 min of arc, 66 per cent contrast presented in a 5° central field). The observed changes (decrease of amplitude and latency) during the course of each *individual* session were regarded as a sign of fatigue. The observed changes (increase of amplitude and latency) during the course of *consecutive* sessions, however, indicate improvement of discrimination by training. The transfer of changes from one eye to the other evinced the post-chiasmic site of processes involved.

INTRODUCTION

Visual recognition requires synthesis of the actual input and visual learning and memory. Unlike the mechanisms involved in the primary visual response there is a paucity of information regarding the processes involved in visual learning. This is not only because of unknown fundamentals about learning and about memory itself but also because of the lack of methods to investigate these processes. Recording the visual evoked cortical potential (VECP) is a possible window to the visual brain and consequently some authors have used this method to investigate one of the more simple forms of learning, habituation (Walter 1964). However, the findings are not unequivocal since it was found that VECPs recorded from wires accurately implanted in the human primary visual cortex did not habituate (Walter 1964). This finding suggests a non-uniform origin of the scalp recorded VECP, i.e., the normal VECP may consist of both habituating and non-habituating components. There is also some disagreement concerning the role of peripheral mechanisms in VECP habituation (Bergamini, Bergamasco, Manbelli & Gandiglio 1965). Despite these difficulties these studies suggest more sophisticated forms of learning as compared with habituation, may be represented by changes in

VECPs. This seems plausible because many reports indicate plasticity in the human visual system, such as the achievement of stereoscopic vision by training of normal subjects (Wittenberg, Brock & Folsom 1969).

The aim of the following study is to investigate the representation of learning processes in the human VECP.

METHODS

Visual cortical potentials evoked by patterned stimuli were recorded in 15 healthy persons (age range 18–25 years). The active electrode was placed on O_1, O_2 and the reference electrode on F_P following the International 10–20 electrode convention. The ground electrode was placed at the right ear lobe. A black and white checkerboard pattern was presented on a TV-screen masked to produce a 5° central field. The subject was placed sitting 1 m in front of the screen fixating the center. Each square of the checkerboard subtended an angle of 19 min of arc. The contrast ratio of the bright and the dark checks was 66 per cent.

The checkerboard pattern reversed 6 times per second. The sweeptime was 5.12 s and the VECP was averaged 48 times. Recording and evaluation was done by means of a PDP 11/40 computer (see Figs. 1 and 2). Each

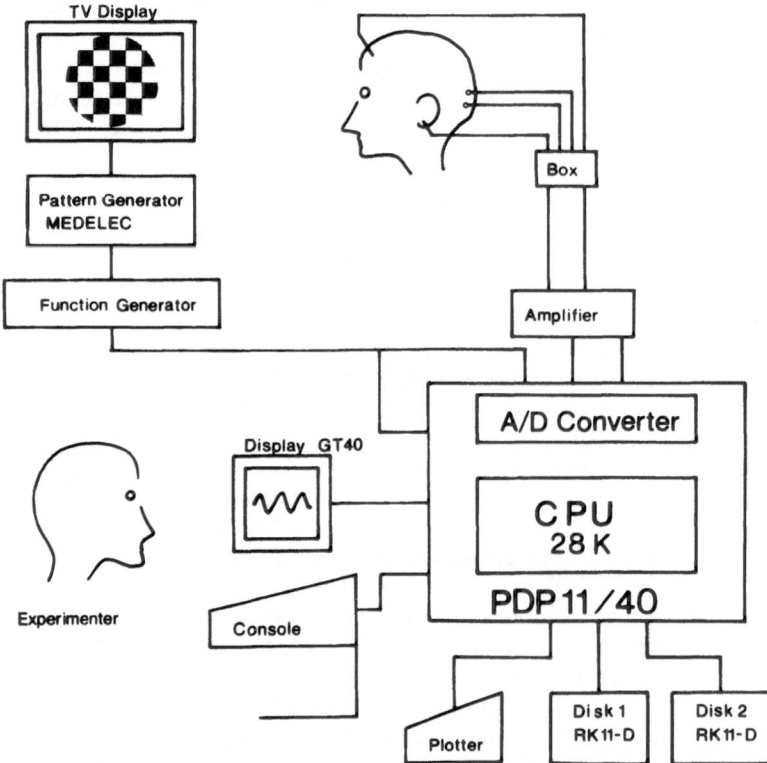

Fig. 1. Schematic flow chart of stimulus and recording apparatus.

418

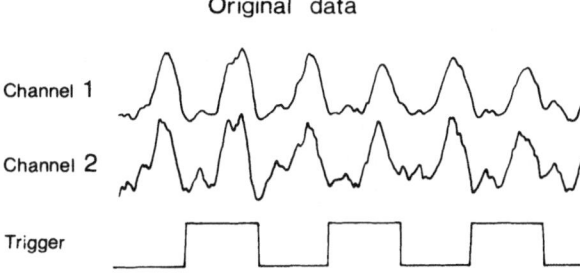

Original data

Channel 1

Channel 2

Trigger

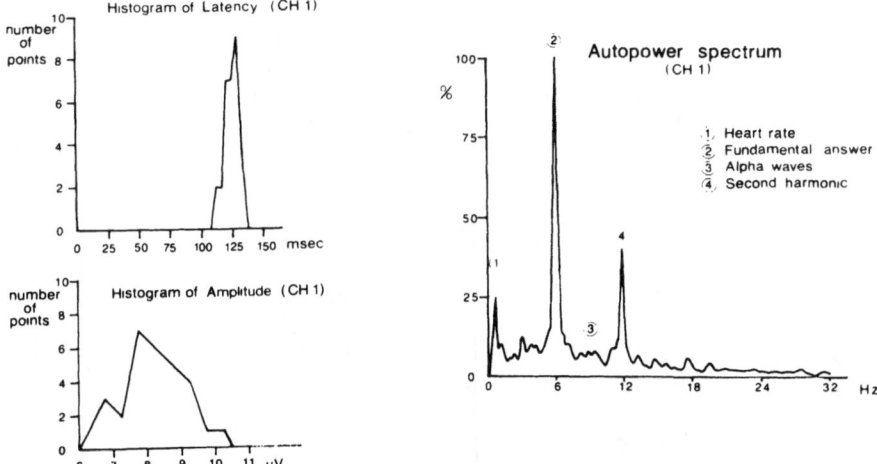

Fig. 2. Above: Original VECP records from O_1 (Channel 1) and O_2 (Channel 2) and data processing. Left: Evaluation of data from O_1 as shown (middle) by the histogram of latencies (ranging from 105 ms to 140 ms) and (below) by the histogram of amplitudes (ranging from 6 μV to 10.5 μV).

At the lower right shown is the autopower spectrum from the above record, indicating peaks corresponding to heart rate (1), stimulus frequency (2), alphawaves (3) and the second harmonic of the stimulus frequency (4).

subject was exposed monocularly to the same stimuli for five hours without interruption, once a week. Before and after each individual session the VECP was recorded, stimulating both the trained and the non-trained eye one after the other, and the visual acuity was checked by using Snellen charts. This procedure was performed over a time period of 4 weeks, i.e., 5 times. Our experimental session started randomly without considering the influence of daily biorhythms.

RESULTS

The present findings of VECP changes due to repetitive stimulation are summarized for one person in Fig. 3. The changes observed in the course of each individual session (upper half of the figure) were a decrease of VECP

419

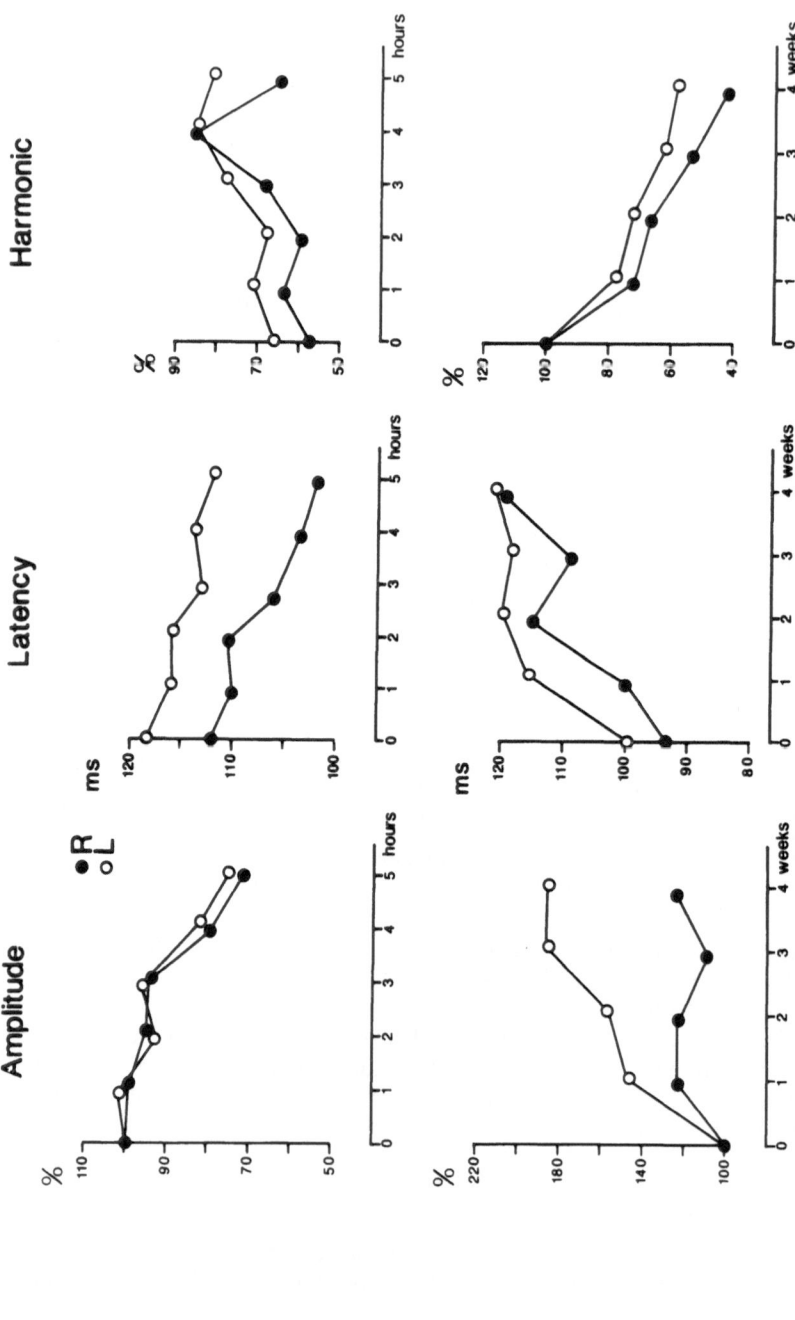

Fig. 3. Graph showing the effect of repetitive stimulation on VECP wave shape. Upper row: Changes of amplitude, latency and second harmonic during 5 hours exposure. Lower row: Changes of amplitude, latency and second harmonic during the course of weekly consecutive sessions. The data refer to the beginning of the individual session.

420

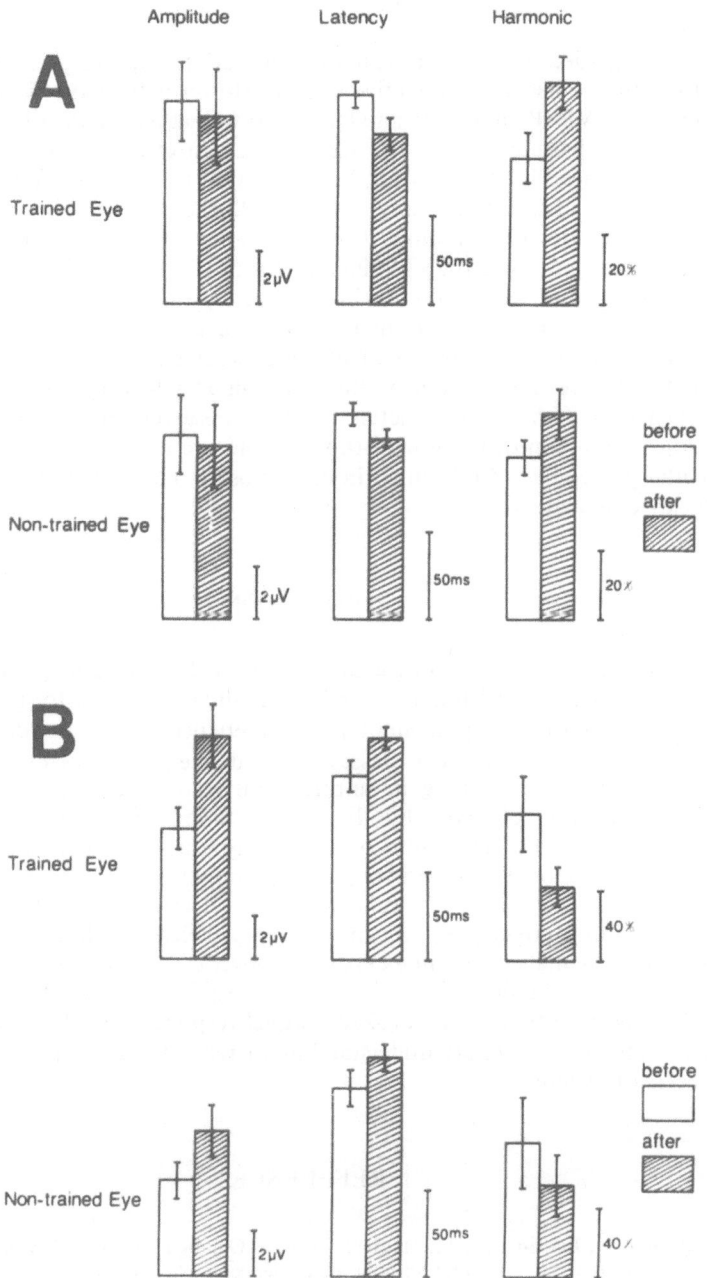

Fig. 4. Changes of VECP amplitude (μV), latency (ms) and harmonic (per cent of fundamental answer) of the trained and the non-trained eye (A) during 5 hours exposure, (B) during the course of weekly, consecutive sessions.

amplitude and latency as well as an increase of amplitude of the second harmonic.

We regarded these as a sign of habituation and fatigue. The changes during the course of consecutive sessions (lower half of the figure) were an increase of VECP amplitude and latency as well as a decrease of amplitude of the second harmonic. We regarded these as an effect of visual training or learning. Since visual acuity has been reported to improve after consecutive presentation of stimuli (Keesey 1960) the Snellen visual acuity was checked before and after each session. The mean value of the Snellen visual acuity of the trained eye was found to increase from 1.2 to 1.5. Using the Wilcoxon-test these values were found to be statistically significant ($P < 0.01$). There was no statistically significant increase in visual acuity in the untrained eye.

The post-chiasmatic origin of changes observed was shown by recording the VECP after stimulation of the non-trained fellow eye. Fig. 4 compares the changes of VECP parameters from 15 observers occurring after stimulation of the exposed eye with those of the eye not exposed to the experimental procedures (A) during 5 hours exposure, (B) during the course of the weekly consecutive sessions.

DISCUSSION

The present results can not be understood without assuming a far reaching plasticity of the visual brain in the human adult. Evidence for this is already obtained from daily ophthalmological experience such as the disappearance of distortions after new eye glasses are used, the improvement of visual and stereo-acuity after training in normal adults and the longterm changes in color perception observed by the use of tinted opthalmic lenses (Hill & Stevenson 1976). The results of this study suggest a plasticity of VECP parameters imposed by repetitive pattern stimulation.

Until now no concept is available in respect to a structural manifestation of the learning-effect presently shown. Nevertheless we should be aware that evoked potentials are time-dependent events. After repeated exposure to patterned stimuli the so-called normal subjects are no longer 'normal' with respect to their visual evoked cortical responses. Further investigations in this area may facilitate understanding of related phenomena including the process of memory.

REFERENCES

Bergamini, L., Bergamasco, B., Manbelli, A.M. & Gandiglio, G. Visual evoked potentials in subjects with congenital aniridia. Electroenceph. clin. Neurophysiol. 19: 394–397 (1965).

Hill, A.R. & Stevenson, R.W.W. Long-term adaptation to ophthalmic tinted lenses. In: Colour Vision Deficiencies III (Ed. G. Verriest) Karger, Basel. 17: 264–272 (1976).

Keesey, V.T. Effects of involuntary eye movement on visual acuity. J. Opt. Soc. Am. 50: 769–774 (1960).

Walter, W.G. The convergence and interaction of visual, auditory and tactile responses in human non-specific cortex. Ann. N.Y. Acad. Sci. 112: 320–361 (1964).

Wittenberg, S., Brock, F.W. & Folsom, W.C. The effect of training of stereoscopic acuity. Amer. J. Optom. 46: 645–653 (1969).

Authors' address:
Dr. B. Degering
Augenklinik
Zentralkrankenhaus
St. Jürgenstrasse
D-2800 Bremen, F.R.G.

K. Yanashima
MPI für Physiol. und Klin. Forschung
W.G. Kerkhoff – Institut
Parkstrasse 1
D-6350 Bad Neuheim, F.R.G.

CONTRAST EVOKED POTENTIALS IN THE EVALUATION OF SUSPECTED MALINGERING

H. WILDBERGER

(*Zurich, Switzerland*)

ABSTRACT

Pattern visual evoked potentials (VEPs) can be used as a test in patients simulating impaired visual acuity. For an objective measurement of visual acuity with VEPs, a scaling method was established using orthoptic filters. Responses from a group of normal subjects to different check sizes were compared with those registered from suspected malingerers. Proof that visual acuity must be better than pretended by the patient is demonstrated easily at lower visual levels only. Under clinical conditions recording evoked potentials to very small check sizes which represent higher visual resolution is not always possible even in normal subjects. The presented results are based on a study of 27 suspected malingerers.

INTRODUCTION

The majority of malingerers pretending impaired visual function show reduced visual acuity. Malingering is suspected in the presence of various contradictory results between psychophysical tests and objective findings. Organic lesions of the visual pathways should be excluded by objective methods such as visual evoked potentials (VEPs) before a patient is called a malingerer. In this case normal or better than expected VEPs are recorded. Using pattern reversal stimulation, the question arises of whether visual acuity better than pretended can be proved. It has to be considered to what degree the VEP would be impaired in the presence of a real organic lesion within the optic pathways.

MATERIALS AND METHODS

Twenty-seven malingerers were observed. In a first group were 17 malingerers (most of them were schoolgirls) without clinical evidence for an organic lesion. In a second more heterogeneous group were 10 adult suspected malingerers with an obvious lesion within the visual system caused by accident or disease. This latter group pretended a more than expected impaired visual acuity often for the non-affected eye as well.

The VEPs were recorded with a television pattern generator as described by Arden et al. (1977). The pattern reversal rate was 2 Hz, the checks subtended visual angles of 38, 19, 9 and 4 minutes of arc and the contrast between bright and dark squares was 50% (for further details see Huber & Wagner 1978). Intending an objective estimation of visual acuity, four normal, well motivated subjects were tested with the four check sizes. A scale of graded orthoptic filters was inserted to reduce the visual acuity to 0.7, 0.5, 0.3, 0.2 and 0.1. Amplitudes were measured from the first surface positive peak to the following negative peak.

RESULTS AND DISCUSSION

All suspected malingerers of the first group had a latency within the normal range of 102.6 ± 6.4 msec (Huber & Wagner 1978) as measured at the peak of the first positive deflection with the 38 min pattern. Symmetric, well defined responses were obtained from both eyes to the 38, 19 and 9 min pattern (Fig. 1). With normal visual acuity amplitudes are largest with checks

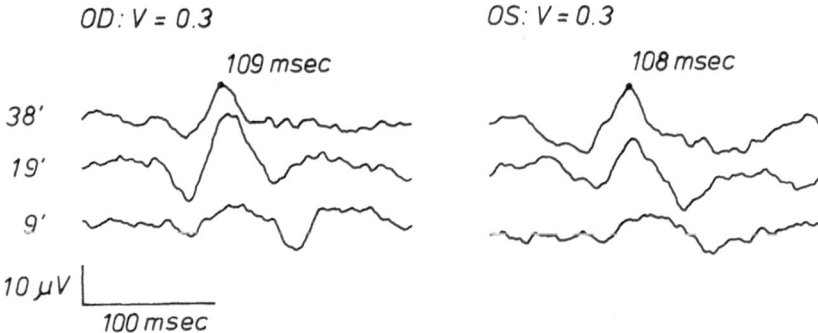

Fig. 1. Suspected malingering: 11 year-old girl pretending a bilateral visual acuity of 0.3. Normal VEP to pattern stimulation with checks subtending visual angles of 38, 19 and 9 min of arc. Amplitude to the 19 min checks is larger than to the 38 min checks.

subtending 10 to 20 min of arc (Harter & White 1970). Infants seem to reach full visual acuity by 6 months if this criterion is applied (Sokol & Dobson 1976). In the first group of 17 malingerers (34 eyes) the 19 min pattern gave greatest amplitudes to 21 eyes, in 4 eyes the 38 and 19 min pattern gave equal resonses, whereas the 38 min amplitudes prevailed in 9 eyes. Even in normal subjects maximal amplitudes can arise from checks larger than 20 min (Sokol 1976). To measure the highest spatial resolution directly, Marg et al. (1976) presented gratings of 30 cycles per degree equal to a visual acuity of 1.0 and they found VEPs even at this level. Other authors have estimated highest resolution indirectly by extrapolation (Campbell and Maffei 1970; Berkley and Watkins 1971). Our scale with orthoptic filters (Fig. 2) gives responses

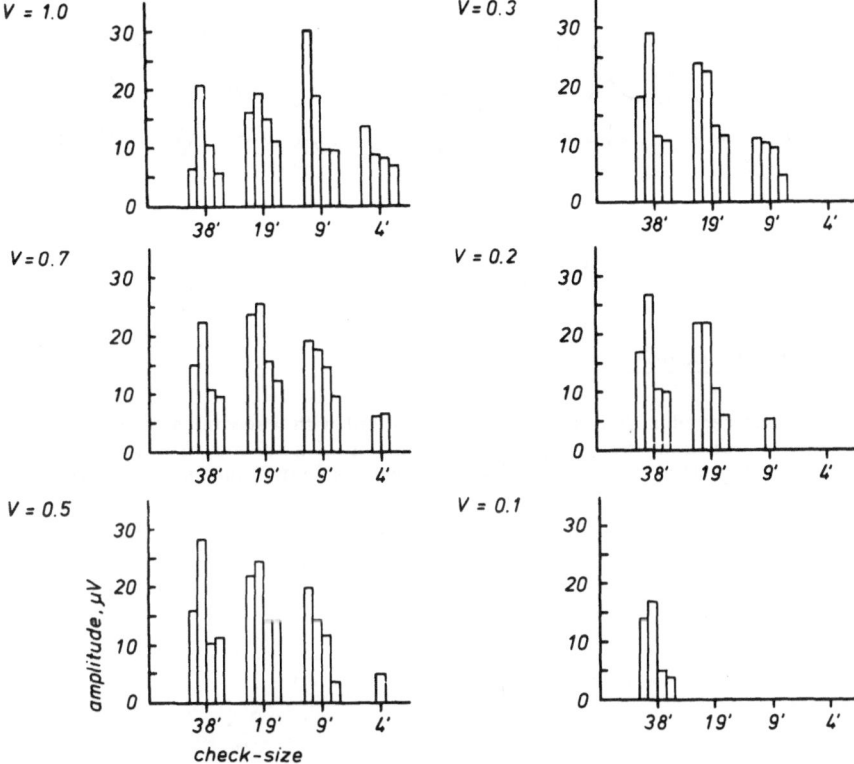

Fig. 2. Gradually reduced visual acuity with orthoptic filters. VEP amplitudes to checks subtending 38, 19, 9 and 4 min of arc from 4 normal subjects. Each bar represents the VEP amplitude of one subject. The VEP amplitudes with large check stimulation (38 min, 19 min) are nearly unaffected by a reduction in visual acuity to 0.2.

to the 4 min pattern down to a visual acuity of 0.5 which is to be expected since 4 min of arc are equal to a visual acuity of 0.25. The presence of a response to the 9 min pattern corresponds to an acuity of at least 0.3, the presence of a response to the 19 min pattern to a minimal acuity of 0.2. The 38 min pattern gives consistent responses also at a visual acuity of 0.1. The quality of the 4 min checks on the TV-screen is limited and the responses are inconstant even in normals and often absent under clinical conditions. For that reason we renounced using the 4 min checks. This means that the presence of a 9 min response proves only that the visual acuity lies between 0.3 and 1.0 without further differentiation. Thirteen out of 17 suspected malingerers of the first group pretended to have a visual acuity between 0.3 and 0.6. In these cases the VEP alone was not able to prove malingering. The scale method was successful in proving a better visual acuity for the remaining 4 patients who pretended to see less than 0.3. For 7 out of 10 malingerers of the second group, however, a visual acuity better than

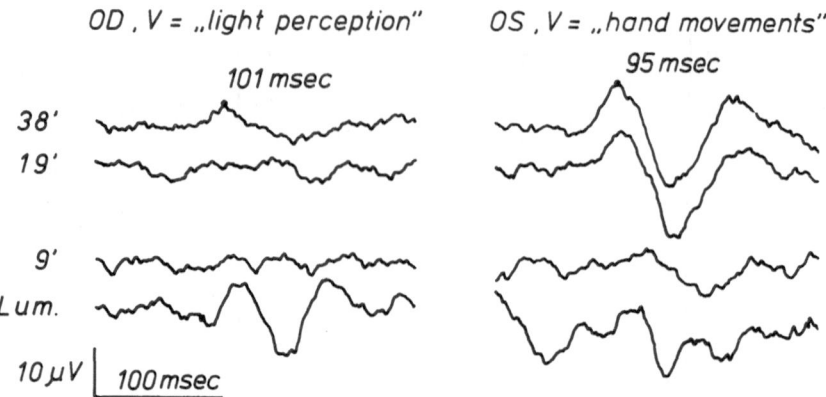

Fig. 3. Suspected malingerer: 50 year old patient with a recovered bilateral posterior cyclitis. VEP from the left eye allows estimation of a minimal visual acuity of 0.3 in contrast to the pretended acuity of hand movements. Lum. = luminance stimulation.

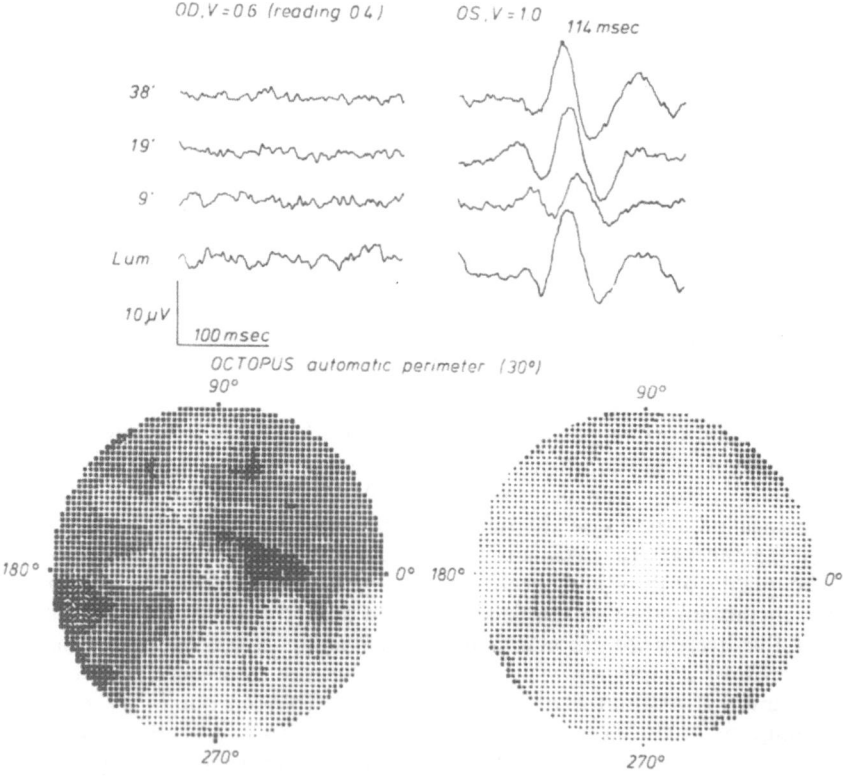

Fig. 4. Recovered optic neuritis of the right eye of a 44 year-old patient with multiple sclerosis. OCTOPUS automatic perimetry tests the central 30 degrees of the visual field (program 31). Non-recordable VEPs at the right with a visual acuity of 0.6.

428

pretended was proved in one or both eyes. Most malingerers with an organic lesion of the visual pathway pretended to see much less than 0.3; this made the demonstration of malingering easier. Fig. 3 shows the VEP of a patient with light perception in the right eye and hand movement in the left eye after a bilateral posterior cyclitis. The VEPs in the right eye are impaired whereas in the left they allow estimation of a minimal visual acuity of 0.3. A clear separation of malingering from a true organic disease with impaired vision is facilitated by the fact that a neuritis or a chiasmal process with a visual acuity of 0.3 for instance gives much more disturbed VEPs than that from an orthoptic filter with the same acuity. Caution, however, is important even in this respect because optic nerve diseases with similar acuities and sensitivities over the posterior pole (measured with the OCTOPUS automatic perimeter) may produce a non-measurable response in one case (Fig. 4) and weak but present responses in another case (Fig. 5). Moreover very small parafoveal or foveal defects with slightly reduced visual acuities seem to produce normal VEP.

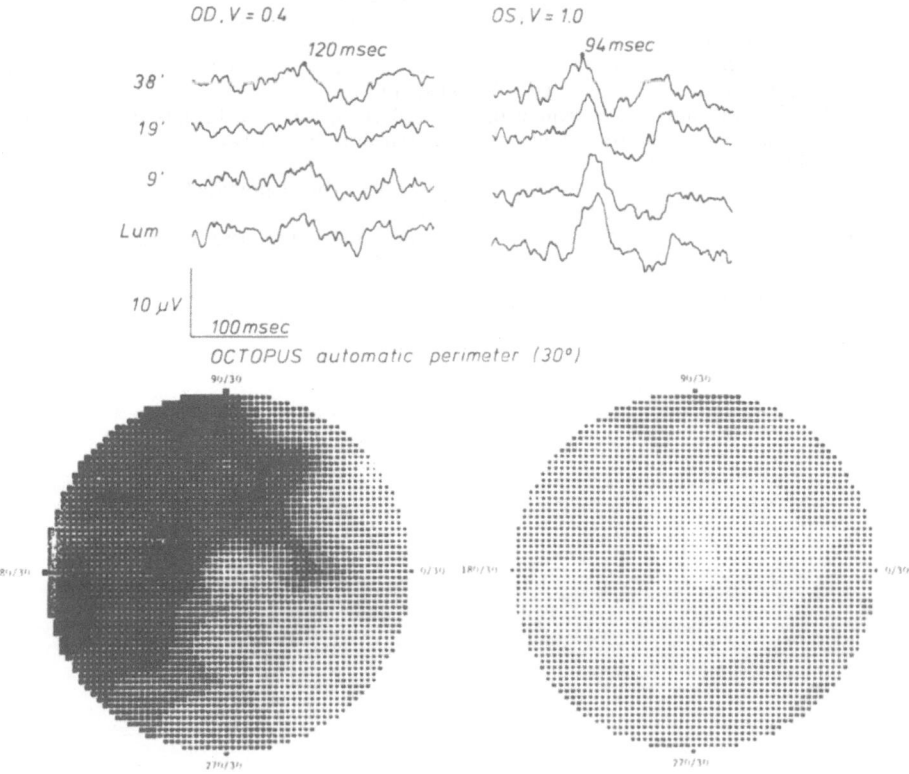

Fig. 5. Recovered vascular papillitis of the right eye of a 61 year-old patient. Same recording methods as in Fig. 4. Small and delayed VEP at right with a visual acuity of 0.4.

429

CONCLUSION

The proof that a visual acuity must be better than pretended by a suspected malingerer is demonstrated with VEPs easily at lower visual levels only. Recording potentials to very small checks representing a higher resolution often fails even in normal subjects under clinical conditions. Only indirect evidence for good visual acuity is then given by the VEP.

REFERENCES

Arden, G.B., Faulkner, D.J. & Mair, C. A versatile television pattern generator for visual evoked potentials. In: Visual evoked potentials in man: new developments (Ed. J.D. Desmedt) Clarendon Press, Oxford. 90–109 (1977).

Berkley, M.A. & Watkins, D.W. Visual acuity of the cat estimated from evoked cerebral potentials. Nature 234: 91–92 (1971).

Campbell, F.W. & Maffei, L. Electrophysiological evidence for the existence of orientation and size detectors in the human visual system. J. Physiol., Lond. 207: 635–652 (1970).

Harter, M.R. & White, C.T. Evoked cortical responses to checkerboard patterns: effect of check-size as a function of visual acuity. Electroenceph. clin. Neurophysiol. 28: 48–54 (1970).

Huber, C. & Wagner, T. Electrophysiological evidence for glaucomatous lesions in the optic nerve. Ophthal. Res. 10: 22–29 (1978).

Marg, E., Freeman, D.N., Peltzman, P. & Goldstein, P.J. Visual acuity development in human infants: evoked potential measurements. Invest. Ophthalmol. Vis. Sci. 15: 150–153 (1976).

Sokol, S. & Dobson, V. Pattern reversal visually evoked potentials in infants. Invest. Ophthalmol. Vis. Sci. 15: 58–62 (1976).

Sokol, S. Visually evoked potentials: theory, techniques and clinical applications. Survey of Ophth. 21: 18–44 (1976).

Authors' address:
Universitäts Augenklinik Zürich
Stadelhoferstr. 42
8001 Zurich, Switzerland

ABSTRACTS

THE INFLUENCE OF 'HIGH' TEMPORAL FREQUENCIES ON THE PUPILLARY REFLEX

K.M. van den Berge
Laboratory of Medical Physics, University of Amsterdam,
Herengracht 196, 1016 BS Amsterdam, The Netherlands

The dynamic pupillary reflex can be described by a frequency characteristic of a third order passive filter having a cut-off frequency of about 1.5 Hz, as a linear approximation. For frequencies of 4 Hz and higher the direct dynamic response is negligible. It is well known that the pupil responds to a continuous stimulus of these high frequencies with a steady-state contraction.

Our investigations have shown interesting related phenomena. When a low frequency stimulus and a continuous 4 Hz stimulus are presented simultaneously, the direct (low frequency) reflex of the pupil is strongly decreased with only small amounts of high-frequency modulation. A decreased response also occurs when the stimuli are presented dichoptically. Suppression of the pupil reflex response by the high frequency stimulus component was measured as a function of both modulation-depth and frequency.

TEMPORAL FACTORS IN THE MACULAR ERG

W.R. Biersdorf
Dept. of Ophthalmology, Univ. of South Florida, and
James A. Haley Veterans Hospital
13000 N. 30th St., Tampa, FL 33612, U.S.A.

Latencies of the macular (4° diameter) ERG and sensitivity of the technique in various diseases have been investigated. The method, previously reported (Biersdorf & Diller, Am. J. Ophthalmol. 68: 296 (1969)) uses a rapidly flickering red test patch against a white surround of rod saturating luminance.

An amplitude ratio between macula and blind spot stimulation is used to control for stray light. In macula degeneration, the sensitivity limit of the test is about 20/60 acuity.

New findings include:

1. In normal subjects, the macular ERG latency is longer than the full-field photopic ERG latency. Values depend on the high pass limit of the amplifiers.

2. In senile macular degeneration, the macular ERG latency is usually not abnormally delayed (83% of 18 eyes).

3. In Stargardt's macular degeneration, the macular ERG latency is usually abnormally delayed. (For 20/40 or worse, 84% of 19 eyes were delayed).

4. In retinitis pigmentosa the sensitivity limit of the macular ERG (amplitude ratio) is about 20/30 (26 eyes). Latencies may or may not be delayed.

THE ELECTRICALLY EVOKED RESPONSE

G.K. Bijl
Dept. of Neurophysiology, University of Groningen,
Groningen, The Netherlands

With a specially designed stimulating and recording system electrically (phosphene) evoked responses were recorded. The system uses opto-coupling to avoid interference between the simulating electrodes and equipment and also to provide safety for the subjects. Examples of recordings of responses evoked by single impulses, double impulses and interrupted sine-waves will be shown.

ELECTROPHYSIOLOGICAL OBSERVATIONS
IN RESPIRATORY DISTRESS SYNDROME

A. Bohár, Á. Farkas, G. Radó, & K. Széll
2nd Dept. of Ophthalmology, Semmelweis University of Medicine,
Maria u. 39, 1085 Budapest, Hungary

Retinal (ERG) and cortical evoked potentials (EP) were measured in healthy premature babies of different gestation time and body weight. These potentials can be considered as a 'development-indicator' for a given age.

The ERG and EP alterations are of prognostic value in respiratory distress syndrome.

MORPHOLOGICAL AND PHYSIOLOGICAL EFFECTS OF DL-α-AMINOADIPIC ACID ON THE RETINA

N. Bonaventure, G. Mack, & G. Roussel
Laboratoire de Neurophysiologie, Centre de Neurochemie du C.N.R.S.,
11 rue Humann, 67085 Strasbourg, France

Electron microscopic studies have shown that an intravitreal injection of DL-α-aminoadipic acid (considered to be a glutamate agonist) selectively destroys the Müller cells in the chicken, rat or frog retina. This destruction is not always irreversible, but mitochondria seem to be especially affected. The physiological effect of this drug was tested by means of the ERG, ganglion cell discharges and tectal evoked potentials. The possible involvement of Müller cells in the origin of the b-wave, as well as in the intraretinal transmission of information is discussed in an attempt to correlate physiological and morphological effects.

RETARDATION OF THE SCOTOPIC ERG B-WAVE BY CHEMICAL INTERACTION OF CEREBRAL-RETINAL MECHANISMS

M. Carapancea
'D. Danielopolu' Institute of Normal and Pathological Physiology,
Bucharest, Rumania

Injections in the rabbit of 1% solutions of strychnine, benzedrine and eserine provoked a non-specific increased latency of the scoptic ERG b-wave. The latency, normally 0.02 sec, consistently and significantly ($p < 0.001$) increased to 0.04 sec for a 20–30 minute period. Within the following 5–6 hours the latency oscillated between 0.02 and 0.03 sec. After 24 hours complete recovery was noted and latency values returned to normal.

The results indicate that central excitation by strychnine, benzedrine and eserine disrupts retinal neurotransmitters. This disruption causes diminished spontaneity of retinal excitability and conductability, resulting in delayed reaction of intraretinal photochmical decomposition and synthesis. The resulting bioelectric interactions lead to a delayed triggering of the ERG. This situation also provides a possible explanation for retinal photoexcitability threshold increases.

ELECTROPHYSIOLOGY AND PHOTOCOAGULATION IN DIABETIC RETINOPATHY

S.S. Declercq & K. Lee
Division of Ophthalmology, Stanford University Medical Centre,
Stanford, CA., 94305, U.S.A.

Patients with diabetic retinopathy and predominantly disc neovascularization without much background disease were enrolled in this study. Each patient received a complete electrophysiological evaluation before and after photocoagulation was performed. The amount of retinal ablation was calculated and correlated with the electrophysiological findings. The results which will be presented at the meeting point towards a large individual variability in photocoagulation tolerance.

PHOTORECEPTOR INNER SEGMENT DEGENERATION AFFECTS B-WAVE SIGNALS IN BACKGROUND ADAPTATION

A. Fulton, K. Manning & S. Schukar
Department of Ophthalmology, Children's Hospital,
Boston, MA 02115, U.S.A.

The hyperbolic stimulus-response functions of the scotopic b-wave show progressive changes during the course of a degeneration of retinal cells which begins in the photoreceptor inner segments of mutant mice (pcd/pcd) within the first post-natal month.

For dark adapted eyes, sensitivity decreased 100 fold between 1 and 10 months; the amplitude of maximum responses began to decline after age 4 months and was accompanied by prolongation of the time to peak of half maximum responses; by age 11 to 12 months ERG responses to brief, blue Ganzfeld flashes were extinguished. Steady backgrounds had less effect on the b-wave sensitivity of pcd/pcd mice than of normal mice; by the third post-natal month the slope of the linear portion of log sensitivity vs log background plots (Weber-Fechner curves) was less than $+0.2$ for pcd/pcd mice but was $+0.9$ for normal mice. The variation of maximum response amplitude by background lights became abnormal after age 4 months when the degeneration is known to involve portions of distal retina in addition to the inner segments.

The observed deterioration of adaptive functions suggests that from very early in the course of this particular degeneration, b-wave signals are processed and transmitted abnormally in the most distal stages of the visual pathway.

Supported in part by K 07 EY 00 107 from NEI, NIH.

FIRST DYNAMIC MEASUREMENTS OF SPECTRAL SENSITIVITIES IN VISUAL SYSTEMS BY FIS (FOURIER INTERFEROMETRIC STIMULATION)

R. Gemperlein
Biophysics Group at the Zoological Institute of the
Ludwig Maximillians University of Munich,
D-8000 Munich, F.R.G.

Analysing the spectral sensitivity of the visual system is typically done by the sequential presentation of single monochromatic stimuli. Each stimulus is applied several times and the response averaged to reduce the signal-to-noise ratio. Fourier interferometric stimulation (FIS) introduces a new technique which allows the simultaneous measurement of all wavelengths with high spectral resolution and in a dynamic fashion. One important advantage of FIS is the high reduction in measurement time. This is especially valuable in research with short lived preparations and in studying time-varying properties. For clinical application measurement periods of 20 sec can produce reliable spectral sensitivity curves from an ERG response to a FIS-stimulus. The experimental set up consists of a computer controlled continuous scanning Michelson interferometer which produces an interferogram which is the Fourier-transform of the light source. This is the stimulus for the system under study. From the stimulus-response pairs the Fourier algorithm allows computation of the spectral sensitivity of the system. The technique is described and the stimulus demonstrated. Results on selected individuals are presented.

A NEW METHOD OF STIMULATION IN VISUAL ELECTROPHYSIOLOGY

Y. Grall, Y. Boiteux & J. Keller
Service Central de Biophysique et de Medecine, Hôpital Lariboisière,
2 rue Ambroise-Paré, 75010 Paris, France

We have undertaken the development of a new method of stimulating the retina by means of a light pencil conducted through optical fibers from the light source to the pupil of the patient's eye. For this purpose, the extremity of the fiber is set in a scleral lens placed on the cornea. This 'contact lens' also contains a measuring electrode for electroretinogram (ERG) which enables the operator to easily perform various investigations (Static ERG, Dynamic ERG, measurement of the retinocortical conduction time). The building and testing of the prototype have now been completed, and the advantages of the system appear to be the following:
1. Recordings are not affected by movements of the patient's head, eyes or eye-lids.
2. Respective positions of the patient and the light source do not interfer making the system very convenient.
3. The results are linked to a precise stimulating wave-length determined by the geometrical characteristics of the optical fiber and by the position and characteristics of the interference filter set between the source and the fiber.

LATENCY AND AMPLITUDE OF THE HYPOKINETIC PUPILLARY RESPONSE IN CASES OF HOMONYMOUS HEMIANOPIA FOLLOWING SUPRATHRESHOLD STIMULI

K.U. Hamann, K.A. Hellner, W. Jensen & P. Oeding
Dept. of Ophthalmology, University Hospital of Hamburg,
Martinistrasse 52, D-2000 Hamburg 20, F.R.G.

The latency and amplitude of the pupillary response in patients suffering

435

from various lesions of the optic radiation was examined. The consensual pupillary light reflex, triggered by the test light of a perimeter was measured and registered with a special TV processor designed for this purpose, the infrared vidicon introduces no delay and the data therefore can be processed in real time. Parameters of the pupillary responses studied in the hemianopic defective and hemianopic normal visual fields are compared and evaluated.

SERUM FACTOR IN MS PATIENTS PRODUCING IN VITRO DEPRESSION OF THE ERG

S. Korol, A. Zwahlen & K. Pournaras
University Eye Clinic, Geneva, Switzerland

Physiological, clinical and experimental studies suggest that other factors (synaptic or antineural) in addition to or independent of demyelination may by playing a role in symptoms occuring in MS. (Namerow, *UCLA Forum* 16: 143 (1972); Bornstein & Crain, *Science* 148: 1242 (1965); Cerf & Carels, *Science* 152: 1066 (1966); Vrain, Bornstein & Lennon, *Exp. Neurol.* 49: 330 (1975)).

To examine these factors experiments were conducted in vitro on isolated perfused frog retinas. Electroretinogram (ERG) recordings were obtained with a micro-electrode before and after changing the nutritional medium for different solutions of test serum. All tests were performed at constant pH and temperature.

Serum obtained from patients with MS during periods of active illness always produced a significant and reversible depression of the b-wave of the ERG. The active factor in the serum appears to depend on the presence of complement (classical pathway). Conversely, serum from MS in remission (N = 4) and from other neurological patients (N = 12) or normal controls (N = 50) has not shown this modification of the ERG in vitro. The results also suggest that, in part, the ophthalmological symptoms of MS may result from synaptic or neuronal block in the visual system. It is hoped that the preparation used in the present experiments will provide a useful clinical test for differential diagnosis in neurological cases.

THE HUMAN ELECTRORETINOGRAM STUDIED WITH PATTERN ONSET-OFFSET STIMULI

M. Korth & V. Reiman
Institut für Physiologie und Biokybernetik der Universität Erlangen-Nürnberg,
Universitätsstrasse 17, D-8520 Erlangen, F.R.G.

Square-wave grating patterns of high contrast were presented under photopic luminance levels in the onset-offset mode using a Maxwellian view stimulator. The general shape of the averaged response following pattern onset consisted of a b-wave and a negative after potential followed by a slowly developing positive plateau-like potential that persisted as long as the pattern was present; no a-wave was observed. Following pattern offset an a-wave was recorded followed by a b-wave and an immediate decrease of the plateau potential. Upon varying the spatial frequency of the pattern from 0.2 to 9.4 c/deg the b-wave following pattern onset had an amplitude maximum at about 3 c/deg, the plateau potential was largest around 5 c/deg. The amplitudes of the a- and b-waves following pattern offset decreased monotonically with increasing spatial frequency. The results might indicate that retinal areas receiving local decreases in luminance make a stronger contribution to the onset response than retinal areas receiving increases in luminance. The reverse seems to hold for the offset response. This view was supported by further control experiments.

In addition to the slow components, fast wavelets were observed on the ascending slope of the b-waves. They were different in number and amplitude at onset and at offset of the pattern and showed characteristic differences below and above a spatial frequency of about 3 c/deg.

ANALYSIS OF ELECTRORETINOGRAMS IN STREPTOZOTOCIN-DIABETIC RATS

W.M. Kozak, L.G. Deneault, S.T. Danowski & T.S. Danowski
Carnegie-Mellon University, Pittsbugh, PA 15213, and
Shadyside Hospital, Pittsburgh, PA 15232, U.S.A.

We investigated the effects of diabetic control on retinal electrophysiology. Electroretiongrams (ERGs) to white and colored flashes were recorded in dark-adapted albino rats before and during three months following intravenous Streptozotocin injections. Non-diabetic (N group) rats served as controls. ERGs obtained under standardized conditions were computer-analysed off-line for amplitudes and latencies of the a, b-waves and wavelets. Diabetic rats were either left without insulin (D-0 group), injected once-a-day with insulin (D-1 group) or injected three times a day (D-3 group) with the same daily insulin dosage as D-1 group.

A-wave amplitudes did not change significantly with time. B-wave amplitudes progressively diminished and their latencies lengthened in the D-0 and D-1 groups whereas in the D-3 and N groups the b-amplitudes increased and their latencies shortened. The ERG wavelets' amplitudes diminished dramatically and latencies lengthened in the D-0 group to both white and colored flashes. Similar changes occurred in the D-1 group, but the amplitude reduction was less pronounced. In the D-3 group, as in the N group, there was no net change of the wavelet amplitudes and latencies during the 3 month period under study. However, wavelets elicited by violet light had progressively diminished in amplitude and lengthend in latency in both D-3 and N groups, whereas the wavelets elicited by red light had increased their amplitudes and shortened latencies during the same period.

Thus, with a better control of diabetes (D-3 group) ERGs behave as in normal rats. Concommitant changes in other indices, such as blood and urine glucose, water intake, body weight and vitreous fluorophotometry are discussed.

Supported by The Juvenile Diabetes Foundation.

ELECTROOCULOGRAMS FROM IN VITRO PERFUSED FELINE AND CANINE EYES

G. Niemeyer

Dept. of Ophthalmology, Universitätsspital,
CH-8091 Zürich, Switzerland

In spite of the clinical value of various EOG tests little is known about the origin of the corneo-fundal potential. This standing potential and its light-induced slow oscillations are similar in man and in other vertebrate species. DC recordings between cornea and posterior pole have been obtained in anaesthetized experimental animals. Since intracellular recordings, ERGs and optic nerve action potentials revealed physiologic responsiveness of the retina and the pigment epithelium in areterially perfused cat eyes (Niemeyer, *Docum. Ophthal.* 39 (1975)), we tested this preparation for EOG activity.

Eyes from anaesthetized cats and dogs were perfused with oxygenated, serum-enriched medium, and dark-adapted ERGs were recorded in a steady-state for 1 hr. Shielded silk-saline-Ag-AgCl electrodes, placed at the cornea and at the sclera close to the optic nerve, recorded DC potentials of 1 to 3 mv. Light steps of 2.3 and 4 log units induced slow, positive oscillations of amplitudes from 1.5 to 3 mv and peak latencies up to 7 min.

These data are comparable to in vivo recordings in various species. Perfused eyes therefore are suitable to study mechanisms involved in the generation of the EOG and provide access to experimental procedures that are not possible in whole animals.

EXTRACELLULAR CONE RESPONSE FUNCTIONS OF THE PRIMATE RETINA

D. van Norren & J.M. Valeton
Institute for Perception TNO, Kampweg 5,
3769 DE Soesterberg, The Netherlands

We developed a bipolar micro-electrode to isolate the cone receptor potential from the local electro-retinogram (LERG) in the rhesus monkey retina. Responses were recorded as a function of electrode depth in the fovea. A component analysis, based on Rodieck's (1973) scheme, showed that the DC-component and the R-component (pigment epithelium) have large contributions to the LERG. With bipolar electrodes these components could be distinguished from the receptor responses.

438

For further evaluation of the bipolar recordings, Na-aspartate was infused into the eye. The results corroborated those of the component analysis.

Finally, DC-recordings to steady state lights were obtained which also reveal retinal and pigment epithelial contributions.

THE EOG AFTER MONOCULAR PERFORATING INJURY AFFECTING THE ERG OF BOTH EYES

R. Rix, F. Emmrich & M.J. Korth
Institut für Physiologie und Biokybernetik der Univ. Erlangen-Nürnberg
Univ. Augenklinik, Universitätstrasse 17, D-8520 Erlangen, F.R.G.

In earlier studies (Rix & Emmrich, *Ber. Dtsch. Ophthalmol. Ges.* 76: 415 (1979)) it was demonstrated that in cases of metallosis oculi of one eye the electroretinogram (ERG) (a- and b-wave, wavelets) was reduced considerably not only in the injured eye but also, to a lesser extent, in the uninjured eye.

In the present study the electro-oculogram (EOG) of both eyes was examined in 23 cases of unilateral perforating injuries caused by metal foreign bodies. Recordings made shortly after the injury and follow-up studies showed that the EOG of the uninjured eye was reduced in most cases, whereas the other eye exhibiting an ERG of decreased amplitude showed a normal EOG. The results indicate that the binocular effect described earlier does not affect the resting potential responsible for the generation of the EOG, but only those structures that generate various components of the light-induced ERG.

THE AMPLITUDE OF THE HUMAN C-WAVE IN RELATIONSHIP TO INTENSITY AND DURATION OF THE STIMULUS

J. Röver, M. Hüttel & G. Schaubele
University Eye Clinic, Killianstrasse 21, D-7800 Freiburg, F.R.G.

Further development of the recording apparatus for DC-ERGs now enables us to use the c-wave as a parameter to diagnose pathologies of the pigment epithelium in clinical routine. As the recording time following the stimulus is comparatively long, it was our aim to find a stimulus which presents a minimal burden to the patient yet remains effective. We therefore tested the relationship of the c-wave to the intensity and duration of the light stimulus. Our investigations showed that the c-wave amplitude is mainly dependent upon the amount of total stimulus energy. Within certain limits the stimulus time and intensity could be varied without changing the c-wave amplitude as long as the light energy remained constant. We found that a stimulus energy of about $6\,cd/m^2$ elicited a distinct c-wave without undue patient discomfort.

ROD AND CONE COMPONENTS OF FAST EOG OSCILLATIONS

P.W. Russell, T. Lawwill & J.R. Nelson
Dept. of Ophthalmology, University of Louisville School of Medicine,
301 E. Muhammad Ali Boulevard, Louisville, KY 40202, U.S.A.

The characteristics of the 'fast components' of the human electro-oculogram were examined, with special emphasis on the separation of photopic and scotopic components. It is known (Kolder & Brecher, *Arch. Ophthal.* 75 (1966)) that periodic alternations in luminance (T = 2.2 minutes) produce a following oscillation in the corneoretinal electrical potential. In the current experiment color-luminance alternations were produced by alternating the position of Wratten filters placed close to the subject's eye as he viewed a large bank of fluorescent lamps. The filters were chosen to provide, for instance, an alternation of *photopic* luminance of 1.5 log units while producing no change in the *scotopic* luminance. Several different combinations of color and luminance were tested. Most data were for one observer, with confirming data for two others. With a large field of view (approximately 60° x 60°) no clear evidence for a photopic contribution to the response could be found. In fact, the amplitude of the peak oscillation was roughly proportional to the logarithm of the step in scotopic luminance, regardless of the magnitude or direction of the photopic luminance step. With a smaller adapting field (11° x 45°) the influence of the photopic system became apparent so that both photopic and scotopic changes affected the fast EOG oscillation.

MICROCOMPUTERS FOR BIOELECTRICAL DATA PROCESSING

G. Schaubele & J. Röver
University Eye Clinic, Killianstrasse, D-7800 Freiburg, F.R.G.

A low cost system for processing bioelectric signals basically consists of a single board 8-bit microcomputer, an A/D-converter, and a terminal. This configuration can be adapted for simple analysis of bioelectric signals in the time domain, including averaging, and latency or amplitude measurements. Sampling rates of 10 kHz or more (to process e.g. myographic signals) demand a 16-bit processor with fast interrupt response time and complete arithmetic instruction set. Equipped with either floppy disc or more than 32 kbyte storage capacity, this system can handle cross-correlation techniques, frequency analysis or more complex digital filtering. Time consuming programming in assembly languge can be avoided at the expense of real-time capability when a 'Basic'-interpreter is used. However, in this case further processing must be done off-line. This disadvantage is overcome by the introduction of 'Pascal' which combines the comfort of a high level language with real-time capability and makes the 'micro' a viable alternative to the far more expensive 'mini'.

CENTER-SURROUND ORGANIZATION OF THE LOCAL ELECTRORETINOGRAM (LERG) OF THE GOLDFISH

N.A.M. Schellart
Laboratory of Medical Physics, University of Amsterdam,
Herengracht 196, 1016 BS Amsterdam, The Netherlands

LERGs recorded with low impedance micropipettes in isolated goldfish retina mainly consist of the P III component to small spot (diameter 0.1–0.5 mm) stimulation; the b-wave is weak compared to the in situ ERG. Response amplitude is nearly linear proportional to the intensity and the area of the stimulus spot. Ricco's law holds up to spots of 0.5 mm^2. In Ricco experiments for spots larger than the Ricco area the response decreases faster as a function of spot size than is predicted by the amplitude-intensity relation, suggesting a more complicated 'receptive field' of the LERG.

Stimulation with an annulus concentric to the electrode roughly yields a sign reversal of the response and a latency increase of about 20 msec. Whereas this response is nearly invariant to electrode depth, the spot response decreases with increasing electrode depth. In the annulus response the P II component predominates. Application of ammonia first affects the surround response (P II), and, more slowly, the center response. Picrotoxin also abolishes the .LERG surround response but has little effect on the center response. The described center-surround structure is most obvious for long wavelengths.

ERP REGENERATION IN NORMALS, ACHROMATS AND RETINITIS PIGMENTOSA

P.A. Sieving & C.A. Fishman
Eye & Ear Infirmary, University of Illinois,
1855 W. Taylor St., Chicago, Il. 60612, U.S.A.

We measured human early receptor potential (ERP) regeneration times and compared them with known values of pigment kinetics from densitometry. We used two methods of bleaching: prolonged 3 minute bleaches and 1 millisecond flash bleaches. Exponential regeneration time constants for two achromats were 418 sec (SD = 61) and 405 sec (SD = 36) after prolonged bleach 196 sec (SD = 62) and 192 sec (SD = 21) after flash bleaches. Comparable values for four normals were 180 to 218 sec for prolonged bleach and 130 to 150 sec for flash bleach. As expected, millisecond flash bleaching yielded faster regeneration than prolonged bleaches. ERP regeneration for achromats is consistent with that of rhodopsin by both bleach methods. The difference in times between normals and achromats is consistent with a predominance of cone pigments in the ERP of normals.

The literature suggests fast ERP kinetics in retinitis pigmentosa (RP). Five female X-linked RP carriers studied with the flash method and three using the prolonged bleach showed decreased ERP amplitudes but normal regeneration. An autosomal dominant RP patient and a sector RP subject both had markedly reduced ERP amplitudes but normal regeneration.

The data support the hypothesis that the human ERP reflects activity of visual pigments. With normal controls, ERP regeneration can be measured clinically in a realistic way by a technique of sequential flash bleaching.

VITELLIFORM MACULAR LESIONS

H.W. Skala

Eye Foundation Hospital, University of Alabama in Birmingham,
1720 Eigth Avenue South, Birmingham, AL 35233, U.S.A.

Until recently, vitelliform macular lesions were considered pathognomonic of Best's vitelliform macular dystrophy, a dominantly-inherited progressive disease characterized by a normal electroretinogram (ERG) and an abnormal electro-oculogram (EOG).

In 1973, Birndorf and Dawson (*Invest. Ophthalmol. Vis. Sci.* 12: 830 (1973)) described a patient with 'typical' bilateral vitelliform lesions whom they felt had Best's dystrophy, but who had a normal EOG. In 1977, Kingham and Lochen (*Am. J. Ophthalmol.* 84: 526 (1977)) described 6 patients with vitelliform lesions and normal (in 11 of 12 eyes) EOG ratios, referring to this fundus picture as vitelliform macular degeneration. Also in 1977, Fishman and co-workers (*Arch. Ophthalmol.* 95: 73 (1977)) described 3 patients with vitelliform lesions and normal EOG ratios. These lesions were called pseudovitelliform macular degeneration.

We present the clinical, fluorescein angiographic and electrophysiologic findings in 2 additional patients with bilateral vitelliform macular lesions and normal EOG ratios, and discuss the characteristics these patients share with the above-reported cases.

As these patients do not appear to have a genetic dystrophy, the term 'vitelliform dystrophy' appears to be inappropriate, as does 'vitelliform degeneration' since the underlying cause is unknown and progression has not been demonstrated. The 'pseudovitelliform' designation merely complicates matters, as these lesions are clinically truly vitelliform. We propose the term 'vitelliform lesion' (which may or may not occur together with the other findings of Best's dystrophy), and propose an etiologic theory for these bilateral, localized lesions.

ELECTROPHYSIOLOGICAL RESULTS IN STARGARDT'S MASCULAR-DYSTROPHY

G. Stadler & G.M. Muschalek
Universitäts-Augenklinik Marburg/Lahn, Robert-Koch-Str. 4,
D-3550 Marburg/Lahn, F.R.G.

Pathological retinal function was investigated with electro-physiological recordings. The ERG results indicate differentiation of
1. benign central bulls-eye retinopathy,
2. classical Stargardt's macular-dystrophy,
3. cone dystrophy, and
4. cone-rod dystrophy.
In groups 2 through 4 ERG oscillatory potentials were either subnormal or extinguished (an exception was found in one case exhibiting normal potentials).

The VER results to checkerboard stimulus in groups 2 through 4 were also strongly altered or not recordable.

Juvenile hereditary macular-dystrophy is not distinguished without thorough electrophysiological examination.

THE EOG AND CHOROIDAL MALIGNANT MELANOMAS

J.A. Staman, C.R. Fitzgerald, W.W. Dawson, M.C. Barris & C.I. Hood
University of Florida, Dept. of Ophthalmology, Box J-284
J. Hillis Miller Health Centre, Gainesville, FL 32610, U.S.A.

Fifty-four patients with a unilateral pigmented choroidal lesion were studied with electro-oculography (EOG). Eighteen of 21 patients with histologically proven (13) or presumed (8) malignant tumors of the choroid had light peak-dark trough ratios $(L/D) \leqslant 150$. Seventeen of 21 patients in the malignant group had an interocular L/D difference $(L/Dd) \geqslant 23\%$, whereas only one of 33 patients with nevi or a condition simulating a nevus had a percent difference of such magnitude. Combining the L/D and L/Dd criteria resulted in a 98% accurate double-blind prediction of the final clinical/pathological results. The EOG is an objective, noninvasive test useful in the diagnosis of choroidal malignant melanomas.

THE EARLY RECEPTOR POTENTIAL (ERP) IN ROD AND IN CONE DOMINATED EYES (CAT, PIGEON)

J. Tanabe & E.R. Lapp
Max-Planck-Institute for Physiological and Clinical Research,
Parkstrasse 1, D-6350 Bad Nauheim, F.R.G.

Early Receptor Potentials (ERP) both in the rod dominated cat's eye and in the cone dominated pigeon's eye were investigated by examining their wave forms, response-to-energy-relationship, time courses of recovery after bleaching, and spectral characteristics. In general the wave forms and time courses of both the cat's and the pigeon's ERP were similar, though the R1 component of the ERP of the pigeon was larger in amplitude than that of the cat; the R2 component of the pigeon's ERP showed a higher threshold than that of the cat. Half recovery of R2 after bleaching (15 min. retinal illumination 0.4×10^6 $1m/m^2$ in the pigeon, 1.2×10^6 $1m/m^2$ in the cat) was much faster (45 sec) in the pigeon than in the cat (8 min). The spectral sensitivity of the R2 component in the cat was similar to the absorption spectrum of visual purple, whereas in the pigeon the highest sensitivity was seen at 560 nm. Both in the cat and in the pigeon scotopic as well as photopic elements have been reported. However, the present results suggest, that in the cat's ERP the R2 component originates from visual purple receptors, whereas in the pigeon merely cones generate the ERP.

THE PEAK LATENCY OF THE LIGHT INDUCED SLOW EOG-OSCILLATION

A. Thaler, H.E. Kolder, S.S. Hayreh & P. Heilig
2nd Dept. of Ophthalmology, Univ. of Vienna, Vienna, Austria, and Dept. of Ophthalmology, Univ. of Iowa, Iowa city, U.S.A.

Experimental occlusion of the central retinal artery in rhesus monkeys caused prolonged latencies of the light induced slow EOG-oscillation. In patients with mild ischemic retinopathy delayed peaks may be the only change in the electro-oculogram. It is suggested therefore that the recording in clinical electro-oculography should be continued until the maximum of the first light oscillation is reached.

STANDARDIZATION OF ELECTRO-DIAGNOSTIC MEHTODS IN OPHTHALMOLOGY

R. Trau, P, Salu & P. Jonckheere
Dept. of Ocular Electrophysiology A.Z., V.U.B. Brussels, Belgium

The present state of standardization of electrodiagnostic methods in clinical ophthalmology was assessed by analyzing replies in response to a questionnaire sent to ISCEV members. The analysis revealed minimal standardization with some general trends. Common tendencies of the respondents included the use of the xenon flash for stimulation, the oscilliscope and averaging for recording, combination testing of ERG's and VER's and some agreement regarding normal ERG and VER values (though with a wide margin of variability).

Suggestions for better standardization in the future are discussed.

GLOBAL VISUAL RESPONSE (GVR)
A NEW APPROACH TO THE STUDY OF VISUAL RESPONSES

R. Trau, P. Salu, P. Jonckheere & R. Leysen
Dept. of Ocular Electrophysiology A.Z., V.U.B., Brussels, Belgium

In previous publications (ISCERG 1977) we described a multichannel averager-recorder that allows the simultaneous recording of the ERG and VER. The study of the simultaneous recordings of several hundred normal and pathological cases during the recent years has shown a consistent synchronism or a definite time link between the ERG and VER waves. This has lead us to consider the ERG and VER not as distinct entities but rather as different local aspect of a unitary response of the visual system as a whole i.e. the global visual response (GVR).

The main features of the GVR are (1) quasi synchronism but opposed polarity between a and b waves and corresponding waves of the VER and (2) synchronism between the late O.P. of the photopic ERG and corresponding waves of the VER. Typical examples are shown and discussed. Possible interpretations are given, based on embryological and anatomical considerations, and on comparisons with electronic circuitry for the treatment of visual data (interconnections, feedback, relays).

MATURATION OF THE PATTERN EVOKED POTENTIAL

L.H. de Vries-Khoe & H. Spekreijse
The Netherlands Ophthalmic Research Institute,
P.O. Box 6411, 1005 EK Amsterdam, The Netherlands

Clear, focussed and aligned sight is important for normal maturation in acuity. Disturbances which are not corrected at a young age, may result in permanently impaired visual function. Our aim is to follow normal visual development by means of the contrast evoked potential, as conventional acuity tests are not appropriate at the critical period.

The stimulus consists of checkerboard patterns with varying check sizes presented on a television screen. To hold the attention of infants and young children familiar programs can be superimposed on the stimulus display.

We have measured the pattern evoked potentials of two hundred and fifty individuals as a function of check size. All of these subjects underwent standard ophthalmic examination prior to testing. This sample includes thirty children from two months to four years of age, one hundred and forty-five children from four to twelve years of age, twenty-four children from twelve to sixteen years of age and forty adults.

To obtain an estimate of visual acuity, we have plotted the amplitude of the contrast evoked potential as a function of check size. Since no contrast evoked potential can be recorded when the pattern is below subjective threshold, we assumed that acuity can be estimated by extrapolation of the

445

plot for decreasing check sizes to zero amplitude. We observed that threshold decreases with age, from about fourteen minutes of arc at the age of two months to three minutes of arc at the age of eight months. The mean threshold diminishes slowly reaching a level of one and a half minutes of arc at puberty. From the age of sixty years the threshold increases again.

COLOR OPPONENCY IN THE CHICKEN ERG REVEALED BY COLOR MIXTURE EXPERIMENTS

N. Wioland & N. Bonaventure
Laboratoire de Neurophysiologie, Centre de Neurochemie du C.N.R.S.,
11 rue Humann, 67085 Strasbourg, France

It was observed that in the chicken ERG (1) white light flashes evoke a b-wave of an amplitude much lower than that evoked by monochromatic flashes of equal brightness (the latter being assessed on the basis of the voltage of the ERG a-wave or of the aspartate isolated PIII component) and (2) the stimulus intensity-voltage function (I–V) of the b-wave for white light flashes saturates at a level much lower than the I–V functions obtained for monochromatic flashes. These observations led to the hypothesis that some color opponency process occurs in the inner retina between different color coding channels; this opponency is present in the b-wave. Color mixture experiments confirmed this hypothesis; an important loss of sensitivy (up to .3 log unit) was observed in the I–V functions for the b-wave when paired monochromatic stimulation was compared to pure monochromatic. Two different opponency mechanisms have clearly appeared: one between green and orange-red which is not evident in the a-wave, the other between green and far-red for which color opponency is already evident in the a-wave as well as in the aspartate isolated PIII component.

CITED AUTHOR'S INDEX

449